The Breastfeeding Atlas

Fourth Edition

Barbara Wilson-Clay, BS, IBCLC, FILCA
Kay Hoover, M Ed, IBCLC, FILCA

418 color photographs and explanatory text

The Breastfeeding Atlas, 4th edition, Copyright © 2008
Fourth Printing, 2012

First Edition 1999
Second Edition 2002
Third Edition 2005

Published by:

BWC/KH Joint Venture
12710 Burson Drive
Manchaca, Texas 78652, USA
Phone: 512-292-7227
Fax: 512-292-7228

Cover photograph by Kay Hoover
Cover and book design by David Wilson-Clay

To contact the authors:

Kay Hoover   Barbara Wilson-Clay
613 Yale Avenue   12710 Burson Drive
Morton, PA 19070-1922 Manchaca, TX 78652
610-543-5995   512-292-7227
kay@hoover.net   bwc@lactnews.com

www.BreastfeedingMaterials.com

Library of Congress Control Number: 2008907994

ISBN 0-9672758-5-7

We dedicate this edition to David Wilson-Clay.

Foreword

As private practice lactation consultants with more than 20 years of clinical experience, Barbara Wilson-Clay and Kay Hoover have seen it all. They generously share the fruits of their clinical experience with us in this 4th edition of *The Breastfeeding Atlas*, their important contribution to the body of lactation knowledge. Anyone who helps mothers to breastfeed or teaches breastfeeding should have this book. Wilson-Clay and Hoover share their experience and skills and give us detailed examples in the form of color photos and case studies. I know how valuable these resources are because I use them in the online breastfeeding class that I teach.

There are other textbooks that cover breastfeeding from "A to Z" -- but none explore clinical observations to such great depth. The authors draw upon their personal observations of the mother and baby as "hands on" investigators. They open our eyes with their cameras, presenting color photographs illustrating almost every conceivable breastfeeding situation.

Because both authors' backgrounds are in education, they think like teachers. It is important to them to make their information accessible even to readers who are not native English speakers. But the book's straightforward language, rich visual illustrations, and thorough index make this a valuable resource for anyone involved in lactation.

Medical and nursing schools often fail to offer their students any clinical experience with breastfeeding during training. *The Atlas* helps to fill that gap to show relevant clinical pathology because, unfortunately, the course of lactation is not always smooth. This book is a guideline for recognizing certain conditions and treating them using evidence-based findings.

More than 18,000 individuals worldwide have passed the International Board of Lactation Consultant Examiners certifying exam and are practicing in hospitals, medical offices, and private practices. It goes without saying (but I will say it anyway) that *The Breastfeeding Atlas* is a must for anyone planning to become a lactation consultant.

I have been a colleague of Wilson-Clay and Hoover for a couple of decades. As dedicated clinicians in daily practice they see every possible problem from simple nipple soreness to the "train wrecks" who come to them as a last resort. This exceptional text is a marriage of clinical expertise, scholarship, and heart. The authors' insights are a remarkable gift to the medical profession at large and to the new mothers and babies whom we serve.

Jan Riordan, EdD, RN, IBCLC, FAAN, FILCA
Author of *Breastfeeding and Human Lactation*

Preface to the Fourth Edition

The explosion of exciting new research in the field of lactation can be daunting to authors who write review texts such as *The Breastfeeding Atlas* -- especially in an era with such emphasis on evidence-based practice. Kay and I pride ourselves on staying current with the literature, and we constantly update our lectures to reflect new studies and techniques. We feel the same obligation to apply equally high standards to our book. Consequently, the new edition contains many new references and some changes in focus.

Some readers may be disappointed to discover we have removed the videos. After experiencing quality control issues with the DVD that was included in the Third Edition, we decided not to enclose the video disk with the book. Eventually we will make those (and additional) video case studies available in more durable packaging. We are eager to provide students with the opportunity to see and learn from films of actual consultations.

Kay and I continue to grow as LCs, enriched by sharing the experiences of the mothers we assist. Thanks to the generosity of all the mothers who have allowed us to photograph them, we continue to pursue our original goal of helping to educate the next generation of LCs.

All photographs, with the exception of Figs. 189 and 190 (courtesy of Susan Gehrman), Fig. 251 (courtesy of Colette Acker, IBCLC), and Fig. 414 (courtesy of Keith Bird) were taken by us. We ask that people respect our work by not violating our copyrights.

We want to thank Anna Swisher, IBCLC, who edited the book for us, and Jan Riordan for her Foreward. The *Atlas* project owes a huge debt of gratitude to David Wilson-Clay for designing and laying out the majority of this edition. His expert photo editing helped make the book useful and the cover beautiful. Kay and I both wish he could have lived to see the publication of the Fourth Edition. David not only loved babies and breast milk, he loved lactation consultants. He thought LCs were the smartest, most dedicated, best people, and he loved being part of the *Atlas* project.

We always wish we could acknowledge by name all the pioneering lactation scientists and consultants who have educated and inspired us. We stand on the foundation they built.

Barbara Wilson-Clay
Kay Hoover
2009

TABLE OF CONTENTS

Introduction

Breastfeeding is a robust, biologically stable activity so central to our evolutionary identity that it names the class of animals to which we belong. Human babies, placed on their mothers' abdomens after birth, share with other mammals the instinctive ability to crawl to the nipple and begin breastfeeding (Righard 1990, Colson 2008). The completion of this journey and a satisfactory first breastfeed might rightly be called the natural culmination of a normal birth. The very survival of our species attests to the fact that for millennia under all sorts of conditions, many of us, gently assisted by our mothers, successfully made that journey.

Uncertainties and even dangers have always surrounded the birth process, and some mothers and babies are more vulnerable than others. Studies show that approximately one third of women experience difficulties initiating breastfeeding, or have babies who exhibit "suboptimal" breastfeeding behaviors in the first week after birth (Dewey 2003, IC NHS UK 2007). Many books describe normal breastfeeding. The goal of this book is to help professionals recognize and manage common and unfamiliar problems. When women encounter feeding difficulties, many do not feel they received adequate support (McLeod 2002). Research suggests that breastfeeding duration can best be increased through "specific advice" (Labarere 2005). Therefore, clinicians must be trained both to respect normal and to recognize deviations from the norm in order to help mothers solve problems in a timely manner.

Pictures are useful teaching aids, and many of the photographs in this book are typical of the cases seen by private practice lactation consultants (LCs). Access to visual images enhances the learning experience and improves counseling and assessment skills.

While *The Breastfeeding Atlas* contains information that will assist the LC in any practice setting, it is important to note that the authors are private practice LCs. The private practice lactation consultant may assist with normal early issues, but is more likely to be involved with mothers who are struggling. Practitioners must be aware that factors that increase the stress of pregnancy or complicate delivery or postpartum recovery may also influence and affect the course of lactation (Chen D. 1998, Hall 2002). The main challenge for all those who are charged with providing support to breastfeeding women will be to distinguish between the mothers and babies with situations that are uncomplicated and those who need special assistance. For such dyads, support must be extended beyond the immediate hospital stay and continue in the community.

Common sense must prevail in making this assessment. The inability to feed is quickly recognized as a symptom of illness or dysfunction when it affects an older child, an elderly person, or even a household pet. However, the poorly breastfeeding infant frequently waits many days before being assisted. This contributes to increased family stress. Early hospital discharge adds to the problem, often sending the breastfeeding mother and baby home before the onset of copious milk production and before feeding is well established. Delays as long as 2 weeks between discharge and the first medical evaluation are common. During this time, well-meaning individuals may try to reassure the new mother, telling her to ignore her accurate perceptions of poor feeding (Ramsay M. 1995).

While rare, some breastfeeding babies suffer harm during these intervals (Rand 2001). This has led to the reporting of sensational stories that have chosen to focus on the risks of breastfeeding (Helliker 1994) rather than on a failure of the health care system to provide adequate follow-up care. The American Academy of Pediatrics recommends that breastfeeding infants be evaluated medically at 2 to 3 days after discharge, so that mothers and babies who are at risk for feeding problems can be identified and helped. A visit at 2 to 3 weeks of age should be routinely scheduled to monitor weight gain and provide "additional support and encouragement to the mother during this critical period" (AAP 2005).

An International Board Certified Lactation Consultant (IBCLC) may be among the team of allied health care providers (HCP) called upon to assist a new mother struggling to initiate lactation. This individual has special expertise in lactation science. The lactation consultant does not seek to replace traditional sources of cultural support, such as advice from family members and peers in the community. No one suggests that every breastfeeding woman needs the assistance of a specialist. However, those women who do experience problems have the right to expert help designed to enable them to continue to breastfeed. Women with more complicated problems may need frequent follow-up until their situation stabilizes.

Why is it so important to go beyond encouragement and to provide effective interventions to remediate breastfeeding problems? Research documents that breastfed infants in developed as well as developing countries have lower rates of morbidity from infectious disease. A study evaluating the effect of breastfeeding on postneonatal mortality found similar reductions in the risk of death. Approximately 720 US infant deaths could be prevented annually with increased breastfeeding (Chen A. 2004). Clearly, even in developed countries, breastfeeding makes a difference in the health of babies.

US Healthy People 2010 goals call for breastfeeding initiation rates of 75 percent, 50 percent continuation at 6 months, and 25 percent breastfeeding at one year (US DHHS 2000). Previously, data on breastfeeding in the US was only obtainable from formula manufacturers. In 2001, the US Centers for Disease Control (CDC) began including breastfeeding-related questions in the National Immunization Survey (NIS). Following the advice of many researchers to clarify the definition of breastfeeding, the NIS survey defines breastfeeding as "only breastmilk and water - not solids or other liquids." NIS breastfeeding information is available for geographic areas within the US and includes socio-demographic characteristics.

While the incidence of any breastfeeding has increased in the US from 68.3 percent in 1999 to 74.2 percent in 2008, the rates of exclusive breastfeeding in the US at 3 months and 6 months are 31.5 percent and 11.9 percent respectively (CDC 2008). These rates fall below target goals and document significantly lower rates of exclusive breastfeeding among black infants and infants born to unmarried mothers. Low rates of duration for exclusive breastfeeding are not unique to the US. A Cochrane Review described breastfeeding rates in many developed countries as "resistant to change" (Britton 2007). Both social and physiological factors appear to influence breastfeeding outcomes. Early use of formula and premature weaning continue to undermine duration goals worldwide.

We are beginning to understand some of the cultural issues that influence early weaning. An Australian study found that 5 percent of women will discontinue breastfeeding prior to hospital discharge because of pre-pregnancy feeding decisions, based on whether their own mother breastfed and on the perception that the baby's father prefers formula feeding (Scott 2001). North American and Australian studies identify embarrassment and concerns about breastfeeding in public as major barriers (Sheeshka 2001). We know that infant feeding disorders appear to be less well tolerated by emotionally fragile mothers or those who lack social support (Abadie 2001). These mothers are at increased risk for early weaning.

Various health care system factors influence breastfeeding in the early postpartum period. As an example, both in-hospital lactation consultation and home visits improve breastfeeding outcomes (Kuan 1999). A retrospective analysis of a financial data base at a US hospital examined the relationship between postnatal home nursing visitation, readmissions, and emergency department care for neonatal jaundice and dehydration in the first 10 days after

birth. The study concluded that a home nursing visit after newborn discharge is a highly cost-effective way to reduce the need for subsequent hospital services (Paul 2004).

The opinions and practices of health care providers also influence women's breastfeeding decisions (Lu 2001, Taveras 2004). Studies indicate that families face frustration caused by inconsistent or non-supportive information from caregivers (Freed 1993, Taveras 2004). However, clinicians complain of limited time to provide preventative care for breastfeeding problems. The need for preventative care suggests that additional resources and assistance should be added to traditional sources of support, at least until the culture of breastfeeding revives.

Without this support, the reality is this: many new mothers in the US wean in the first week postpartum (Hall 2002). Many others wean between 1 and 4 weeks (Lewallen 2006). They quit because of difficulties in getting the baby to latch on, sore nipples, and concerns about low milk production. They wean because they are returning to school or work and have not received information that enables them to continue breastfeeding.

The US Preventative Services Task Force (2003) analyzed available data to evaluate effective types of breastfeeding assistance. The task force affirmed the importance of early maternal contact with newborns, rooming in, and the avoidance of unnecessary formula supplementation. Commercial discharge packs including formula samples are associated in their report with reducing the rates of exclusive breastfeeding.

Now that researchers have begun to identify the reasons why women wean, interventions can be designed to help remove these barriers.

For decades, lack of funding for community breastfeeding support has limited both promotion and intervention efforts. At long last, the economic benefits of breastfeeding and the societal consequences of not breastfeeding are being quantified. A US Department of Agriculture study concluded that a minimum of $3.6 billion annually would be saved if the prevalence of exclusive breastfeeding increased from current rates to the Surgeon General's goals (Weimer 2001). This figure underestimates the total possible savings, since it accounts for only otitis media, gastroenteritis, and necrotizing enterocolitis. Cost analysis is a useful tool to assist in breastfeeding advocacy, especially in legislative efforts to effect policy changes to remove breastfeeding barriers (Wilson-Clay 2005).

Globally, the cost analysis of not breastfeeding includes other issues such as the cost of buying formula, fuel costs of heating and cleaning bottles, and environmental costs related to formula production, distribution, and container waste processing. These studies also include increased adverse effects on maternal as well as child health outcomes (International Women Count Network 2000). Economic data can only assist in strengthening the argument that support for breastfeeding is an important and cost-effective way to impact public health (Wright 1998, Kramer 2001).

The lactation consultant works on the front lines of breast-feeding support. Whether an LC specializes in normal or special situations, she or he must be sensitive to factors that signal a need for more help (Dewey 2003). These factors may include better prenatal education, earlier identification of risk factors for early weaning, and closer postpartum monitoring of the breastfeeding mother and her baby. A Cochrane Review describes evidence that breastfeeding education has a significant positive effect on increasing initiation rates compared to routine care (Dyson 2005). Giving birth at a hospital that employs an IBCLC is associated with increased likelihood of breastfeeding at discharge for full term and for premature babies (Castrucci 2006, Castrucci 2007). Community-based care completes the safety net that must be in place to help women achieve their breastfeeding goals.

To evaluate breastfeeding effectively requires a clear understanding of how the anatomy, physiology and psychology of the mother and the baby interact during lactation, and how the events of lactation may be affected by complications during pregnancy, delivery and the post-partum period. The purpose of this text is to provide photo illustrations of various clinical breastfeeding situations to assist health care providers, lactation students, and lactation consultants in identifying common and uncommon breastfeeding-related conditions. Its goal is to broaden the assessment skills of those who support breast-feeding mothers and babies, in order to make them more effective in the important work of protecting breastfeeding and supporting optimal infant health.

A Note from the Authors About Clinical Photography

Both authors have been asked: How do you approach a woman about taking such intimate photographs?" Tact is the key. Sometimes a woman's situation is so distressing that it is best to forego the request to take a picture. In some cases, the woman's cultural background and issues related to modesty preclude such a request. However, many women are extremely generous when informed that a photo of their problem might be useful in helping other women in the future, or when they learn that the photo will be used to educate HCPs who assist with breastfeeding.

On numerous occasions, mothers have heard about the authors' interest in clinical photography and have invited them to take pictures.

Both of the authors are sensitive to privacy issues and aware of concerns about the exploitation of clients. Generally, some accommodation has been made in return for use of the photo. Often, if taken during the course of a consultation, the consultation fee was waived or reduced. Some mothers received a model fee.

Photographers must have a Consent To Photograph form that clarifies issues of use. The form used by the authors explains that the photograph will be used for educational purposes and to promote breastfeeding. All individuals whose photos are included in this text signed the consent form. In most cases, macro lenses or close-up views have been used, and there are generally no identifying features. Names are not used, in accordance with the ethical requirement to protect the confidentiality of the client.

Photographs, Intellectual Property, and Copyright Law

The IBLCE Code of Ethics states that the IBCLC must: "Understand, recognize, respect, and acknowledge all intellectual property rights, including but not limited to copyrights (which apply to written material, photographs, slides, illustrations, etc.), trademarks, service marks, and patents" (IBLCE 2004).

Photographs, like written work, belong to their creators. Clinical photographs are challenging to acquire, in part because the opportunity to obtain a specific image depends upon chance. The authors waited many years to capture certain images. Secondly, because these photographs are taken in the context of clinical settings, the lighting is often suboptimal. Babies wiggle and fidget. Some shots, especially views of the oral cavity, are extremely difficult to capture. Many tries may produce only one useable shot.

Consequently, it is distressing when photographers learn that their work has been photocopied, reproduced, and even distributed without permission and without photo-graphic credit. Such use violates copyright law and the IBLCE Code of Ethics. To help educators, the authors have put the images from this text on a CD, and provide limited permission to import the photographs into PowerPoint presentations and to print accompanying black and white handouts. Users may not insert photos into new materials such as books, patient handouts, on-line presentations, or the like. Please obtain prior written permission from the authors before using photos in any type of print publication.

A planned CD of the 4th edition of The Breastfeeding Atlas will feature all the photos in this text, plus bonus shots not shown in the book that depict normal breastfeeding mothers and babies.

*Orders: **www.lactnews.com***

Aadie V, Andre A, Zaouche A, et al. Early feeding resistance: a possible consequence of neonatal oro-oesophageal dyskinesia. *Acta Paediatrica* 2001; 90(7):738-45.

American Academy of Pediatrics (AAP) Section on Breastfeeding. Breastfeeding and the use of human milk. *Pediatrics* 2005; 115(2)496-506.

Britton C, McCormick FM, Renfrew MJ, et al. Support for breastfeeding mothers. *Cochrane Database of Systematic Reviews* 2007, Issue 1.

Castrucci BC, Hoover KL, Lim S, et al. A comparison of breastfeeding rates in an urban birth cohort among women delivering infants at hospitals that employ and do not employ lactation consultants. *Journal of Public Health Management Practice* 2006; 12(6):578-585.

Castrucci BC, Hoover KL, Lim S, et al. Availability of lactation counseling services influences breastfeeding among infants admitted to neonatal intensive care units. *American Journal of Health Promotion* 2007; 21(5):410-415.

Centers for Disease Control (CDC). *Breastfeeding Report Card-United States*, 2008. Division of Nutrition, Physical Activity, and Obesity, National Center for Chronic Disease Prevention and Health Promotion, Centers for Disease Control and Prevention, Atlanta, GA, US, 2008. www.cdc.gov/breastfeeding/data

Chen A, Rogan W. Breastfeeding and the risk of postneonatal death in the United States. *Pediatrics* 2004; 113(5):e435-439.

Chen D, Nommsen-Rivers L, Dewey K, et al. Stress during labor and delivery and early lactation performance. *American Journal of Clinical Nutrition* 1998; 68(2):335-344.

Colson SD, Meek JH, Hawdon JM. Optimal positions for the release of primitive neonatal reflexes stimulating breastfeeding. *Early Human Development* 2008; 84(7): 441-449.

Dewey K, Nommsen-Rivers L, Heinig M, et al. Risk factors for suboptimal infant breastfeeding behavior, delayed onset of lactation, and excess neonatal weight loss. *Pediatrics* 2003; 112(3):607-619.

Dyson L, McCormick F, Renfrew MJ. Interventions for promoting the initiation of breastfeeding. The Cochrane Database of Systematic Reviews 2005; Issue 3.

Freed G. Breast-feeding: time to teach what we preach. *Journal of the American Medical Association* 1993; 269(2):243-44.

Hall R, Mercer A, Teasley S, et al. A breast-feeding assessment score to evaluate the risk for cessation of breast-feeding by 7 to 10 days of age. *Journal of Pediatrics* 2002; 141(5):659-64.

Helliker K. Dying for milk. *Wall Street Journal* (1994, July 22), A1, A4.

Information Centre, National Health Service, UK (IC NHS UK). Infant Feeding Survey 2005. Ch 4, pg. 133. May 14, 2007. http://www.ic.nhs.uk/statistics-and-data-collections/health-and-lifestyles/infant-feeding-survey-2005. Accessed December 21, 2007.

International Board of Lactation Consultant Examiners (IBLCE). The Code of Ethics: International Board Certified Lactation Consultants. Falls Church, VA: IBLCE, 2004. www.iblce.org. Accessed December 29, 2007.

International Women Count Network and World Alliance for Breastfeeding Action, Women & Work Task Force. *The Milk of Human Kindness.* London and Philadelphia: Crossroads Books, 2000.

Kramer M, Chalmers B, Hodneff E, et al. Promotion of breastfeeding intervention trial (PROBIT): a randomized trial in the Republic of Belarus. *Journal of the American Medical Association* 2001; 285(4):413-420.

Kuan N, Britto M, Decolongon J, et al. Health system factors contributing to breastfeeding success. *Pediatrics* 1999; 104(3):e28.

Labarere J, Gelbert-Baudino N, Ayral A-S, et al. Efficacy of breastfeeding support provided by trained clinicians during an early, routine, preventive visit: a prospective, randomized, open trial of 226 mother-infant pairs. *Pediatrics* 2005; 115(2):139-146.

Lewallen L. A review of instruments used to predict early breastfeeding attrition. *Journal of Perinatal Education* 2006; 15(1):26-41.

Lu M, Lange L, Flusser W, et al. Provider encouragement of breastfeeding: evidence from a national survey. *Obstetrics and Gynecology* 2001; 79(2):290-295.

McLeod D, Pullon S, Cookson T. Factors influencing continuation of breastfeeding in a cohort of women. *Journal of Human Lactation 2002; 18(4):335-343.*

Paul I, Phillips T, Widome M, et al. Cost-effectiveness of postnatal home nursing visits for prevention of hospital care for jaundice and dehydrations. *Pediatrics* 2004; 114(4):1015-1022.

Ramsey M, Gisel E. Neonatal sucking and maternal feeding practices. *Developmental Medicine and Child Neurology* 1996; 38(1):34-47.

Rand S, Kolberg A. Neonatal hypernatremic dehydration secondary to lactation failure. *Journal of the American Board of Family Practice* 2001; 14(2):155-158.

Righard L, Alade M. Effect of delivery room routines on success of first breast-feed. *Lancet* 1990; 336(8723):1105-1107.

Scott J, Landers M, Hughes R, Binns C. Psychosocial factors associated with abandonment of breastfeeding prior to hospital discharge. *Journal of Human Lactation* 2001; 17(1):24-30.

Sheeshka J, Potter B, Valaitis R, et al. Women's experiences breastfeeding in public places. *Journal of Human Lactation* 2001; 17(1):31-38.

Taveras E, Ruovei L, Grummer-Strawn L, et al. Opinions and practices of clinicians associated with continuation of exclusive breastfeeding. *Pediatrics* 2004; 113(4):e283-290.

US Department of Health and Human Services, Healthy People 2010. Conference Edition – Volumes I and II. Washington, DC: Public Health Service, Office of the Assistant Secretary for Health, Jan. 2000, pp. 2, 47-48.

US Preventative Services Task Force. Behavioral interventions to promote breastfeeding: recommendations and rationale. *Annals of Family Medicine* 2003; 1(2):79-80.

Weimer J. The economic benefits of breastfeeding: a review and analysis. Food and Rural Economics Division, Economic Research Service, U.S. Department of Agriculture. Food Assistance and Nutrition Research Report No. 13. 1800 M St. NW, Washington, DC 20036-5831, March 2001.

Wilson-Clay B, Rourke J, Bolduc M. Learning to lobby for pro-breastfeeding legislation, *Journal of Human Lactation* 2005; 2(2):191-200.

Wright A, Bauer M, Naylor A, et al. Increased breastfeeding rates to reduce infant illness at the community level. *Pediatrics* 1998; 101(5):837-844.

Infant State and Infant Assessment

Learning to "read" the baby is one of the great challenges each new parent faces. It is a skill the feeding specialist also requires. The concept of infant "state" provides a useful system that helps practitioners and parents classify infant behavior. The LC also must learn to assess infant tone, movement, and color, and to identify unusual body posture or physical anomalies that may affect feeding. These observations can help explain why a baby is having difficulty feeding. Behavior and body language often provide clues to the problem, which may then be addressed. It is important to understand that an underlying medical condition may create feeding problems that resist modification until the infant is treated or matures.

The Stable Baby

What does a stable infant look like? Heidelise Als describes state stability as the manifestation of appropriate sleep patterns, rhythmical and robust crying, and the ability to self-quiet. Parents find these babies to be consolable. They reward their caregivers with focused, "shiny-eyed alertness," and animated, responsive facial expressions (Als 1986). When given the opportunity, these infants can usually latch onto the breast with minimal assistance. Feeding generally is enjoyable for mother and baby.

The Stressed Baby

Infants who are stressed behave in characteristic ways. Their behaviors include: whimpering, strained fussing, gaze aversion, or staring. Their parents describe irritability, crying, inconsolability, worried alertness, and restlessness. Motor activity, the way these babies use their bodies, reveals stress (Als 1982). Stress cues may manifest as *hypotonia* (the baby is flaccid or limp) or *hypertonia* (the baby is rigid or stiff). Stressed babies flail their arms and legs. They stiffen, splay their fingers, startle frequently, arch, grimace, and twitch. The mildly stressed infant may begin to yawn, sneeze, or hiccup. The severely stressed baby may vomit, gasp, cry, gag, show skin color changes, and, in extreme cases, experience seizures.

Because it can be difficult to separate stress-related cues from certain neurological disorders, the persistence of significant stress cues should be reported to the baby's doctor. If the baby acts stressed only at feeding time, something about feeding feels overwhelming and requires focused evaluation.

Alertness as an Indicator of Infant State

Brazelton's work (1984) looks at state from another angle, identifying variations in levels of infant alertness. Feeding can take place in four of these states, but not in deep sleep or during intense crying. Individual babies may feed better in one state than another.

Infant States
- deep sleep
- light sleep
- drowsy
- quiet alert
- active alert
- crying

The gestational age, maturity, neurological status, and health of an infant affect state stability and influence which level of alertness will predominate. Premature babies spend a great deal of time asleep. Conditions such as jaundice may make babies lethargic or irritable and affect their availability to feed. Babies who are injured or ill may "tune out," or experience such discomfort that they lack focus for feeding. It is important to observe a baby who is breastfeeding poorly for an entire feeding. The point at which a baby begins to act stressed during a feeding may indicate the cause of the stress. Such observations help determine what interventions might be needed.

The Sleepy Baby

Excessive infant sleepiness may have various causes. Sleepiness may be associated with neuromaturation. Preterm and small-for-gestational-age infants show less organized state behavior, act sleepy, and often give indistinct feeding cues (Buckley 2006). Sometimes medications may cause sleepiness. For example, hydrocodone is a narcotic commonly used in nursing mothers to manage postpartum pain. While moderate dosages appear acceptable during breastfeeding, several case reports describe excessive sedation of newborns. Infants who display excessive lethargy should be referred for medical examination (Anderson 2007).

The baby who is sleepy at the beginning of a feed may need assistance moving into a more alert state. Some babies will feed better if blankets are unwrapped, since small reductions in ambient temperature can improve alertness (Elder 1970). However, parents need to be taught to identify signs of thermal stress such as shivering and skin mottling. Preterm infants, particularly, may have difficulty with thermal regulation (Raju 2006). If not held skin-to-skin, they require protection from cold and should be re-wrapped after feeding.

Some babies may be roused by being undressed and placed in an upright position. Or try laying them flat and rolling them gently from side to side. Some parents may try talking to them in animated tones or playing lively music. A well-lit room is more stimulating than a dark one. Light stroking touches can be useful, although the baby's response to light touch should be closely observed. Some infants, particularly those with sensory defensiveness disorders, cannot tolerate light touch and will become agitated and distracted by it.

The baby who falls asleep before completing a feed may have very different issues. Stamina may be the problem, and the mother may need to alter her approach to feedings. Many small, short feeds help compensate for the baby's inability to sustain a feeding of normal length. The infant may need temporary complementary feeds of pumped milk to increase caloric intake.

The Hypersensitive Baby

For babies who have difficulty making smooth transitions between states, or who are hypersensitive, decreasing stimuli may be useful. Dimming the lights and providing quiet will create a calmer environment for the baby who cannot tolerate distractions. Firm touch is preferable to light touch, which is ticklish and may provoke a stress reaction. The irritable, disorganized baby might profit from the containment provided through swaddling in a flexed position and from rhythmic rocking. This type of baby may feed much better when warm, drowsy, and relaxed.

Views of Infant State

The infant in **Fig. 1** is in a state of *deep sleep*. While the mother may be ready to feed, the infant does not easily rouse. Note the good color, excellent facial tone and symmetry of this 7 day-old. A well-defined philtrum (the "dimple" between the upper lip and the nose), the bowed upper lip, and the ability to maintain lip closure indicate good facial tone. The baby has rounded cheeks, indicating the presence of well-developed subcutaneous fat pads. Good cheek tone helps stabilize sucking.

Contrast the appearance of the infant in **Fig. 2**. This infant is also in a deep sleep state. However, this infant is slightly jaundiced. Note the inability to maintain lip closure during sleep. This may be an indication of poor facial

tone, or perhaps the infant has nasal congestion requiring mouth breathing. Both poor facial tone or blocked breathing may contribute to feeding difficulty.

The infant in **Fig. 3** is in a *light sleep* state. Her eyes are closed, but her hand-to-mouth behavior indicates she may be receptive to feeding.

The 6 week-old baby in **Fig. 4** is *drowsy*. He is enjoying *non-nutritive sucking* (NNS).

Contrast the facial expression of the obviously stressed baby in **Fig. 5**. This drowsy baby is also engaged in NNS. However, the baby's frown indicates that there is something unpleasant about the experience. It may be the taste of soap on his dad's just-washed hand, or perhaps the size or depth of penetration of the thumb has triggered the gag reflex. The frown and grimace are behavioral stress cues, and the parent correctly responded by removing his thumb.

The bright-eyed baby boy in **Fig. 6** is 4 days old and demonstrates a vibrant state stability. His calm, focused facial expression is typical of an infant in the *quiet alert* state. Following an unmedicated delivery, this baby went to the breast within moments of birth and fed vigorously. He recovered his birth weight by Day 3. Here he exhibits an early feeding cue, raising his hand to his mouth.

The infant in **Fig. 7** is 6 days old. Note the kicking feet and the hand that reaches for the crib toy. The infant is in the state described as *active alert*. His body language demonstrates good muscle tone and eye-hand coordination. This baby demonstrates the capability to enthusiastically engage with his environment (Klaus 1985).

Fig. 8 provides a visual example of an alert infant demonstrating motoric stress cues. That is, his body language reveals tension and distress. Note the shaved area on the head and other evidence that this baby has undergone recent medical procedures. Thus, the infant may have little patience or tolerance for unpleasant experiences. A diaper change, exposure to cold, or perhaps the lack of containment while lying on the bed has resulted in the baby's worried look. His fingers are splayed, his toes are curling, and his arms and legs are rigid.

Fig. 9 also illustrates a stressed infant who is 3 weeks old and still 3 oz (85 g) below her birth weight. Infants who fail to thrive often present with anxious facial expressions and manifest a "worried alert" state. They may lack the energy to cry and appear apathetic (Lawrence 2005).

Crying is a stress cue. It can be a normal response to hunger, undressing, diaper changing, or to any form of handling that startles the baby. Inconsolable crying may be a sign that the baby is ill (Short 2004).

The infant in **Fig. 10** is *crying*. Note the elevated, retracted tongue tip. Babies cannot safely swallow while crying, so they raise their tongues to protect their airways. It is important to calm a crying baby before attempting to feed. Also notice the thin cheeks and deep creases under the eyes that indicate lack of subcutaneous fat pads in the cheeks. The upper lip lacks definition – a possible sign of poor lip tone. Poor lip and cheek tone may interfere with the baby's ability to form a strong seal at breast.

The infant shown in **Fig. 10** may be premature or have experienced intrauterine growth retardation (IUGR). His feeding ability may be compromised by his relative lack of development (Lawrence 2005). Excessive crying may be a sign of hunger. Breastfeeding generally improves as such infants gain weight, size, and stamina. Temporary complementary feeds of mother's own pumped milk may be required.

In **Fig. 11** a satiated baby demonstrates a rather "drunken" appreciation for a good feed. One can see the remains of a wet burp dribbling from the corner of her mouth. In contrast, a baby vomiting from illness, bowel blockage, or reflux generally appears to be distressed. Infants with these problems generally do not grow normally. Their poor growth becomes an important clue distinguishing them from the baby who gains well and who is a "spitter." A baby merely burping up after a large feed generally does not appear to be worried or in pain. Pointing out the difference in state behavior serves to reassure the parents. Note this baby's symmetrical features, chubby cheeks and well-defined lips. These are all signs of a normal baby.

Assessing the Skin

Visual evaluation of the newborn includes assessment of the skin. Parents and lactation consultants may sometimes encounter infants who have unusual rashes. The infant in **Fig. 12** has a newborn rash. Newborn rash moves around. It seems to fade and then darken within minutes. The LC who noticed the rash was working in a hospital and asked the neonatologist to take a quick look. She was reassured to hear that it was only "normal newborn rash."

The infant in **Fig. 13** however, was ill and required hospitalization. *Petechiae* (red rash) may be a sign of neonatal sepsis (Short 2004). In neonates, symptoms of *sepsis* (infection) are nonspecific. Sepsis may present with a subtle clinical picture in neonates with only one or two signs present in an otherwise "well" baby. LCs provide a safety net for infants discharged within 48 hours. Because

neonates may develop sepsis prior to the first well-baby check-up, rashes, low body temperature, fever, or excessive lethargy should be reported immediately to the baby's health care provider to ensure medical evaluation.

Normal infant skin temperature should feel warm and dry to the touch. Newborns during the first 2 days who are not held in skin-to-skin contact with their mother may have difficulty maintaining thermal stability (Anderson 2003). Many infants are over-dressed and kept so warm that they are difficult to rouse. Being too warm may increase the risk of SIDS (Davis 2004). Some parents may not be able to identify signs of cold stress, and are unaware that their infant is not wearing enough clothing. They will need help learning to recognize signs such as mottling, shivering, or bluish coloration of the skin as indicators that their baby is cold.

The infant in **Fig. 14** shows symptoms of cold stress. The marbled look of her skin is called *mottling*. Sepsis, especially in the preterm infant, may present as hypothermia. Acute difficulty in maintaining proper body temperature can be as serious as fever and is also a sign of infection. The infant in **Fig. 14** was undressed for weighing and got chilled. LCs should place such babies (wearing hats) skin-to-skin with their mothers. Cover both with blankets to trap body heat to stabilize the baby's temperature. The skin color of the baby in **Fig. 14** soon returned to normal.

Babies with Birth Trauma

In assessing infants, it is important to identify a history of physical trauma that may complicate the baby's ability to feed. Trauma may be apparent or may be revealed by taking a history and discovering, for example, that the birth required forceps or vacuum extraction (Caughey 2005). Infants experience pain and express their reaction to it in their behavior. Increased parental holding and breastfeeding can assist the infant in managing pain (Carbajal 2003, Gray 2002). Parents should be encouraged to contact the baby's doctor to report any concerns.

A forceps delivery after a long labor has left the 3 day-old baby in **Fig. 15** bruised and distressed. Discharged from the hospital without ever having established breastfeeding, this infant is difficult to rouse and chooses to tune out most of the time. The baby is producing scant wet diapers and is not stooling. Positioning the baby at breast is difficult. She appears to be in pain when her head is turned or touched in certain ways. Using a spoon to feed the baby expressed colostrum encouraged her to open her eyes. Once awake, she took the breast for brief periods, although sucking was not vigorous.

Breastfeeding in a side-lying position was the least stressful for the baby in **Fig. 15**. Lying on the bed increased the baby's postural stability without putting as much pressure on her head as was likely if she were fed in cradle position. At follow-up on Day 5, the baby still demonstrated poor stamina. She fell asleep before she took in a normal amount of milk (as determined by pre- and post-feed intake weights on a sensitive electronic scale). Her mother had begun using a hospital-grade pump to bring in and protect her milk supply. The pumped milk was used to jump-start the baby at the beginning of feeds and to top her off with extra calories until her injuries began to heal. By Day 12, she seemed to "wake up," as her mother put it. From that point on, breastfeeding was effective and enjoyable for both mother and baby.

The one week-old baby seen in **Fig. 16** experienced an extremely stressful birth. Observe the abrasion on his head from a vacuum extraction. The baby was in so much pain that he cried during most of his waking moments. Note his arched back and his clenched, defending arm. This infant refused to go to breast in spite of numerous interventions. His mother was instructed to pump her milk and deliver it in a Special Needs Feeder ™ (formerly called a Haberman Feeder). This special bottle, often used in feeding infants with cleft palate, is designed with a valve and a controllable flow rate, and does not require the use of suction. Special bottles can be useful when feeding agitated babies whose crying creates an aspiration risk. The parents can also use regular bottles with pacing techniques (see Ch. 14).

The baby in **Fig. 16** was placed in a flexed position, with his hips up against his mother's abdomen. This position helps control the baby's tendency to arch away. Note how the mother has been instructed to place her supporting hand at the base of the baby's neck where it will not touch his wounded head. Over time, as the baby recovered from the birth trauma, the mother began to transition the baby to some breastfeeding. The baby continued to be partially bottle-fed with a standard bottle after his mother returned to work.

The 5 day-old infant seen in **Fig. 17** shows scalp bruising from a fetal monitor. Bruising increases the risk of developing jaundice (AAP 2004). This mother was incorrectly taught to latch the baby by shoving the baby's head into her breast. The baby responded by crying and struggling during latch-on. After the mother was taught to bring the baby's shoulders close to her without touching the head, latch-on was more effective. The baby no longer associated latching on with pain. From then on, breast-feeding improved.

Assessing the Head and Neck for Asymmetries and Torticollis

Localized cranial molding is common in newborns. The rate of occurrence is 13 percent in singletons, and 56 percent of twins exhibit some degree of cranial asymmetry. Risk factors for localized cranial molding include assisted vaginal delivery, prolonged labor, primiparity, infant birth position and male gender (Peitsch 2002). Infants with abnormal head shape and cranial asymmetry (*plagiocephaly*) require careful evaluation. Unusual head shape has an association with an increased risk of *torticollis* (twisted neck) and range-of-motion limitations that may impact breastfeeding (Hummel 2005, Walls 2006). Infants with such issues may respond as if in pain when placed in feeding positions that stress the muscles in the neck and shoulders. Parents often misinterpret the infant's signals of distress (which may include breast refusal on one or both sides) to mean that the baby dislikes breastfeeding.

Muscular spasms or rigidity may contribute to jaw clenching, or influence the baby to prefer the breast he can turn toward most easily. Limitations in range-of-motion, rigidity caused by muscle spasm, and pulling to one side all can impair the baby's ability to create tight lip seal. Poor lip seal impacts the baby's ability to maintain suction. If the baby employs compensations to remedy deficits caused by inability to maintain seal and create suction, the mother may experience sore nipples. The baby's compensations (such as jaw clenching) feel painful. Mothers in such situations often say: "My baby has a strong suck," when, in fact, the suck is weak and the *compensations* are uncomfortable.

The infant in **Fig. 18** spent the final weeks of gestation in breech position, and required a cesarean delivery. Because of his intrauterine position, the baby's ear is flattened level with his skull. Over time the ear position will probably normalize and will not create problems. However, the flattened ear is a *marker* indicating that this baby was unable to move freely in the womb. That issue may have repercussions as it may affect whether or not the baby has full range-of-motion or has acquired torticollis (Hummel 2005). On a positive note, observe how the infant in **Fig. 18** maintains a closed lip position during sleep. This suggests that this infant has good lip tone. The LC evaluates both strengths and weaknesses in each infant assessment.

The 4 day-old infant in **Fig. 19** has a very narrow head. She experienced cranial molding and bruising during a long second stage of labor, that lasted approximately 3 hours. The infant's early breastfeeding behavior was lethargic. The LC visited on Day 4 and observed that lactogenesis II had been delayed longer than 72 hours (the time period considered to be normal for this event). Delays in copious milk production have been attributed to stressful labor with a long second stage (Chen 1998, Dewey 2003). The infant had lost 8 percent of her birth weight and appeared jaundiced, but alert during the consultation. She had an adequate number of wet diapers, but few soiled diapers. The LC explained to the parents that soiled diapers provide a more accurate indication of adequate intake and explained that delayed passage of meconium contributes to an increased risk of jaundice.

The mother's nipples were badly abraded. She also had a history of previous breast surgery. Within the past year, an intraductal papilloma had been excised from her right breast. The LC observed a laterally located incision scar visible at the areolar edge from 10 o'clock to 12 o'clock. The breast tissue under the scar was lumpy and tender to the touch, and the baby seemed to have greater difficulty nursing on that side. The LC corrected the latch and the mother reported immediate improvement in her level of comfort. A test weight indicated that the baby took 30 ml of milk from the left, but only 4 ml from the scarred right breast.

Because of the multiple infant and maternal risk factors in this case, the LC recommended "insurance pumping" and suggested that the parents offer pumped milk to the baby until the diaper output increased. Gentle cleansing and topical antibiotic cream helped heal the mother's nipples, and she did not progress to mastitis. Pumping and improved latching helped bring in the milk and thoroughly drain the surgically affected right breast. The baby recovered well from the stressful delivery, and soon began breastfeeding happily. Stool counts rapidly increased permitting withdrawal of all interventions within 2 days. The baby regained her birth weight by Day 10 and breastfed for 18 months at last follow-up.

Fig. 20 shows a photo of 6 week-old twins. The twin on the right requires surgery to correct prematurely fused cranial sutures and allow room for the brain to grow normally. This is a dramatic example of cranial malformation.

The head of the infant in **Fig. 21** was engaged low in the mother's pelvis during the latter weeks of pregnancy. During the delivery she sustained a *cephalohematoma* (a collection of effused blood that forms under the tissue that covers the skull). Infants with this type of birth trauma are at higher risk for poor early feeding activity because pain can create disorganized feeding behavior and bruising can contribute to development of jaundice. Infants who are jaundiced and in pain may be sleepy and difficult to feed. Measures may be needed to protect the mother's milk supply, and the infant may require temporary supplements of pumped milk.

Breast Preference

Occasionally a mother will complain that her baby will take one breast while refusing the other. Several possible factors can contribute to unilateral breast refusal. The baby may have a painful muscle injury or torticollis (Hutchinson 2004). A broken clavicle can create similar discomfort. Sometimes one nipple lacks elasticity and is difficult to grasp, leading the baby to prefer the one that is more manageable.

One of the authors (KH) maintained contact with a mother whose baby would only breastfeed while lying on his right side. The mother discovered that she could breastfed him in the football hold on one breast, and in cradle position on the other breast. After 5 months, he became willing to lie on his left side and would accept both breasts in the cradle position. At a year he was diagnosed with sensory integration dysfunction. There are case reports of babies who rejected one breast because they were blind in one eye. They preferred to nurse on the breast that allowed them see their mothers while feeding (Harm 2001). Similarly, infants who are deaf in one ear may become upset when their hearing ear is blocked.

Infant Pain and Stress

Fig. 22 pictures the heel of an infant born at 37 weeks gestation who is being monitored for hyperbilirubinemia. Frequent heel sticks, or other unpleasant stimuli resulting from necessary medical care may cause some infants to develop patterns of sensory defensiveness that may affect feeding. For instance, infants who have been vigorously suctioned, or who have been intubated, may have injured vocal cords (indicated by raspy cries) and sore throats. They may be anxious about oral penetration whether from a long maternal nipple, a bottle teat, finger, or pacifier. This may manifest as an easily activated gag reflex.

Lumbar punctures (spinal tap), circumcision and intramuscular injections provide other examples of the types of painful experiences that may cause babies to shut down and become difficult to rouse for feeding. While new guidelines have been developed to help in the management of neonatal pain, such management is hampered by a lack of awareness among health care professionals and parents that babies do experience pain.

If a procedure is painful to adults, it should be considered painful to newborns. Because neural inhibitory mechanisms are lacking in preterm infants, they are at risk for increased sensitivity to pain compared to older children and adults. Repeated noxious stimuli can lead to chronic neuropathic states, resulting in normally innocuous stimuli being perceived as painful. Consequently, it is important to minimize and manage neonatal pain in order to promote normal growth and development (Duhn 2004).

As in adults, adequate treatment of pain may be associated with decreased clinical complications. Anand's (2001) guidelines recommend three types of interventions:

- **Environmental:** reducing noise and light; grouping medical procedures to allow babies rest periods.
- **Behavioral:** breastfeeding or breastmilk should be used to alleviate pain in neonates undergoing painful procedure. When not possible, use swaddling, glucose and pacifiers (Carbajal 2003, Gray 2002, Shah 2006).
- **Pharmacological:** appropriate use of anesthetics and analgesics as ordered by the physician.

Jaundice

Neonatal jaundice is common, occurring in most newborns (Brown 1993, Herschel 2004). It typically resolves within the first week after birth unless calories are restricted. However, because of the risk of bilirubin toxicity, infants should be monitored to screen for those who might develop severe hyperbilirubinemia, bilirubin encephalopathy or kernicterus (AAP 2004). Risk factors for exaggerated neonatal jaundice include a positive Coombs' test and ABO incompatibility, starvation, dehydration, and vacuum assisted delivery (Bertini 2001). The presence of cephalo-hematoma or significant bruising is also considered a risk factor (AAP 2004).

Lethargy and poor arousal negatively impact feeding. These are common problems for the baby with hyper-bilirubinemia. The lactation consultant may be called upon to support the mother whose infant needs more milk intake in order to reduce bilirubin levels. It is beyond the scope of this book to undertake a thorough examination of all the issues related to jaundice; however, it must be emphasized that poor caloric intake contributes to and may result from jaundice. An aim of therapy with such babies is to increase stooling, since the major route of excretion of bilirubin is in the bowel movements. To increase stooling, calories must be increased. Insuring 8-12 effective feedings per 24 hours is advised (AAP 2004). The mother may need to pump to protect her milk supply. She can supplement with her own milk, if needed.

Compare the skin color of the 4 day-old Caucasian baby in **Fig. 23** with his father's arm. This baby is jaundiced on the face, trunk, and palms. As bilirubin levels increase there is a *cranio-caudal* (head to foot) progression of jaundice discoloration of the skin.

The family of the infant shown in **Fig. 23** had been keeping the drapes closed. Taking the baby from a dimly lit room into sunlight helped the parents identify that their baby's jaundice had worsened. Identifying this problem helped explain why the baby was so sleepy, and motivated the parents to begin interventions to improve her milk intake.

Pressing a finger on the skin of a baby and observing the underlying color of the skin can identify the presence of jaundice (AAP 2004, Short 2004). See **Figs. 24** and **25**.

Visual inspection of infants to gauge their bilirubin level is felt to be unreliable, particularly in non-Caucasian populations. Serum levels provide more accurate information. With infants leaving the hospital within a few days of birth, before physiologic bilirubin levels typically peak, new recommendations advise that all neonates receive bilirubin screening prior to hospital discharge (AAP 2004).

Many US newborns are discharged at 48 hours postpartum. While US public health guidelines recommend follow-up on Days 3 to 5 when bilirubin levels are most likely to peak (AAP 2004), some infants do not see a pediatrician or visit a clinic for several weeks. The community-based lactation consultant may be contacted by a mother concerned with poor breastfeeding behavior or inadequate infant stooling. The LC may observe jaundice that requires evaluation. The lactation report should describe the visual appearance of jaundice on the baby's body and alert the health care provider to the need for early follow-up. If such reports are typically mailed rather than faxed, the LC in this case may wish to phone the health care provider.

Fig. 26 pictures an infant wearing a fiber optic device to lower the bilirubin concentration. Using this "bili blanket" permits the baby to be held and breastfed during treatment, does not require that the baby's eyes be protected, and allows the baby to receive treatment at home.

In **Fig. 27** an infant with ABO incompatibility receives the more traditional form of phototherapy with special lights over the bed requiring eye patches. This treatment temporarily disrupts holding and may alter feeding frequency. Keeping the mother and infant in close proximity may be one way to ensure frequent breastfeeding. Breastfeeding and breastmilk feeds are not contraindicated when a baby is jaundiced, although the baby may be difficult to rouse and may feed poorly. The milk supply in such situations requires protection with additional pumping. The parents require reassurance that the baby's jaundice will safely resolve with appropriate care (Kemper 1989).

Als H. A synactive model of neonatal behavioral organization: development in the premature infant and for support of infants and parents in the neonatal intensive care environment. *Physical and Occupational Therapy in Pediatrics* 1986; 6:3-53.

Als H. Toward a synactive theory of development: promise for the assessment and support of infant individuality. *Infant Mental Health Journal* 1982; 3(4):229-243.

American Academy of Pediatrics (AAP), Clinical Practice Guidelines, Subcommittee on Hyperbilirubinemia. Management of hyper-bilirubinemia in the newborn infant 35 or more weeks of gestation. *Pediatrics* 2004; 114(1):297-316.

Anand K. The International Evidence-Based Group for Neonatal Pain: Consensus Statement for the Prevention and Management of Pain in the Newborn. *Archives of Pediatric and Adolescent Medicine* 2001; 155(2):173-180.

Anderson G, Moore E, Hepworth J, et al. Early skin-to-skin contact for mothers and their healthy newborn infants *The Cochrane Database of Systematic Review* 2003; Issue 4.

Anderson PO, Sauberan JB, Lane JR, et al. Hydrocodone excretion into breast milk: the first two reported cases. *Breastfeeding Medicine* 2007; 2(1):10-14.

Bertini G, Dani C, Tronchin M, et al. Is breastfeeding really favoring early neonatal jaundice? *Pediatrics* 2001; 107(3):e41.

Brazelton T. *Neonatal Behavioral Assessment Scale*. Philadelphia, PA: J.B. Lippincott, 1984.

Brown L, Arnold L, Allison D, et al. Incidence and pattern of jaundice in healthy breast-fed infants during the first month of life. *Nursing Research* 1993; 42(2):106-110.

Buckley KM, Charles GE. Benefits and challenges of transitioning preterm infants to at-breast feedings. *International Breastfeeding Journal* 2006; 1:13.

Carbajal R, Veerapen S, Couderc S, et al. Analgesic effect of breastfeeding in term neonates: randomized controlled trial. *British Medical Journal* 2003; 326(7379):13-15.

Caughey AB, Sandberg PL, Zlatnik MG, et al. Forceps compared with vacuum: rates of neonatal and maternal morbidity. *Obstetrics & Gynecology* 2005; 106(5 Pt 1):908-912.

Chen D, Nommsen-Rivers L, Dewey K. Stress during labor and delivery and early lactation performance. *American Journal of Clinical Nutrition* 1998; 68(2):335-344.

Davis K, Parker K, Montgomery G. Sleep in infants and young children: Part one: Normal sleep. *Journal of Pediatric Health Care* 2004; 18(2):65-71.

Dewey K, Nommsen-Rivers L, Heinig MJ, et al. Risk factors for suboptimal infant breastfeeding behavior, delayed onset of lactation, and excess neonatal weight loss. *Pediatrics* 2003; 112(3):607-619.

Duhn L, Medves J. A systematic integrative review of infant pain assessment tools. *Advances in Neonatal Care* 2004; 4(3):126-140.

Elder M. The effects of temperature and position on the sucking pressure of newborn infants. *Child Development* 1970; 41(1):95-102.

Gray L, Miller L, Philipp B, et al. Breastfeeding is analgesic in healthy newborns. *Pediatrics* 2002; 109(4):590-593.

Harm LS. In your words; not quite perfect. *American Baby* 63(2):58, 2001.

Herschel M, Gartner L. Jaundice and the Breastfed Baby, in J Riordan. *Breastfeeding and Human Lactation (3rd edition)*. Boston. MA: Jones and Bartlett, 2004; pp. 311-321.

Hummel P, Fortado D. Impacting infant head shapes. *Advances in Neonatoal Care* 2005; 5(6):329-340.

Hutchison BL, Hutchinson LA, Thompson JM, et al. Plagiocephaly and brachycephaly in the first two years of life: a prospective cohort study. *Pediatrics* 2004; 114(4):970-980.

Kemper K, Forsyth B, McCarthy P. Jaundice, terminating breastfeeding, and the vulnerable child. *Pediatrics* 1989; 84(5):773-78.

Klaus M, Klaus P. *The Amazing Newborn*. Reading, MA: Addison-Wesley Co.,1985.

Lawrence RA, Lawrence RM. *Breastfeeding: A Guide for the Medical Profession (6th edition)*. Philadelphia, PA: Elsevier Mosby, 2005; pp. 427-443.

Peitsch W, Keefer C, La Brie R, et al. Incidence of cranial asymmetry in newborns. *Pediatrics* 2002; 110(6):e72.

Raju TN, Higgins RD, Stark AR, et al. Optimizing care and outcome for late-preterm (near-term) infants: a summary of the workshop sponsored by the National Institute of Child Health and Human Development. *Pediatrics* 2006; 118(3):1207-1214.

Shah PS, Aliwalas LL, Shah V. Breastfeeding or breast milk for procedural pain in neonates. *The Cochrane Database of Systematic Reviews* 2006; Issue 3.

Short M. Guide to a systematic physical assessment in the infant with suspected infection and/or sepsis. *Advances in Neonatal Care* 2004; 4(3):141-153.

Walls V, Glass R. Mandibular asymmetry and breastfeeding problems: experience from 11 cases. *Journal of Human Lactation* 2006; 22(3):328-334.

Notes:

Orofacial Assessment and Feeding Reflexes

It is important to assess the infant's facial tone and structures because deficits or anomalies will affect ability to feed. Observation of feeding reflexes also will provide information about *why* a baby may not be breastfeeding well or gaining weight appropriately. While it is beyond the LC's scope of practice to diagnose or remedy all these problems, the LC must be able to identify weaknesses. These observations should be included in the routine report to a primary care provider according to guidelines in the International Board of Lactation Consultant Examiners' Code of Ethics (IBLCE 2004).

Experienced LCs have found it useful to form relationships with Speech-Language Pathologists (SLP), Physical Therapists (PT), Occupational Therapists (OT), and other practitioners trained to assess neuro-muscular performance. Many useful insights can be obtained from their professional journals, which often contain information about oral-motor function helpful to the LC. These other professionals serve as important referral resources for families, even if they lack specific information about breastfeeding. Collaborations between specialties create opportunities for the LC to educate other health care professionals (HCPs) about normal breastfeeding behavior. The LC remains available to adapt information for developing feeding plans that prioritize the use of human milk. The optimal outcome is that the baby can feed normally. Normal infant feeding, for our species, is defined as breastfeeding.

Assessment of the Oral Structures

Oral structures change over time with maturation and growth. Changes in the first 4 to 6 months of life can be dramatic. Both structure and function can be affected by prematurity, injury, congenital malformation, neurological deficit, or illness. Each of these occurrences can negatively affect breastfeeding (Ogg 1975).

The Lips

The baby uses the lips to draw the breast into the mouth (Wolf 1992). The lips work with the tongue to form a tight seal around the breast (Genna 2008). Lip seal facilitates the creation of negative pressure (suction) inside the mouth. Poor lip seal impairs the amount of suction the baby can create and maintain. Frequent loss of suction requires that the baby constantly re-latch. Feeding becomes tiring and the baby may discontinue the feed early. Unless the available residual milk is expressed and fed to the baby, weight gain may be poor and the milk supply at risk for down regulation.

When the lips are smoothly flanged around the breast, they help stabilize the position of the breast in the baby's mouth. Poor lip seal reflects poor motoric and muscular control of the lips. However, before assuming that poor lip tone is the reason a baby loses the breast, be sure to assess breast support and positioning. Deficits in these areas can cause the infant to release the breast. Certain conditions related to low muscle tone or weakness (prematurity, extreme weight loss, neuromuscular issues, or illness) can make it difficult for a baby to maintain good lip seal.

Both decreased and excessive lip tone can be problematic. Assess the lips by observing the baby's ability to open, round (see **Fig. 39**), and shape the lips. The infant should be able to maintain a closed lip position awake and asleep, and to control saliva secretions. It is unusual for infants to drool until the onset of teething (Morris 1977). While it is normal for a teething baby to drool, excessive drooling in a young infant can indicate that the infant is having difficulty swallowing. Drooling is a warning sign that the infant may be easily overwhelmed by large volumes of fluid and should prompt closer assessment for fatigue aspiration.

Gentle digital pressure against the lips should generate some resistance. In other words, the baby's lips should be responsive to touch. The LC should observe the baby's ability to seal on a finger, the breast, or a bottle teat. Remember that for some infants with weak facial tone, it will be easier and require less effort for them to seal on narrow objects. Some infants who appear to seal well on a finger or narrow bottle teat tire quickly when trying to sustain a seal on a wide-based object such as a breast.

Uniform lip seal should be visually assessed. Sometimes, what appears to be a problem at the lips is actually a jaw or tongue issue that affects lip seal. For example, jaw asymmetry can make it impossible for an infant to seal the lips uniformly. Poor jaw grading (opening too wide) may break lip seal and result in loss of suction. Inability of the tongue to form a central groove can also create a break in the seal at the corners of the mouth.

Clicking or Smacking Sounds and Milk Leaking

Weak lip seal may result in loss of milk during feeding, or be revealed by intermittent breaks in suction with resultant clicking or smacking sounds. Leaking milk during breast or bottle-feeding may be a sign that a baby cannot sustain good lip seal. Milk leaking and noisy feeding may also indicate weakness of the muscles of the soft palate, a sub-mucosal cleft palate, tongue-tie, or other oral anomaly.

Intermittent breaks in lip seal do not always indicate weak lip tone or a structural anomaly. Breaking the seal may also be a strategy that a baby *deliberately* employs when trying to manage a milk flow rate that is too rapid. Thus, mothers with strong let-down reflexes may observe clicking or smacking sounds and milk leaking during breast-feeding. Their baby has learned to release the seal in order to slow down the milk flow rate.

When assessing infants who are smacking or leaking milk, it is important to look at the whole picture. If the infant is gaining weight robustly and the milk supply is ample, the smacking sounds are probably not an indication of a problem. On the other hand, if an infant is gaining poorly, and having difficulty completing feeds, smacking sounds and milk leaking may reveal dysfunction.

The Philtrum

A bow shaped upper lip and well-defined *philtrum* (the groove between nose and upper lip) are indicative of good lip tone. Infants with thin cheeks often have very flat philtrums (**Fig. 28**). As their cheeks fill out, the philtrum becomes more developed. Total absence of a philtrum may be an indication of fetal alcohol syndrome.

Lip Retraction

Lip retraction is a compensation a baby may employ to hold onto the breast when lip tone is weak (**Fig. 29**). Lip retraction may contribute to the formation of sucking blisters (**Fig. 30**). Often described as "normal," sucking blisters might better be characterized as "common." The creation of blisters or calluses on skin is always a sign of frictional trauma. The rough calluses formed can cause irritation to the nipples, generally at the base of the nipple. Mothers can gently use a finger to help flange the lip. They can also apply a light coat of purified lanolin to the baby's lips to help soften and heal the skin.

Therapeutic Exercises to Strengthen Lip Tone

The brief use of firm pressure stimulus (tapping, stretching, stroking) of the *orbicular oris* muscle around the lips prior to feeding, as in **Fig. 31,** may improve tone and help strengthen the baby's ability to form a competent lip seal (Alper 1996). Use of a finger, bottle teat, or a pacifier with a round-shaped nipple to play "tug of war" with the baby is an exercise that can assist in strengthening lip tone.

The Cheeks

Subcutaneous fat deposits in the cheeks provide structural support for oral and pharyngeal function. Cheek stability influences lip seal (Wolf 1992). Premature or low birth weight infants often demonstrate immature development of subcutaneous fat pads in their cheeks. By placing a gloved finger inside and a thumb outside a baby's cheek (**Fig. 32**), the LC can assess the thickness of subcutaneous fat deposits. Thin cheeks contribute to difficulty creating sufficient suction, owing to the extra effort required to create a vacuum in a larger than normal intra-oral space. Collapsing cheeks create an appearance of "dimpling." Observation of dimpling during feeding suggests cheek instability or loss of suction.

Low tone (hypotonia) can contribute to poor cheek stability. The use of external counter-pressure can improve cheek stability by decreasing the intra-oral space (see **Fig. 351** and **Fig. 352**, the Dancer hand position). As the baby gains weight, the fat deposits in the cheeks will increase, generally resulting in improved feeding stability.

The Jaws

The jaws provide stability for the movements of the tongue, lips, and cheeks (Wolf 1992). Normal jaw movements are rhythmic and graded. In other words, the jaw excursions are neither too wide nor too narrow during feeding. Opening and closing motions are smooth, and regular. Arrhythmical jaw movements and inconsistent degree of jaw excursions signify disorganization of sucking. Jaw asymmetry and abnormally wide jaw excursions break the seal at breast with resultant loss of suction. The infant may clench the jaws to hold onto the breast, causing pain for the mother. Milk intake suffers. This pattern is described as a *dysfunctional suck* (Palmer 1993).

If the baby cannot open wide enough, latching is difficult. When the latch is narrow and shallow, jaw closure occurs on the nipple shaft, increasing the risk of sore nipples. Sometimes, a baby with weakness of the tongue or lips will compensate by using excessive jaw clenching as a strategy to hold the breast in the mouth. Providing support for the jaw helps such a baby (see **Fig. 48**). The Dancer hand position not only reduces the intra-oral space, but also provides support for the baby's chin.

The position of the adult jaw is normally neutral, with lower and upper gums approximating. Infants have somewhat receding lower jaw structures because the lower jaw development is less than 40 percent complete at birth. Head circumference increases by an average of 5 cm during the first 5 months after birth, and the lower jaw begins to move anteriorly at a rapid pace (Ranly 1998).

The forward growth of the *mandible* (lower jaw) during the first 3 years of life changes the profile, typically correcting the somewhat receding chin normally observed in the infant. Some infants have significantly receding chins, true *retrognathia*. This characteristic can be familial or associated with specific chromosomal disorders.

Fig. 33 shows an infant with a receding chin. Note also the slight anomaly in the development of the ear. Receding chin may also result from intrauterine positioning that prevents the jaw from growing forward (as in certain breech presentations).

Observe the marked jaw asymmetry of the 8 day-old infant pictured in **Figs. 34** and **35**. His position in utero negatively affected the development of the shape of his head and pushed his jaw to the side. The infant was unable to latch successfully onto the breast. The LC and mother observed cheek dimpling as he fed. Use of a nipple shield failed to improve his sucking His mother pumped her milk for 4.5 months, but he never transitioned to the breast.

Receding chin and arched palate (which may also be seen in such cases) pose physical challenges to breastfeeding that are difficult to overcome. They may be markers for oro-esophageal motor control problems that lead to neonatal feeding resistance (Abadie 2001). Repositioning is one of the few interventions that might help when the infant has a receding chin. It is important to position the baby with his head tilted back, so that the lower jaw extends into and indents the breast. This will help to compensate for a receding chin and may help prevent jaw closure on the nipple shaft (see **Ch. 17** for more discussion related to receding chin).

Asymmetries of the jaw can be associated with abnormal jaw development, asymmetrical muscle tone, injury, torticollis, or facial nerve paralysis associated with forceps delivery (Smith 1981, Wall 2006). Neck position can influence jaw function. If the head is hyperflexed, free range of motion of the jaw will be inhibited. Feeding is facilitated when the mother provides appropriate postural support that flexes the baby at the hips and supports the head in a neutral or extended position.

The Tongue

The tongue draws in the nipple and breast tissue and helps seal the oral cavity. It must be able to lift to compress the breast against the palate. The degree of lift is important because it determines the distance that the tongue will then drop, creating negative pressure (a vacuum). It is the creation of suction via this mechanism that moves milk from the breast. The tongue also must be mobile enough to form a central groove to control the direction of fluids

during swallowing, or the baby will be at increased risk of aspiration (Wolf 1992).

The normal tongue is soft rather than rigid, and is capable of the elastic maneuvers described above (see **Ch. 16** for a full discussion of range-of-motion issues related to tongue function). The tongue is thin rather than thick and bunched, and the tip is rounded (Ogg 1975). Tongue tone should be excellent and may be assessed with gentle digital pressure on the mid-section of the tongue. The tongue should resist when pressed, pressing back up against the finger. When a gloved finger is inserted pad side up to assess for sucking ability, the tongue should extend over the lower gum, cup around the digit, and move rhythmically with pressure against the finger.

If the tongue cannot move properly, the baby cannot breathe, suck, or swallow efficiently. Conversely, problems with free range-of-motion of the body or issues related to swallowing and breathing may make the baby compensate by using abnormal tongue movements.

Abnormal presentations of the tongue include *ankyloglossia* (tongue-tie), short, bunched, retracted, or flat tongue (one that cannot easily form a central groove). Tongue protrusion can result from low tone and chromosomal disorders such as Down Syndrome. One of the authors (BWC) has observed tongue asymmetry as the result of forceps injury that affected the nerves of the tongue.

Abnormally high muscle tone can cause tongue retraction. As the head pulls back and the baby arches from the effects of hypertonia, the tongue drops back. Flexion of the baby at the hips may help control such arching, but the more immediate question may be to ask: why is the infant arching?

Some infants with airway obstructions such as *tracheomalacia* may arch to try to hold open a collapsing trachea. It can be dangerous to deliver large volumes of milk rapidly when an infant demonstrates arching behavior and abnormal tongue function. Pacing techniques help prevent aspiration when an infant is being alternatively fed.

Tongue-tip elevation can make insertion of the breast difficult (see **Fig. 44**). A nipple shield is often a useful temporary device to help a baby drop the tongue into the correct position for breastfeeding.

The Palate

The palate provides stability to the structures of the mouth (Wolf 1992). The bony *hard palate* opposes the tongue, forming a surface against which the tongue can compress the breast. The *soft palate* is a muscular flap that lifts during swallowing to seal off the opening to the nasopharynx to prevent milk from entering the nose. It drops when the posterior tongue rises to form a sealed oral cavity during sucking. A sealed oral cavity facilitates creation of negative pressure and suction (Ramsay 2004b).

The angle of the slope of the palate should be smooth and moderate, and both palates should be intact, with no evidence of a cleft. The shape of the hard palate should accommodate the tongue (Bosma 1977). Familial narrow, arched, or grooved palates can occur. Palate shape may be influenced by intrauterine breech position that prevents the tongue from elevating to spread and shape the developing palate. In a similar way, tongue-tie may prevent the tongue from shaping the palate during fetal development.

BWC has observed that infants with tongue-tie will often have high or bubble palates. Observe the bubble shape of the palate of the 2 week-old infant pictured in **Fig. 36**. He was born with a tongue-tie and was unable to breastfeed. His visible frenulum membrane was clipped on Day 5 and has healed well. However, he still cannot lift his tongue above the midline when his mouth is open wide. Lack of full range of motion is an indication that his tongue is still abnormally adhered to the floor of the mouth. This characterizes a Stage 4 tongue-tie and requires more extensive surgery to remediate (Genna 2008). For a full discussion of ankyloglossia, see **Ch. 17**.

Long periods of intubation can create grooves in the palate or contribute to narrow, arched palates (Wolf 1992). Babies with conditions such as Turner Syndrome often present with grooved (channeled) hard palates (see **Figs. 364, 408-409**).

Stamina influences muscle performance. Poor stamina may lead to *fatigue aspiration* when a weak baby begins to lose control of soft palate muscle function. Loss of ability to seal the rear of the oral cavity may not be evident at first. It becomes more noticeable as the feeding progresses and the baby tires. If aspiration occurs because of a cleft of the soft palate or because of a muscle stamina problem, the baby may sound congested or have stuffy breathing. Parents or HCPs may observe excess nasal debris from aspirated milk that has accumulated in the nose.

More information about clefts of the palate can be found in **Ch. 18**.

The Nose

The nasal passages should be assessed (Alper 1996), and unusual breathing noted. Congested breathing during and after feeds may be a sign of aspiration. Organisms prioritize breathing over eating, and some instances of early feed termination or outright breast rejection may be connected with inability to breathe adequately while feeding. On rare occasions, abnormally small nasal openings are observed. The 4 week-old infant in **Fig. 37** has abnormally small nares. His mother had been attempting to breastfeed him, but each time she held him firmly at her breast, he panicked and fought to push away. The LC concluded that when his mouth was full of breast, his nostrils were not sufficiently large to permit him to adequately breathe.

The LC observed similar behavior when the baby drank from a bottle. He pushed away after a few gulps and struggled to catch his breath (see **Fig. 330**). Feedings were miserable for both mother and baby until the LC demonstrated external pacing techniques (see **Ch. 14**).

Within 24 hours of instituting paced bottle-feeding, this baby calmed down for feedings. His mother reported that it was like feeding "a totally different baby." Neither the LC nor the pediatrician considered referring this infant to a pediatric Ear Nose and Throat specialist (ENT) for evaluation of the narrow-appearing nasal passages. However, when the baby was assessed for sleep apnea and snoring at 9 months, the ENT remarked that it would have been possible to enlarge the small nasal passages with a dilation procedure at an earlier age when the cartilage was malleable.

As previously mentioned, nasal congestion in the absence of respiratory illness may be related to fluid aspiration during feedings. Debris may accumulate in the nose, causing congestion. If the parents report or the LC identifies audible nasal congestion, an alternative explanation may be that the baby is having difficulty managing a forceful milk ejection. The baby may also have difficulty *coordinating* sucking and swallowing with breathing.

In cases where obstructed nasal breathing is observed, the mother may be able to assist the baby if she changes to a more upright nursing position or softens the breast before the baby feeds. Expressing a small amount of milk reduces the spray pressure of the first milk ejection (let-down reflex), making it easier for the baby to cope with the milk flow rate. She may need to allow the baby to release the breast periodically in order to rest. If the mother is supplementing, she may find it necessary to assume more responsibility for the pace of feedings, matching the delivery of milk to the baby's breathing. This helps the baby reorganize his breathing and assists the baby in learning how to self-pace (see **Ch. 14**).

Respiratory distress in the infant requires evaluation by a medical professional. Swallowing disorders and conditions such as reflux contribute to respiratory distress and often impact breastfeeding. Diagnostic tests are available to evaluate infants with breathing or swallowing disorders. As infants grow and mature, some conditions (such as reflux) may resolve. Other infants will require treatment with medication or occupational therapy.

Feeding Reflexes

Normal infants are born with reflexes that assist with feeding. These reflexes include:

- Swallowing
- Sucking
- Rooting
- Gagging
- Coughing

Prematurity, injury, illness, or congenital disorders may affect feeding reflexes. If a feeding reflex is depressed or hyperactive, a baby may have difficulty feeding normally. The LC's assessment should include observation of the presence or absence of functional feeding reflexes.

The Swallowing Reflex

Swallowing develops early in fetal life (12-14 weeks gestation) with ingestion of amniotic fluid. The volume of the fluid, the delivery of fluid to the back of the tongue, and the reaction of chemical receptors in the larynx and pharynx trigger swallowing in the infant (Woolridge 1986, Wolf 1992).

Abnormalities of the tongue and palate interfere with safe swallowing and are risk factors for aspiration. Swallowing dysfunction is distressing. It feels like drowning! Infants who have difficulty safely swallowing may develop aversive reactions to feeding. Poor weight gain may result.

The Sucking Reflex

Sucking behavior has been observed in utero as early as 13 weeks gestation (Hafstrom 2000). By 28 weeks, disorganized and random mouthing patterns are observed. By 32 weeks, stronger sucking with a burst-pause pattern begins to occur. By 34-35 weeks gestational age, some infants can sustain a stable sucking rhythm that allows them to feed effectively (Brake 1988). However, feeds at this stage are generally brief and late preterm infants fatigue quickly (Meier 2007).

Sucking is stimulated by touch pressure on the lips and tongue (Wolf 1992), and by stroking of the posterior palate near the junction of the hard and soft palates (Woolridge 1986, Ramsay 2004b).

Sucking is categorized into two modes: nonnutritive (NNS) and nutritive (NS). NNS develops earlier and matures at about 37 weeks. NNS sucking patterns change with maturity. Both the number of sucks in each burst and suction pressure increase as the baby develops. Bursts of NNS are more rapid than NS, and appear to affect behavioral state. NNS has been observed to decrease stress in preterm infants. Preterm infants experience reduced length of hospitalization when given opportunities for NNS (Premji 2000). Premji suggests that NNS may also play a role in stimulating fibers in the oral cavity that activate the vagal nerve, influencing the levels of gastrointestinal hormones that affect digestion.

NNS can occur as the baby sucks on a pacifier, a finger, or an emptied (just pumped) breast (Narayanan 1991). It is characterized by rapid, shallow sucking and a lack of swallowing. The rate of sucking is 6-8 sucks for each swallow.

Nutritive sucking occurs solely in the presence of fluid transfer and is more organized (Glass 1994). The sucking rate is slower than in NNS. Some breath holding (brief *apnea*) occurs during NS because of the pauses for swallowing. Breathing rate increases during the pauses between sucking bursts (Geddes 2006).

The terms NNS and NS are often used incorrectly to describe *effective* versus *ineffective* suck. The LC must recognize that within a breastfeeding session, sucking rates are variable and the baby may alter back and forth between NNS and NS depending upon the milk flow rates before, during, and after each milk ejection.

Ultrasound is a noninvasive method of breast examination previously used primarily to detect breast abnormalities in nonlactating women. Milk ejection can be visualized by ultrasound techniques. Visualization verifies that milk flow rate is low before milk ejection occurs. This is because women's breasts lack milk cisterns. Human milk is not stored in large ducts close to the nipple. In fact, milk appears to reflux or flow in reverse back up into the smaller ducts and ductules of the breast for storage between milk ejections. Therefore milk is not readily available unless released by the milk ejection (Ramsay 2004a). Clinicians have described the baby's rapid sucking pattern during the initial part of a breastfeed as "start-up" or "call-up" sucking. Rapid sucking appears to help trigger the letdown or milk ejection reflex. Ramsay observed that a typical milk ejection lasted for approximately 1.5 minutes, during which time the baby's sucking rate was observed to change to the slower NS pattern. The higher milk flow rates during milk ejection necessitate a slowing of the sucking rate to accommodate the need of the infant to breathe after swallowing.

The normal, term infant maintains coordinated, sustained NS. The LC may describe this to parents by pointing out that infants generally feed in sucking bursts of 10-30 sucks before pausing briefly to rest (Palmer 1993). Then they launch into another vigorous burst of sucking. This pattern is repeated several times, and correlates well with what Ramsay's (2004a) ultrasound studies reveal: multiple milk ejections occurring during normal breastfeeds.

Many parents verbalize concerns about infants "using the breast as a pacifier." They do not know that significant amounts of intake occur during the later part of a breastfeed, when the breast feels less full and the sucking rate slows. While the mother may not sense all the milk ejections (Ramsay 2004a), the baby is still obtaining milk. Test weighing confirms that some milk transfer continues to occur even during "comfort sucking."

It is useful to discuss infant sucking and to help parents of normal infants interpret the baby's breastfeeding behavior. However, it is critical for LCs to remember that research demonstrates that observation alone is not sufficient to assess intake in the *at-risk* infant. Whenever an infant experiences feeding difficulties or there is concern about intake, an accurate scale should be used for assessment (Meier 1994, Sachs 2002).

Abnormal Suck

McBride (1987) described types of abnormal sucking. Abnormal suck can lead to impaired intake and growth. The LC must be able to distinguish between babies who are sucking effectively and those whose sucking rhythms and patterns reveal dysfunction.

An absent or diminished suck might indicate:

- Central nervous system immaturity, prematurity
- CNS abnormality (various trisomies)
- Prenatal CNS insults such as exposure to drugs
- Asphyxia, trauma, stroke, sepsis
- Congenital problems (heart disease, hypothyroidism)

A weak suck might indicate:

- CNS abnormalities associated with hypotonia: One of the authors (KH) observed changes in her son's sucking ability at nine months. His increasing low tone and feeding difficulties eventually led to the diagnosis of a brain tumor (**see Fig 356**).
- Myasthenia gravis or infant botulism
- Medullary lesions
- Abnormalities of the muscles: weak oral and buccal musculature

An uncoordinated suck, marked by mistiming of normal motions or by interference from hyperactive reflexes might indicate:

- History of asphyxia
- Perinatal cerebral insults
- CNS malformations

The variability of sucking patterns over the course of a normal feed should not be confused with the feeding behavior characteristic of a baby who is *unable* to suck nutritively. This infant typically goes to breast with closed eyes and appears unable to sustain normal nutritive sucking episodes. Short, shallow, choppy jaw excursions, lack of swallowing, and flat behavioral affect are indications that the baby is unable to effectively transfer milk. Test weights are critical to verify this impression. Interventions will be required to ensure protection of intake and of milk production.

The Rooting Reflex

The rooting reflex helps the baby locate the nipple. Rooting behavior is present at birth and extinguishes between 2 to 4 months of age, although some experts feel it may persist longer in breastfed infants (Morris 1977). If the rooting reflex is absent or is diminished, it may signal poor tactile receptivity or poor neural integration. If the rooting reflex is hyperactive, the baby may be easily distracted and become frustrated while trying to latch.

The Gag Reflex

The gag reflex protects the baby's airway from large objects. Though usually triggered by pressure to the rear of the tongue, it is stimulated at a more shallow depth in the mouths of young infants (Wolf 1992). Some infants gag with touch pressure on the mid-tongue. The gag reflex is hyperactive in some infants, and constant activation of the gag can create feeding aversion. Those most at risk include the infant whose mother has unusually long nipples, infants repeatedly subjected to invasive procedures or insensitive feeding practices, or infants coping with rapid milk ejection.

If the gag reflex is initiated mid-tongue, the baby may refuse to draw the nipple tip deeper toward the juncture of the hard and soft palates. As a result of a shallow latch, the baby pinches the nipple, causes the mother pain, and fails to obtain sufficient milk from the breast. Because a shallow gag reflex may be a developmental issue, only time and sensitive feeding practices will remedy the problem.

The Cough Reflex

The cough reflex protects the baby from aspiration of fluid into the airway (Wolf 1992). The cough reflex may be immature in preterm and even some term infants, leading to a phenomenon described as "silent aspiration." Instead of coughing to clear fluids from the airway, the baby will hold his breath and attempt to swallow. Any cessation of breathing longer than 20 seconds is described as apnea. Brief apnea is protective, but prolonged apnea contributes to *bradycardia* (a slowing of the heart rate) and to oxygen desaturation and cyanosis. Coughing can be an important clinical sign. Coughing *during* feeding is generally a response to descending fluids (a swallowing problem). Coughing *between* feeds might be in response to ascending fluids (indicating gastroesopohageal reflux).

Learning to "See" the Baby

The following section seeks to help develop clinical observation skills.

The baby in **Fig. 38** has nevus simplex, often called "stork bites" on his face. These skin discolorations are common in newborns and will fade over time.

The baby in **Fig. 39** demonstrates good lip rounding as she interacts with her mother in quiet alert state. Note the excellent facial tone, the well-defined philtrum and the bow in the upper lip. This infant has full, rounded cheeks that help stabilize the muscles of the lips. There is good facial symmetry with no evidence of droop or weakness.

Fig. 40 pictures a 14 day-old infant with hypertonic (excessive tone), "purse string" lips. Note the excessive tension around her lips. At the time of the consultation, the baby had not latched, and the parents had difficulty inserting even their fingers or bottle teats into the baby's mouth. This infant was not able to breastfeed in spite of numerous interventions. After several weeks of pumping and bottle-feeding, the discouraged mother discontinued the lactation.

Contrast the hypertonic infant in **Fig. 40** with the infant in **Fig. 41** who demonstrates generalized *low* facial tone. This 17 day-old infant is still below birth weight and unable to sustain a latch at breast. Note her thin cheeks (revealed in part by the deep creases under her eyes) and the lack of definition of both the upper lip and philtrum. Most strikingly, the baby is unable to bring her lips into a closed position. Her tongue protrudes. Because of her low facial tone, the baby was unable to form a seal at breast and could not generate suction. Pumped milk was bottle-fed to this infant to help her gain strength and energy.

Her mother elected to obtain Cranial Sacral Therapy (CST), a form of soft tissue massage therapy, to help improve the baby's facial tone. Additionally, the mother performed oral-motor strengthening exercises with the baby on a daily basis (see **Fig. 31**).

Fig. 42 shows the same infant at 5.5 weeks after receiving her fifth session of CST. She has gained weight well with bottle-feeds, but still has never breastfed. **Fig. 42** shows the infant achieving lip closure for the first time. Increased weight gain and oral-motor exercise have improved her cheek tone. The lips and philtrum are now well-defined. The baby experienced her first effective breastfeeding following therapy that day (**Fig 43**), and within a week, she was exclusively breastfeeding and gained weight normally. In **Fig. 43** the mother is using the technique of breast compression to help increase the milk transfer. Breast compression helps the weak baby obtain a greater volume and higher calorie milk (Stutte 1988).

Lip, cheek, and jaw tone can be evaluated asleep or awake, on a bottle or at the breast. In **Fig. 44** a jaundiced, 4 day-old infant demonstrates poor facial tone during deep sleep. She cannot maintain lip closure. Note her elevated tongue tip and the sucking blister on the upper lip. Her habitual tongue-tip elevation blocked the nipple from entering her mouth each time her mother attempted to latch her to the breast. Due to the ineffective latch, the baby attempted to grab the nipple with her retracted lips, causing a friction callous. Lip retraction may be a compensation for low tone, or may reflect excessive tone that prevents the baby from comfortably flanging the lips.

Compensatory behaviors or weaknesses may be revealed when a baby is supplemented via alternative feeding methods. Watching the baby feed from a bottle or feeding tube device may provide helpful clinical insights into why the infant cannot breastfeed. Lip retraction can be observed during bottle-feeding, as in **Fig. 45**. This infant is grimacing, thus providing a stress cue indicating that the experience is unpleasant.

The jaundiced preterm baby in **Fig. 46** manifests the general low tonality that is common in premature infants. He spills milk during bottle-feeding and has difficulty sustaining a latch at breast. Weak lip seal creates breast and bottle-feeding difficulties, and may result from immaturely developed subcutaneous cheek fat pads. Thin cheeks, weak lip seal, and low muscle tone are factors contributing to increased lactation risk among preterm and late-preterm infants (Meier 2007).

Jaw asymmetry is apparent in the infant pictured in **Fig. 47**. Note the droop on the left side of his face involving the lips and cheek as well as the jaw. These features suggest there may be dysfunctional sucking ability (Palmer 1993). This boy received CST for over a year, along with other forms of physical therapy. At 2 years old, his facial asymmetry was less apparent, although his parents were told he will eventually need orthodontia.

In the case of an infant with physical anomalies or structural deformities, early identification of the impact upon feeding is crucial. It is necessary, in such circumstances, to recommend more aggressive measures to protect the milk supply. Neglecting to begin pumping during the important milk calibration phase (the first few weeks postpartum) may contribute to what Woolridge (1992) calls an "acquired low milk supply."

Jaw Support

The mother of the infant in **Fig. 48** has placed her finger under the baby's chin to help stabilize jaw excursions that are too wide. This infant loses the breast when his jaw swings too wide, causing a break in the lip seal. The firmly placed finger helps grade the width of the jaw excursion, preventing the baby from opening too wide. The mother keeps the supporting finger forward under the bony part of the chin. If she places her finger under the soft part of the baby's chin, it may choke the baby.

Depressed Reflexes

Depressed feeding reflexes may be an indication that a baby is unable to feed normally. If a baby becomes apathetic only when the mother attempts to latch, this may be a stress cue. A baby who consistently manifests low reflexive arousal may be ill, affected by medications, have CNS depression or injury, or have a sensory-based feeding problem (Palmer and Heyman 1993).

The week-old infant in **Fig. 49** demonstrates a depressed rooting reflex. Taking her clothes off (**Fig. 50**) to help her rouse reveals that this is a normal baby with a normal rooting reflex who was merely in the wrong state for effective feeding. In this case, moving the baby into a more alert state resolved the problem (see the discussion of state behavior in **Ch. 2**).

Feeding Affect

Normal infants feed robustly. They generally go to breast with open eyes and feed with apparent enjoyment. Contrast this with the distressed expression of the 37 week gestational age infant in **Fig. 51** whose mother's long, large diameter nipples trigger a gag reflex each time the baby tries to latch. This preterm baby needed 6 weeks of

weight gain and maturation before she was able to manage her mother's nipples. The mother, a busy physician, returned to work at 4 weeks postpartum. Once reassured that this "fit" problem would resolve over time, she pumped and bottle-fed the baby. Her nipples competed well with bottle teats, and once the baby was able to breastfeed, the mother continued to breast and bottle-feed until the baby was 18 months old (see **Ch. 10** for a detailed discussion of the effect of nipple size on breastfeeding).

Oral Aversion

Repeated trauma to the oral and pharyngeal regions may alter an infant's sensory perceptions, creating avoidance behavior or aversion (Palmer and Heyman 1993). Swallowing dysfunction or an upper-airway obstruction may disrupt oral feeding and create aversive behaviors that interfere with establishing normal feeding (Miller 2007).

The 6 week-old infant born at term pictured in **Fig. 52** experienced a month-long stay in the NICU as the result of a serious lung infection. He was intubated for several weeks and developed sensory defensiveness. He refused the breast and was extremely difficult to bottle-feed as well. His parents were trained to gavage feed him during the night, and most of his milk intake occurred while he slept. Because the original airway obstruction has since resolved, he can be described at this point as having a *non-organic*, *behaviorally-based* feeding problem.

The LC and an OT worked together with the parents to help this baby overcome his oral defensiveness. Here the LC shows the mother how to use a pacifier to play with the baby's lips. The pacifier (or a finger) is gradually penetrated to increasing depth, but only as the infant will permit it. Note the interested, relaxed facial expression. The pacifier is removed if the infant begins to look or act stressed. Therapeutic exercises with a pacifier can be useful for infants with tone problems as well. This activity helps the baby grip with lips and tongue, and it gives the baby the opportunity to strengthen the muscles of the soft palate during non-nutritive sucking. The goal is to improve breastfeeding ability.

Torticollis

Torticollis refers to a contracted state of the muscles of the neck, producing a twisting of the neck and unnatural position of the head (van Vlimmeren 2006). The 12 day-old, term infant pictured in **Fig. 53** developed torticollis, presumably from her breech position in the womb. Note the slight facial asymmetry, the pull of the head to the left, and the baby's general physical rigidity.

The baby was initially unable to breastfeed. She could not form lip seal because excessive muscle tension on the left side of her neck interfered with her jaw alignment. This is illustrated in **Fig. 54** where she is pictured bottle-feeding. Note the gape and break in seal at the corner of her mouth as her head pulls towards the affected side. Hip flexion is being used to improve postural stability at the neck, head, and lips. Over time, physical therapy helped reduce this child's muscle spasms and improved the range of motion of her head and neck. She was able to partially breastfeed by 4 weeks of age, assisted by a nipple shield that helped compensate for her weak ability to create seal and suction. By age 2, physical therapy had successfully resolved her problems, and her physical appearance normalized.

Unusual Presentations

The infant in **Fig. 55** has an ear tag. An isolated ear tag is a minor anomaly consisting of a rudimentary bud of ear tissue, often with a core of cartilage, usually located just in front of the ear. Isolated ear tags are felt to be benign. However, since the ears and the kidneys form at about the same period of intrauterine development, infants with ear tags are generally screened for renal anomalies (Kohelet 2000). The infant in **Fig. 55** was medically evaluated prior to discharge and the parents were reassured to learn that their baby did not have a kidney anomaly. The baby previously discussed in **Fig. 33** has an unusually shaped ear, and also was screened to rule out renal anomalies.

The presence of 2 or more minor anomalies in a child increases the probability of a major malformation. Patients with *auricular* (ear) anomalies should be assessed carefully for accompanying *dysmorphic* (abnormally formed) features, including facial asymmetry (Wang 2001). Whenever an infant has difficulty breastfeeding, underlying anomalies and illness must be ruled out.

The infant in **Fig 56**, who appears to be wearing a vest has a large hairy *nevus*. A nevus is a type of mole or birthmark. Like a mole, it can become cancerous, so changes in appearance should be reported to a physician. This condition does not affect breastfeeding.

Congenital dermal melanocytosis is pictured in **Fig. 57**. Formerly called *Mongolian spots*, this type of birthmark is a benign bluish or bruised appearing mark, typically located on the lower back or buttocks. Sometimes mistaken for signs of abuse, it may fade over time, or may persist for years. This type of birthmark is most often observed in infants with Asian or African ancestry.

Epstein's Pearls, seen in **Fig. 58**, are small white epithelial cysts usually found in the midline of the palate in newborn infants. Sometimes mistaken for oral thrush, these benign cysts do not spread and typically disappear a few weeks after birth (Marmet 2008).

The 6 week-old infant in **Fig. 59** has a *hemangioma* on her lip. A hemangioma is a red or purple-colored skin marking that develops shortly after birth. Most are painless and benign, and some will disappear or fade as the child grows. This infant is clearly growing well, and her hemangioma, while it disfigures her lip, does not interfere with her breastfeeding ability.

The 2 infants sleeping side-by-side in **Fig. 60** are *discordant* twins meaning there is a difference >10 percent in their respective birth weights. One infant weighs 7 lbs (3192g). His sister weighs 5 lbs 2 oz (2337g). This photo emphasizes the necessity of individual assessment. The male twin was breastfeeding well, and gaining approximately 1 oz (28.3g) a day. His sister was not gaining. The mother of these twins needed help to see that feeds would have to be individualized to ensure that the weaker twin received sufficient intake. It helped to feed the twins sequentially, as opposed to simultaneously. The female twin needed supplementary calories for several weeks until she, too, breastfed robustly. Eventually, the mother was able to breastfeed both babies simultaneously (see **Ch. 13** for more on managing twins).

Hand Hygiene

We offer a brief note on the use of gloves by the authors (as seen in photos throughout *The Breastfeeding Atlas*). The use of examination gloves remains controversial in the field of lactation. The argument revolves around the issue of whether use of gloves "medicalizes" breastfeeding assistance.

In recent years, proponents of evidence-based care have emphasized the importance of utilizing research to support clinical practice. Hand hygiene has been singled out as the most important measure in preventing *nosocomial* infections (infections acquired in health care settings) (Lam 2004). And yet, research indicates that health care provider compliance with hand hygiene is poor (Harbath 2001). This issue is of special concern with regard to preterm and ill babies, who are particularly vulnerable to nosocomial infection (Hanrahan 2004). Whatever the gestational age of their baby, all new mothers have the right to know that their caregivers are scrupulous about hand hygiene.

During hospital, clinic, and home visits, the LC may come in contact with other children (often with respiratory symptoms) and with pets. It is easy to transmit organisms on the hands and under fingernails (Pittet 2001, CDC 2002). Scales, clip boards, pens, and other surfaces may also become contaminated with viruses or bacteria (Hanrahan 2004). These objects should be routinely cleaned with sterilizing wipes between patients. Observance of infection control practices has become even more critical with the spread of antibiotic-resistant strains of bacteria, including Methicillin-resistant *Staphylococcus aureus* (MRSA). MRSA infections among postpartum women may manifest as mastitis, and are associated with increased risk of progression to breast abscess (Saiman 2003, Reddy 2007).

MRSA infections in hospitalized infant populations have been documented in neonatal special care units and pediatric departments (Kitajima 2003). Community acquired MRSA has also been documented with increasing frequency resulting in hospital readmission of young infants (Fortunov 2007). Infants may be exposed by carrier medical staff, family members, and even pets. Therefore, it is best for mothers to hold and breastfeed immediately after birth in order to colonize their infants with normal bacteria; to room-in with their infants; and to minimize non-essential interventions by staff. Mothers should remind caregivers to wash their hands prior to handling the infant.

LCs in all practice settings should wash their hands carefully before and after consultations. Alcohol-based hand cleansers may be used to clean the hands. For infant oral exams and for examination of breasts or nipples when open sores are present, the LC should wear non-latex gloves or finger cots (see **Fig. 32**).

Abadie U, Andre A, Zaouche A, et al. Early feeding resistance: a possible consequence of neonatal oro-oesophageal dyskinesia. *Acta Paediatrica* 2001; 90(7):738-745.

Alper M. Dysphagia in infants and children with oral-motor deficits: assessment and management. *Seminars in Speech and Language* 1996; 17(4):283-309.

Bosma J. Structure and Function of the Infant Oral and Pharyngeal Mechanisms, in J Wilson, ed. *Oral-motor Function and Dysfunction in Children.* Chapel Hill, NC: University of North Carolina at Chapel Hill, 1977; May 25-28, p. 46.

Brake S, Fifer W, Alfasi G, et al. The first nutritive sucking responses of premature newborns. *Infant Behavior and Development* 1988; 11:1-9.

Center for Disease Control (CDC). Guidelines for Hand Hygiene in Healthcare Settings. *Recommendations and Reports* 2002; 51(RR16):1-44. Available at: http://www.cdc.gov/mmwR/preview/mmwrhtml/rr5116a1.htm. Accessed Oct. 16, 2007.

Fortunov R, Hulten K, Hammerman W, et al. Evaluation and treatment of Community-Acquired *Staphylococcus aureus* infections in term and late-preterm previously healthy neonates. *Pediatrics* 2007; 120(5):937-945.

Geddes D, McClennen H, Kent J, et al. Patterns of respiration in infants during breastfeeding. Proceedings of the 13th International Conference of the International Society for Research in Human Milk and Lactation Sept. 22-26, 2006; Niagara-on-the-Lake, Ontario, Canada.

Genna CW. *Supporting Sucking Skills in Breastfeeding Infants.* Boston: Jones and Bartlett, 2008; pp. 181-200.

Glass R, Wolf L. Incoordination of sucking, swallowing, and breathing as an etiology for breastfeeding difficulty. *Journal of Human Lactation* 1994; 10(3):185-189.

Hafstrom M, Kjellmer I. Non-nutritive sucking in the healthy pre-term infant. *Early Human Development* 2000; 60(1):13-24.

Hanrahan K, Lofgren M. Evidence-based practice: examining the risk of toys in the microenvironment of infants in the neonatal intensive care unit. *Advances in Neonatal Care* 2004; 4(4):184-201.

Harbath S, Pittet D, Grady L, et al. Compliance with hand hygiene practice in pediatric intensive care. *Pediatric Critical Care Medicine* 2001; 2(4):311-314.

International Board of Lactation Consultant Examiners. Section 9, *Code of Ethics for International Board Certified Lactation Consultants,* International Board of Lactation Consultant Examiners (IBLCE), Falls Church, VA, 2004.

Kitajima H. Prevention of Methicillin-resistant *Staphylococcus aureus* infections in neonates. *Pediatrics International* 2003; 45:238-245.

Kohelet D, Arbel E. A prospective search for urinary tract abnormalities in infants with isolated preauricular tags. *Pediatrics* 2000; 105(5):e61.

Lam B, Lee J, Lau Y, et al. Hand hygiene practices in a neonatal intensive care unit: a multimodal intervention and impact on nosocomial infection. *Pediatrics* 2004; 114(5):e565-e571.

Marasco L, Marmet C, Shell E. Polycystic ovary syndrome: a connection to insufficient milk supply? *Journal of Human Lactation* 2000; 16(2):143-148.

Marmet C, Shell E, Genna CW. Infant Anatomy for Feeding, in R Mannel, P Martens, M Walker (editors), *Core Curriculum for Lactation Consultants.* Boston: Jones and Bartlett, 2008; pp. 209-221.

McBride M, Danner S. Sucking disorders in neurologically impaired infants: assessment and facilitation of breastfeeding. *Clinics in Perinatology* 1987; 14(1):109-130.

Meier P, Engstrom J, Crichton C, et al. A new scale for in-home test-weighing for mothers of preterm and high risk infants. *Journal of Human Lactation* 1994; 10(3):163-168.

Meier PP, Furman LM, Dengenhardt M. Increased lactation risk for late preterm infants and mothers: evidence and management strategies to protect breastfeeding. *Journal of Midwifery and Women's Health* 2007; 52(6):579-587.

Miller CK, Willging JP. The implications of upper-airway obstruction on successful infant feeding. *Seminars in Speech and Language* 2007; 28(3):190-203.

Morris S. Sensorimotor Prerequisites for Speech and the Influence of Cerebral Palsy, in J Wilson, ed. *Oral-motor Function and Dysfunction in Children.* Chapel Hill, NC: University of North Carolina at Chapel Hill, 1977; May 25-28, pp. 123-132.

Narayanan I, Mehta R, Choudhury D, et al. Sucking on the 'emptied' breast: non-nutritive sucking with a difference. *Archives of Disease in Childhood* 1991; 66(2):241-244.

Ogg L. Oral-pharyngeal development and evaluation. *Physical Therapy* 1975; 55(3):235-241.

Palmer M. Identification and management of the transitional suck pattern in premature infants. *Journal of Perinatal and Neonatal Nursing* 1993; 7(1):66-75.

Palmer M, Heyman M. Assessment and treatment of sensory-versus motor-based feeding problems in very young children. *Infants and Young Children* 1993; 6(2):67-73.

Pittet D. Improving adherence to hand hygiene practice: a multidisciplinary approach. *Emerging Infectious Diseases* 2001; 7(2):234-240.

Premji S, Paes B. Gastrointestinal function and growth in premature infants: is non-nutritive sucking vital? *Journal of Perinatology* 2000; 20(1):46-53.

Ramsay D, Kent J, Owens R. Ultrasound imaging of milk ejection in the breast of lactating women. *Pediatrics* 2004a; 113(2):361-367.

Ramsay D, Mitoulas L, Kent J, et al. Ultrasound imaging of the sucking mechanics of the breastfeeding infants. Proceedings of the 12th International Conference of the International Society for Research in Human Milk and Lactation, Sept. 10-14, 2004b; Queen's College, Cambridge, UK.

Ranly D. Early orofacial development. *Journal of Clinical Pediatric Dentistry* 1998; 22(4):267-275.

Reddy P, Qi C, Zembower T, et al. Postpartum mastitis and Community-acquired Methicillin-resistant *Staphylococcus aureus*. *Emerging Infectious Diseases* 2007; 13(2):298-301.

Saiman L, O'Keefe M, Graham P, et al. Hospital transmission of Community-acquired Methicillin-resistant *Staphylococcus aureus* among postpartum women. *Clinical Infectious Diseases* 2003; 37(15 Nov):1313-1319.

Sachs M, Oddie S. Breastfeeding - weighing in the balance: reappraising the role of weighing babies in the early days. *MIDIRS Midwifery Digest* 2002; 12(3):296-300.

Smith JD, Crumley RL, Harker LA. Facial paralysis in the newborn. *Otolaryngology, Head and Neck Surgery* 1981; 89(6):1021-1024.

Stutte P, Bowles B, Morman G. The effects of breast massage on volume and fat content of milk. *Genesis* 1988; 10(2):22-25.

van Vlimmeren LA, Helders PJ, van Adrichem LN, et al. Torticollis and plagiocephaly in infancy: therapeutic strategies. *Pediatric Rehabilitation* 2006; 9(1):40-46.

Wall V. Mandibular asymmetry and breastfeeding problems: experience from 11 cases. *Journal of Human Lactation* 2006; 22(3):326-334.

Wang R, Earl D, Ruder R, et al. Syndromic ear anomalies and renal ultrasounds. *Pediatrics* 2001; 108(2):e32.

Wolf L, Glass R. *Feeding and Swallowing Disorders in Infancy.* Tucson, AZ: Therapy Skill Builders, 1992; pp. 25-29,106-108, 114-122.

Woolridge M. The 'anatomy' of infant sucking. *Midwifery* 1986; 2(4):164-167.

Woolridge M. The Analysis, Classification, Etiology of Diagnosed Low Milk Output. Conference Presentation, La Leche League of Texas Area Conference. July, 1992; Houston, TX.

Notes:

Infant Diapers: Stools, Urine, and Vaginal Discharge

Many clinicians and new parents are aware that infant bowel output is a reasonable way to estimate milk intake in the breastfeeding newborn (Dewey 2003, Shrago 2006). Consequently, "Parents should be encouraged to record the urine and stool output during the early days of breastfeeding in the hospital and at home to facilitate the evaluation process" (AAP 2005). Clinics and hospitals often provide parents with log forms to monitor the number of diapers changed each day in the first week postpartum. However, because of inexperience in judging what a "normal" infant bowel movement looks like, parents may become confused when interpreting these logs.

Some parents worry that their baby is constipated, has diarrhea, or they may think that a normal vaginal discharge is a sign of illness. Breastfeeding mothers may conclude that changes in bowel or urine color indicate that their diet is adversely affecting the baby's digestion. Anticipatory guidance helps assuage such fears. Weight checks remain the best indicator of adequate milk intake whenever there is confusion about what the diaper counts indicate. The AAP recommends all infants be weighed 2 to 3 days following hospital discharge. Close follow-up may be required for infants whose stooling patterns deviate from the expected norms and whose mothers experience delays in the onset of copious milk production.

Normal Appearance of Stools

A baby's first stools are black tar-like meconium (**Fig. 61**). Within a few days of birth, the stools lighten in color to greenish brown (**Fig. 62**). Early transition to yellow stool is associated with less infant weight loss and earlier weight gain (Shrago 2006). Long, stressful labor or cesarean delivery may delay *lactogenesis stage II*, the onset of copious milk production (Chen 1998, Dewey 2003). A delay in the onset of lactogenesis II is defined as >72 hours without signs of increased milk production. Fewer than 4 stools daily by Day 4 *and* delayed onset of lactogenesis II are risk factors for inadequate lactation (Nommsen-Rivers 2008). If an infant has low diaper counts and fails to produce yellow stools by day 7, a follow-up weight check should be obtained in the HCP office.

Well-feeding breastfed infants typically stool frequently. **Fig. 63** shows the 24-hour output of a term newborn on Day 3.

Fig. 64 shows transitional stool that has lightened almost to yellow. This baby's mother had a cesarean delivery, a possible risk factor for delayed lactogenesis. It took this baby several more days than is expected for the stool color changes to occur. In this case, the volume of stool being produced and the transitioning color are both good indications that the volume of milk has increased and that the baby is now removing milk effectively.

Research has demonstrated the validity of maternal perception of the timing of lactogenesis stage II, commonly referred to as the milk "coming in" (Chapman 2000). Because women can reliably identify whether or not this event has occurred, it is important to ask the mother if her milk has "come in." This is a useful screening question with important public health implications because delayed lactogenesis II is a risk factor both for shorter breastfeeding duration and greater infant weight loss by Day 3 (Perez-Escamilla 2001). Sleepy infants, especially of first-time mothers, may understimulate early milk production, increasing their risk for hypernatremic dehydration with associated risk of seizure and even death (Ozdogan 2006).

Parents need specific information that lack of stooling in the first week postpartum is a risk factor. They also need information about how to categorize stool output. Some parents fail to distinguish between small stains and substantial stooling. This can cause confusion if the aim of telephone follow-up is to screen for markers of poor feeding. Specific verbal or graphic representations of appearances of expected infant stool and urine patterns better assist parents in communicating problems to their HCP.

Fig. 65 provides a graphic comparison of the sizes of 2 transitional-colored bowel movements. By Day 4, it is normal for babies to produce 4 or more stools in the course of 24 hours; some large and some small. Caregivers should request a weight check if a parent reports that a newborn fails to stool during any 24-hour period, or if all the daily bowel movements are small. **Fig. 66** shows a coin comparison to provide parents with a vocabulary to describe the size of bowel movements. In order for the stool to "count," it must be larger than 24 mm, about the size of a US quarter (Shrago 2006).

Quick passage of meconium is not only a marker for less weight loss, it is a marker for lower risk of developing jaundice (de Carvalho 1985, Yamauchi 1990). In a study of 358 Nigerian mothers exclusively breastfeeding their term infants, mothers averaged 13 feeds each 24 hours during the first 7 days. High frequency of breastfeeding was associated with rapid passage of meconium and lower neonatal serum bilirubin levels on Days 3 and 7 (Okechukwa 2006).

While it is important to avoid alarming the mother whose baby is feeding adequately in spite of slightly low diaper counts, it is also important not to falsely reassure the inexperienced mother whose baby may be breastfeeding poorly. The key public health message is that adequate intake in the healthy neonate *typically* is associated with frequent stooling (Nyhan 1952, Neifert 1996, AAP 2005). Conversely, since breastfed newborns are seldom constipated, scant stooling should be reported to the HCP as a red flag for poor feeding (Caglar 2006). A rare cause of lack of stooling in a newborn infant is a malrotation of the intestines (bowel blockage) or Hirschsprung's disease.

Composition and Appearances of Stools

The most important determinants of the composition of infant gut microbes are: mode of delivery, type of infant feeding, gestational age, infant hospitalization, and antibiotic use by the infant. "Term infants who were born vaginally at home and were breastfed exclusively seemed to have the most 'beneficial' gut microbiota (highest numbers of bifidobacteria and lowest numbers of *C difficile* and *E coli*)" in their stool (Penders 2006).

The normal stools of breastmilk-fed babies occasionally look watery (**Fig. 67**). Constant watery, explosive stools may be a sign of milk oversupply.

Sometimes the stools of a breastfed baby resemble mustard mixed with sesame seeds (**Fig. 68**). At other times, stools may appear to contain curds (**Fig. 69**) and will be bright yellow like the stool of this 6 day-old baby.

Maternal vitamins, certain vegetables, flavored fruit drinks *et cetera* can stain a mother's milk, causing temporary discoloration of the bowel movement and of urine (Lawrence 2005). **Fig. 70** pictures the diaper of a 3 week-old infant whose mother had just begun taking a new vitamin compound. Previously bright yellow, the temporary appearance of green-colored stool in an otherwise healthy infant is not generally a cause for concern.

Scant research has been done looking at the bowel output of the older breastfed infant. Anecdotal reports suggest that some infants older than 2 months stool infrequently. So long as general health and weigh gain continues to track at reference standards, infrequent stooling in the older infant is not considered to be a problem. However, many breastfeeding mothers continue to observe frequent stooling, often with each diaper change.

The diapers in **Fig. 71** represent the 24-hour output of a 13 lb 4 oz (5999 g) 8 week-old male. His birth weight was 7 lb 11 oz (3480 g).

Urination

Urination is a marker for adequate hydration, but is less clinically accurate at predicting adequate lactation performance (Nommsen-Rivers 2008). In general, parents can expect 3 to 5 urine soaked diapers by 3 to 5 days of age (AAP 2005). Parents using disposable diapers may have difficulty assessing the degree of wetness. When instructing parents about monitoring wet diapers, suggest putting a facial tissue or piece of toilet paper into the disposable diaper in order to better detect when the baby has urinated. Another tip is to encourage parents to put 3 tablespoons (45 cc) of water into a diaper and compare its weight to that of a dry diaper. The baby should produce at least 6 wet diapers of this weight each day by Day 7. Some parents find it easier to monitor urination by using cloth diapers, especially during the first week.

Brick Dust Urine

Brick dust urine (indicative of the presence of uric acid crystals) can be seen in the diapers of some infants in the first few days after birth. It is sometimes mistaken for a small stain of blood. Red-tinged urine is not necessarily an abnormal sign during the first 3 days. However, if there is a delay in the onset of copious milk production > 72 hours, or the baby is unable to access available milk, uric acid crystals in the diaper may be a sign of poor milk transfer and dehydration (Neifert 1996, Caglar 2006).

The infant whose diaper is pictured in **Fig. 72** was born prematurely at 37 weeks gestational age, weighing 6 lb 1 oz (2750 g). On Day 2.5, the baby weighed 5 lb 12 oz (2579 g). For a full-term baby this would not be an unusual weight loss. This 37 week-gestational-age baby, however, did not have extra fat stores on which to draw. Because he was not feeding functionally, his weight loss and rising bilirubin levels put him at risk for dehydration. The appearance of jaundice and the presence of brick dust urine contributed to the decision to begin supplementing the baby with pumped milk until he could more efficiently remove milk from the breast. The baby's urine began to lighten in color 12 hours after supplementation was begun. Within another 12 hours it was clear in color, indicating his hydration status had improved and was now normal.

A diaper containing concentrated or dark urine is a probable indication that the baby is not taking in sufficient volumes of milk and requires further evaluation.

Abnormal Stools

Some breastfed infants stool each time they feed. Because of the frequent stooling pattern, parents need reassurance that diarrhea in the breastfed baby is accompanied by other signs of illness, such as fever and malaise, foul-smell, or blood in the stool. Such signs should be reported to a doctor, midwife, physician's assistant, or nurse practitioner.

Human milk protects young infants from diarrhea. Risk increases when weaning foods are introduced at 6 months of age. Parents in some environments may need instruction about food safety when they begin complementary feeding in order to minimize their infant's exposure to food-borne pathogens (WHO 1993).

Parents need to be informed that babies older than 6 weeks may stool less frequently than newborns; however, their stools will remain loose and unformed. Sudden changes in stooling patterns can be a marker for illness. For example, one of the first signs of infant botulism is lack of stooling (Stiefel 1996). If a parent reports a sudden change in stooling, ask questions about the baby's condition. Is the baby active and alert? If the infant is constipated, having diarrhea, feeding poorly, or seems weak and "floppy," the HCP should be contacted immediately and the symptoms reported.

Blood in the Stools

Blood in the stool (**Fig. 73**) can have multiple causes.

- small anal fissures
- infection (Arvola 2006)
- sensitivity to something in the mother's diet
- a reaction triggered by a food or drug the baby is *directly* ingesting
- internal bleeding from another cause

The appropriate reaction to the discovery of blood in the stool is referral to the primary HCP for evaluation. Modern tests are about 90 percent accurate in localizing the bleeding site. The most common reason for bright red blood that coats, but is not mixed with the stool, is bleeding in the anorectal area. Darker blood or blood more mixed in with the stools may indicate bleeding from a site higher in the intestinal tract (Silber 1990). While alarming to parents, blood in the stool often occurs in infants who are otherwise well and growing normally. Blood in the stool of the breastfed baby has been attributed to cow milk allergy. New research suggests that cow milk allergy may have been over diagnosed in the past. Rectal bleeding in infants often resolves without definitive diagnosis, leading some to describe it as a "benign and self-limiting disorder" (Arvola 2006).

Vaginal Discharge

A baby girl may have a bloody vaginal discharge (**Fig. 74**). This is caused by withdrawal of maternal hormones from the baby's system after birth and generally will subside within a few days. White vaginal discharges (**Fig. 75**) are also common. Persistent or foul-smelling discharge should be reported to the HCP, along with persistent diaper rashes that do not resolve with usual measures of airing, frequent diaper changes, and applications of non-irritating diaper ointments and creams.

American Academy of Pediatrics (AAP) Section on Breastfeeding. Breastfeeding and the use of human milk. *Pediatrics* 2005; 115(2):496-506.

Arvola T, Ruuska R, Keranen J, et al. Rectal bleeding in infancy: clinical, allergological, and microbiological examination. *Pediatrics* 2006; 117(4):e760-768.

Caglar MK, Ozer I, Altugan FS. Risk factors for excess weight loss and hypernatremia in exclusively breast-fed infants. *Brazilian Journal of Medical and Biological Research* 2006; 39(4):539-544.

Chapman D, Perez-Escamilla R. Maternal perception of the onset of lactation is a valid, public health indicator of lactogenesis stage II. *Journal of Nutrition* 2000; 130(12):2972-2980.

Chen DC, Nommsen-Rivers L, Dewey KG, et al. Stress during labor and delivery and early lactation performance. *American Journal of Clinical Nutrition* 1998; 68(2):335-344.

de Carvalho M, Robertson S, Klaus M. Fecal bilirubin excretion and serum bilirubin concentrations in breast-fed and bottle-fed infants. *Journal of Pediatrics* 1985; 107(5):786-790.

Dewey K, Nommsen-Rivers M, Heinig MJ. Risk factors for suboptimal infant breastfeeding behavior, delayed onset of lactation, and excess neonatal weight loss. *Pediatrics* 2003; 112(3):607-619.

Lawrence RA, Lawrence RM. *Breastfeeding: A Guide for the Medical Profession (6th edition)*. Philadelphia, PA: Elsevier Mosby, 2005; pp. 349-350.

Neifert M. Early assessment of the breastfeeding infant. *Contemporary Pediatrics* 1996; 13(10):142-166.

Nommsen-Rivers LA, Heinig MJ, Cohen RJ, et al. Newborn wet and soiled diaper counts and timing of onset of lactation as indicators of breastfeeding inadequacy. *Journal of Human Lactation* 2008; 24(1):27-33.

Nyhan WL. Stool frequency of normal infants in the first week of life. *Pediatrics* 1952; 10(4):414-425.

Okechukwu AA, Okolo AA. Exclusive breastfeeding frequency during the first seven days of life in term neonates. *Nigerian Postgraduate Medical Journal* 2006; 13(4):309-312.

Ozdogan T. Hypernatremic dehydration in breast-fed neonates (letter) *Archives of Disease in Children* 2006; 91(12):1041.

Penders J, Thijs C, Vink C, et al. Factors influencing the composition of the intestinal microbiota in early infancy. *Pediatrics* 2006; 118(2):511-521.

Perez-Escamilla R, Chapman D. Validity and public health implications of maternal perception of the onset of lactation: an international analytical overview. *Journal of Nutrition* 2001; 131(11):3021S-3024S.

Shrago LC, Reifsnider E, Insel K. The neonatal bowel output study: indicators of adequate breast milk intake in neonates. *Pediatric Nursing* 2006; 32(3):195-201.

Silber G. Lower gastrointestinal bleeding. *Pediatrics in Review* 1990; 12(3):85-92.

Stiefel L. In Brief - Hypotonia in infants. *Pediatrics in Review* 1996; 17(3):104-105.

World Health Organization (WHO). Contaminated food: a major cause of diarrhoea and associated malnutrition among infants and young children. *Facts for Infant Feeding*. 1993; 3:1-4.

Yamauchi Y, Yamanouchi I. Breast-feeding frequency during the first 24 hours after birth in full-term neonates. *Pediatrics* 1990; 86(2):171-75.

Notes:

Appearances of Human Milk

Lactogenesis describes the 3-stage process by which the mammary gland develops the capacity to secrete milk, begins copious milk production, and maintains production over time. *Lactogenesis stage I* refers to the mid-pregnancy maturation of the gland. Small amounts of milk produced during this phase may accumulate in the ducts. Some women may leak milk during pregnancy.

A normal event signaling full maturation of the process, referred to as *lactogenesis stage II,* occurs 30-40 hours postpartum (Arthur 1989, Neville 2001). This is commonly described as the milk "coming in." When the onset of copious lactation has not occurred by 72 hours postpartum, lactogenesis stage II is characterized as "delayed" (Dewey 2003). Even in well-motivated populations, delays are common. Delays appear to be associated with sub-optimal neonatal breastfeeding behavior, and with maternal factors such as primiparity, prolonged labor, instrumented delivery, cesarean birth, retained placenta, hypo-androgenism, hypertension, maternal diabetes, excessive blood loss use of non-breastmilk fluids, and maternal obesity (Hall 2002, Dewey 2003, Sert 2003, Rasmussen 2004). Dewey reported that 22 percent of mothers studied experienced delays >72 hours (33 percent of primiparas *vs* 8 percent of multiparas). Chapman found 35 percent of women experience delayed onset of lactogenesis (Chapman 1999).

Delays in the onset of copious milk production have obvious implications for the infant, including risk of greater postpartum weight loss and longer periods for recovery of birth weight than is considered optimal (Nommsen-Rivers 2008). Failure to lactate is an important clue for health conditions that should signal the need for further medical evaluation of the mother (Sert 2003, Villaseca 2005).

Normal Milk Volumes

Please Note: Researchers in the following studies report milk production volumes in both milliliters (ml) and grams (g). Grams, milliliters and cubic centimeters (cc) are essentially equivalent. One ounce (oz) equals 28.3 g, cc, or ml.

Volumes of colostrum are normally low on Day 1, especially in primiparous mothers. However, Wang (1994) described the physiological capacity of the newborn stomach as only 6 ml on the first day and 12 ml on the second day after birth. Wang states, "Although the amount of colostrum secreted is not voluminous, it can still meet the needs of the newborn."

Neville (1988) looked at milk production in a group of 13 multiparous women, following them *longitudinally* (over

time) for 6 months. Her study describes low volumes of milk production on Days 1 and 2, with the mean total for Day 2 of about 175 ml/day (6 oz). Milk production in this group rose rapidly on days 3 and 4 to about 500 ml/day (17.6 oz), and reached levels of about 750 ml/day (26.5 oz) by the end of the first week postpartum. By 6 months these mothers averaged production levels of about 800 ml/day (28 oz).

Villalpando (1996) observed that Day 3 milk production averaged about 360 ml in a group of 30 women. All their infants regained birth weight within 74 hours post birth.

Hill (2005) observed greater challenges in establishing lactation in mothers pumping for preterm infants compared to mothers whose breastfeeding infants directly stimulated the breasts. The nursing mothers' milk output continuously increased over time, while milk output tended to decline or remain stable in mothers who were exclusively pumping. Other research suggests that women delivering preterm infants at less than 28 weeks may not experience full glandular development of the breast. Issues related to premature birth, therefore, may reduce milk production and delay the onset of lactogenesis II (Henderson 2004, Henderson 2008).

Hurst and Meier summarize issues regarding assisting mothers of preterm infants in *Breastfeeding and Human Lactation* (Riordan 2005). They recommend that mothers of non-nursing preterm infants establish a robust supply in early lactation (750-1000 ml/day). Pumping frequently in the early days may provide a hedge against observed decreases in production over time in pump-dependent mothers. Therefore, it is important, if possible, to ensure a robust milk supply at the time of the infant's discharge from the special care nursery.

Hill and Aldag (2005) studied milk production in preterm and term mothers and observed that milk output on Days 6 and 7 is highly associated with Week 2 milk output, and moderately associated with Week 6 output. The same researchers identified similar predictors of term infant feeding outcomes in a longitudinal study of healthy singletons. Milk output during Weeks 1-6 was predictive of feeding type at Week 12 (Hill 2007). If mothers perceived their milk supply was low during the calibration phase, or if they stimulated their breasts fewer than 7.8 times daily, they were more likely to be supplementing their infants at Week 12.

Available research speaks strongly to the need for appropriate *early* support of mothers who are exclusively pumping. Similar levels of support must be provided for mothers with real or perceived insufficient milk supply. Women need accurate, careful guidance in milk supply calibration for the critically sensitive period during the first 2 weeks postpartum. Failure to stimulate sufficiently during this phase may prevent these mothers from establishing adequate lactation.

Kent (1999) confirmed earlier research findings that once established, milk production is relatively constant over the first 6 months of lactation. Using sophisticated imaging techniques, Kent observed that average 24 hour milk production from *each breast* in a group of 8 women was 453.6 ± 20.1 g. This level of production is consistent with previous research by Hartmann (1995) describing 24 hour milk production of 798 ± 216 g at 1 month and 837 ± 190 g a day at 6 months. What is striking in all these studies is the wide range in milk production. Kent observed a range of 440-1220 g/day.

Individual milk production appears to be consistent over a 24 hour period. Lai (2004) reported a novel method of determining a mother's intrinsic hourly rate of milk production which can then be projected over a 24-hour period. The technique has been further refined and simplified (Hale 2008). The mother is instructed to pump hourly for 4 times. The volume of milk pumped from the first 2 pumpings is not considered in the calculation. Add together the volume of the milk from the third and fourth pumping and multiply by 12 to get the 24 hour milk production. Using this method to calculate a woman's production capacity is less intrusive than 24 hour test-weighing.

Available milk production averages and ranges suggest rough norms, but it is important to remember that there is great individuality in the feeding patterns of each mother-baby pair (Dewey 1986). In general, healthy women appear to be able to produce adequate quantities of milk. Infant *intake* is also variable depending on the individual baby. After the first month postpartum, infant appetite is more significant in regulating the milk supply than is maternal production capacity (Woolridge 1982, Kent 1999). Night feeds are common in the early months and comprise a substantial proportion of the daily intake for most infants (Kent 2004).

Several researchers (Kent 2004, Engstrom 2004) report differences, sometimes dramatic, in milk volume production between left and right breasts.

Milk Nutrient Variations

Milk nutrients vary between women and in the same woman according to stage of gestation, stage of lactation,

time of day, degree of breast fullness, and maternal diet (Czank 2007). Obtaining an adequate maternal health history screens for significant issues that may affect milk nutrient values. A maternal history of vegan diet or previous bariatric surgery, for example, may influence maternal levels of vitamin B12, creating deficiencies in the milk (Stefanski 2006). Vegan status and multiparity may result in zinc deficiencies that manifest in the infant as persistent diaper rashes and poor weight gain. The LC must screen clients adequately to identify such issues.

Preterm infants may require protein supplementation to permit normal bone mineralization. Mothers providing milk for their own preterm infants may also require assistance in learning to harvest hind milk to improve infant weight gain (Slusher 2003). Owing to variances between women in the caloric value of their milk, milk donated to milk banks should be tested for fat content. Targeted pooling of high calorie milk (rather than random pooling) may better ensure the growth of preterm infants receiving donor milk (Updegrove 2005).

Milk Color Variations

Human milk comes in a variety of colors. *Colostrum* may be clear (**Fig. 76**), bright yellow (**Fig. 77**), white (**Fig. 78**), orange/pink (**Fig. 79**), or even light brown (**Fig. 80**). KH has seen dark brown milk. Babies probably drink colored milk at their mothers' breasts fairly frequently, but we never see it unless the mother is pumping. Some foods, vitamins, medicine, and flavored drinks color milk without doing harm (Lawrence 2005).

The orange/pink colored milk in **Fig. 79** is attributed to dried blood in the milk ducts that washes out as lactation begins. This is called "rusty pipe" syndrome and is well known in the dairy industry. The coloration may be the result of bleeding inside a milk duct. It is safe to feed pink or orange milk to the baby. Small amounts of blood are not harmful, although parents may find it disturbing and some prefer to discard the milk.

Hand expression can be an effective way to obtain colostrum to feed to a non-nursing newborn. Often mothers are able to express drops of colostrum into a spoon to offer to the infant (**Fig. 81**). They may need reassurance that the amounts of colostrum, although small, are physiologically normal and sufficient for Day 1.

Fig. 81 shows about 0.6 ml of colostrum, which is about the size of a newborn's swallow (Lawrence 2005). Eight to 10 swallows of this size would provide sufficient intake at a feeding during the first 24 hours for a full-term, medically stable newborn.

Figures 76-81 show the first expressions of milk from mothers who are less than 24 hours postpartum. Notice in **Fig. 78** that the amount of milk this 18 year-old mother pumped at her first expression was 56.6 ml or 2 oz! **Fig. 80** shows this mother's first 3 pumpings at 2-hour intervals. The milk yield decreased over the first 3 pumpings, and the light brown color became lighter each time. The lightening in color suggests that a flushing action is clearing debris from the ducts that has stained the colostrum. Over time, milk typically turns whiter and increases in volume.

Figures 76-80 represent unusually large amounts of milk for the first expression, and provide useful illustrations of milk color. Many primiparous mothers may only obtain a few drops of milk at their first attempt at expression. Casey (1986) found the total volume of milk produced on the first postpartum day to be 3 to 32 ml. When women express a large amount (7 ml or more) during the first expression attempt, anticipatory guidance is prudent because the next time or 2 they may express less milk. The volume will increase gradually over the next few days.

Fig. 82 shows 70.7 ml (2.5 oz) pumped by a primiparous woman on Day 3. The yellow color suggests that this is transitional milk. The color and volume of this pumped milk are consistent with typical Day 3 milk appearance.

Fig. 83 documents the typical color change that occurs when milk matures. This mother has pumped in the middle of the night of Day 2. She obtained 32 ml of yellow-stained colostrum. By morning of Day 3, when she pumped off enough milk to help soften her engorged breast, the milk had assumed the whitish color typical of mature milk. Note the thin, transparent quality of this foremilk.

Fig. 84 shows two containers of milk from a woman during *lactogenesis stage III,* the on-going maintenance of milk production over the course of lactation. The mother was asked to express a small amount of milk before breastfeeding her baby and another small amount once her baby had finished feeding. The milk has been allowed to separate, providing a graphic illustration of the difference in the fat content of foremilk and hindmilk. Research suggests that when the breast is full, the volume of fluid dilutes the cream content of the milk (Daly 1993).

Arthur P, Smith M, Hartmann P. Milk lactose, citrate and glucose as markers of lactogenesis in normal and diabetic women. *Journal of Pediatric Gastroenterology and Nutrition* 1989; 9(4):488-496.

Casey CE, Neifert MR, Seacat JM, et al. Nutrient intake by breastfed infants during the first five days after birth. *American Journal of Diseases of Children* 1986; 140(9):933-936.

Chapman DJ, Pérez-Escamilla R. Identification of risk factors for delayed onset of lactation. *Journal of the American Dietetic Association* 1999; 99(4):450-454.

Czank C, Mitoulas LR, Hartmann PE. Human Milk Composition - Fat. in *Hale & Hartmann's Textbook of Lactation.* Amarillo, TX: Hale Publishing 2007; pp. 56-58.

Daly S, Di Rosso A, Owens R, et al. Degree of breast emptying explains changes in the fat content, but not fatty acid composition, of human milk. *Experimental Physiology* 1993; 78(6):741-755.

Dewey K, Nommsen-Rivers L, Heinig MJ. Risk factors for suboptimal infant breastfeeding behavior, delayed onset of lactation, and excess neonatal weight loss. *Pediatrics* 2003; 112(3 Pt 1):607-619.

Dewey K, Lonnerdal B. Infant self-regulation of breast milk intake. *Acta Paediatrica Scandia* 1986; 75(6):893-898.

Engstrom J, Meier P, Zuleger J, et al. Comparison of volume of milk pumped from the right and left breasts in mothers of very low birthweight (VLBW) infants. Poster at the 12th International Conference of the International Society for Research in Human Milk and Lactation. Sept. 10-14, 2004; Queen's College, Cambridge, UK.

Hall R, Mercer A, Teasley S, et al: A breast-feeding assessment score to evaluate the risk for cessation of breast-feeding by 7 to 10 days of age. *Journal of Pediatrics* 2002; 141(5):659-64.

Hale T. Personal communication, Feb. 2, 2008.

Hartmann P, Sherriff J, Kent J. Maternal nutrition and the regulation of milk synthesis. *Proceedings of the Nutrition Society* 1995; 54:379-389.

Henderson JJ, Hartmann PE, Newnham JP, et al. Effect of preterm birth and antenatal corticosteroid treatment on lactogenesis II in women. *Pediatrics* 2008; 121(1):e92-e100.

Henderson JJ, Simmer K, Newnham PJ, et al. Impact of very preterm delivery on the timing of lactogenesis II in women. Proceedings of the 12th International Conference of the International Society for Research in Human Milk and Lactation. Sept. 10-14, 2004; Queen's College, Cambridge, UK.

Hill P, Aldag J, Chatterton R, et al. Comparison of milk output between mothers of preterm and term infants: the first 6 weeks after birth. *Journal of Human Lactation* 2005; 21(1):22-30.

Hill PD, Aldag JC. Predictors of term infant feeding at week 12 postpartum. *Journal of Perinatal & Neonatal Nursing* 2007; 21(3):250-255.

Hurst N, Meier P. Breastfeeding the preterm infant. in J Riordan. *Breastfeeding and Human Lactation (3rd edition).* Sudbury, MA: Jones and Bartlett. 2005; pp.367-406.

Kent J, Cregan M, Mitoulas L, et al. Frequency, volume and milk fat content of breastfeeds of exclusively breastfed babies. Poster at the 12th International Conference of the International Society for Research in Human Milk and Lactation. Sept. 10-14, 2004; Queen's College, Cambridge, UK.

Kent J, Mitoulas L, Cox D, et al. Breast volume and milk production during extended lactation in women. *Experimental Physiology* 1999; 84(2):435-447.

Lai C, Hale T, Simmer K, et al. Hourly rate of milk synthesis in women. Poster at the 12th International Conference of the International Society for Research in Human Milk and Lactation. Sept.10-14, 2004; Queen's College, Cambridge, UK.

Lawrence RA, Lawrence RM. *Breastfeeding: A Guide for the Medical Profession (6th edition).* Philadelphia, PA: Elsevier Mosby, 2005; pp. 261, 349-350.

Neville M. Anatomy and physiology of lactation. in Schanler R ed. *The Pediatric Clinics of North America.* Philadelphia: WB Saunders 2001; 48(1):13-34.

Neville M, Keller R, Seacat J, et al. Studies in human lactation: milk volumes in lactating women during the onset of lactation and full lactation. *American Journal Clinical Nutrition* 1988; 48(6):1375-86.

Nommsen-Rivers LA, Heinig MJ, Cohen RJ, et al. Newborn wet and soiled diaper counts and timing of onset of lactation as indicators of breastfeeding inadequacy. *Journal of Human Lactation* 2008; 24(1):27-33.

Rasmussen K, Kjolhede C. Prepregnant overweight and obesity diminish the prolactin response to suckling in the first week postpartum. *Pediatrics* 2004; 113(5):e465-470.

Sert M, Tetiker T, Kirim S, et al. Clinical report of 28 patients with Sheehan's Syndrome. *Endocrine Journal* 2003; 50(3):297-301.

Slusher T, Hampton R, Bode-Thomas F, et al. Promoting the exclusive feeding of own mother's milk through the use of hindmilk and increased maternal milk volume for hospitalized, low birth weight infants (<1800 grams) in Nigeria: a feasibility study. *Journal of Human Lactation* 2003; 19(2):191-198.

Stefanski J. Breast-feeding after bariatric surgery. *Today's Dietitian* 2006; 8(1):e47.

Villalpando S, Flores-Huerta S, López-Alarcón M, et al. Social and biological determinants of lactation. *Food and Nutrition Bulletin* 1996; 17(4):328-335.

Updegrove KK: Human milk banking in the United States. *Newborn Infant Nursing Review* 2005; 5(1):27-33.

Villaseca P, Campino C, Oestreicher E, et al. Bilateral oophorectomy in a pregnant woman: hormonal profile from late gestation to post-partum: case report. *Human Reproduction* 2005; 20(2):397-401.

Wang YF, Shen YH, Wang JJ, et al. Preliminary study on the blood glucose level in the exclusively breastfed newborn. *Journal of Tropical Pediatrics* 1994; 40(3):187-188.

Woolridge M, Baum J, Drewett R. Individual patterns of milk intake during breast-feeding. *Early Human Development* 1982; 7(3):265-272.

Positioning and Latch-on Technique

Latching onto the breast is an instinctive skill of the normal newborn. Most robust, term infants can eventually self-attach if placed skin-to-skin with their mothers in a conducive environment. Best practices for breastfeeding thus emphasize early and unrestricted contact for breastfeeding, rooming-in, and avoidance of artificial teats unless medically indicated.

Many experienced LCs view the demonstrated ability of a baby to latch to the breast with minimal assistance to be an important assessment criterion. Given the innate capabilities of newborns to self-attach, it is important to advise mothers to get comfortable and to wait until they request or appear to require help with positioning and attachment rather than offering such help routinely (Colson 2005). If the mother and baby appear to be managing well, the LC primarily encourages and provides anticipatory guidance. Such guidance may include tips on how to more optimally position the baby and care for tender nipples. It is useful to provide information on using diaper counts and timing of engorgement as markers for adequate feeding.

In the case of *compromised dyads*, especially when the baby cannot latch, more active assistance may be required to bring the baby to breast and to protect the milk supply until breastfeeding normalizes.

All hospital and birthing personnel need to have a *basic* understanding of how to help mothers bring their infants to breast. The lactation consultant requires a more *sophisticated* understanding of the anatomy and physiology of breastfeeding in order to effectively assist compromised dyads. The following overview is a synopsis of positioning and latch information from experts (Gunther 1945 and 1955, Newton 1967, Woolridge 1986a and 1986b, Savage-King 1992, Glass 1994, Neifert 1995, Wiessinger 1998, Royal College of Midwives 2000, Glover 2000, Smilie 2007, Colson 2008). Ultrasonographic studies have expanded our understanding of the mechanics of breast-feeding (Ramsay 2004, Ramsay 2005, Jacobs 2007, Geddes 2008).

The Mechanics of Sucking

The baby locates the breast guided by nipple coloration and scent (Varendi 1994, Prime 2007). Touch on the face stimulates the rooting reflex, causing the baby to seek the nipple, open wide and latch. With all of his lip surface in contact with the breast, the baby grasps and draws in the breast tissue.

Suction holds the breast in the mouth and elongates the breast tissue to form a "teat." This teat extends to within approximately 5 mm of the junction of the hard and soft palates (Ramsay 2004, Jacobs 2007). During normal, painless sucking, the position of the teat in the mouth has been observed to move (Jacobs 2007). The dropping of the posterior tongue creates negative pressure in the oral cavity. The strong vacuum generated appears to be the primary mechanism of milk removal by the infant (Ramsay 2004, Geddes 2007).

Less than 10 ml of milk is available to the infant prior to the milk ejection (Prime 2007). Nipple stimulation triggers the mother's milk ejection reflex (the let-down), facilitating milk transfer and thorough breast emptying. A mother experiencing significant stress may have inhibited milk ejection, and her infant may not receive full feeds.

Because the infant must be able to draw in enough breast tissue to manipulate the teat, flat and inverted nipples, or severely engorged breasts may prove problematic. The infant must have a fully mobile tongue in order to suck and swallow normally; a tongue-tied infant may be challenged to breastfeed. Similarly there may be problems when the mother has large diameter or her nipples are difficult for the baby to manipulate.

Primitive Neonatal Reflexes

There appears to be great variability in normal breast-feeding behavior. *Primitive neonatal reflexes* (PNRs) refer to reflex responses (rooting, sucking, swallowing), spontaneous behaviors, and reactions to environmental stimuli that may trigger normal breastfeeding responses in mothers and babies (Colson 2008). So-called *Biological Nurturing* methods emphasize skin-to-skin holding of newborns and semi-reclined feeding positions, activating PNRs and assisting infant-self attachment to the breast.

Normal infants cared for in this manner may need little help with positioning. Compromised dyads may need much more active assistance with positioning. Stable head position improves jaw control, influences swallowing, and reduces the risk of aspiration. Stability of the head is influenced by trunk alignment, particularly the stability of the pelvic area (Redstone 2004). Pelvic stability is the reason breastfeeding experts often emphasize hip flexion. Normal infants may be able to compensate for misalignment of body position during feeding. Children with birth injury, neurodisabilities or other weaknesses may not be able to overcome misalignment.

Visual Images of Positioning

Pulling on the baby's jaw or manipulating the baby's head to achieve correct positioning is ineffective and distracts the baby. Correctly orienting the baby to the breast can be more easily done by realigning the placement of the baby's body relative to the mother. At the start of the latch-on sequence in any position chosen, the baby's body is held close, with the mother's arms providing boundaries and support. The baby's head will tilt and the mouth will open wide in order to reach for the nipple. Extension of the head permits the receding lower jaw of the infant to fit tightly against the breast (see **Figs. 112** and **116**).

Mothers should ignore advice to push on the baby's head. Pushing the baby's head will flex the head forward, driving the nose into the breast. Burying the nose obstructs breathing and prevents the baby from looking at the mother. Additionally, if the upper jaw makes first contact with the breast, it is akin to biting an apple with your chin tucked into your neck. Hyperflexion at the neck inhibits jaw opening and prevents comfortable swallowing.

Women breastfeeding in the cradle position are often instructed to place the newborn's head in the crook of their arm. The crook of the arm naturally falls *beside* the body and may be too far to the side of the mother's body for a small baby. When the infant's head "over-shoots" the nipple target, the baby has to bend his head forward, tucking his chin into his chest in order to locate the nipple. Breathing, swallowing, and wide jaw excursions are inhibited.

Fig. 85 shows a poorly positioned baby, whose frustration has resulted in crying and breast rejection. The blankets are in the way, and the mother has resorted to "chasing" the baby with her breast, trying to push it into his mouth. Distortion of the shape of the breast may result in poor milk transfer by collapsing the easily compressible milk ducts (Ramsay 2005, Geddes 2007).

In **Fig. 86**, the same woman has made several changes resulting in a successful latch. The blankets have been removed, allowing the mother and baby to sense one another more acutely. The baby's body is rotated, so that he no longer has to struggle to turn his head in order to find the nipple. The mother has brought the baby's head onto her forearm, which orients the baby to the front of her breast. This allows her to line up the baby so that her nipple touches his nose. Now the baby has to extend his head slightly during latch-on, so that he leads with his chin. This places the chin tightly against the breast. When the chin is tucked into the breast, the nose will be slightly tipped away from

the breast, helping to maintain an open breathing passage. The mother's hand supports the weight of the breast.

Fig. 87 shows a baby lined up with the nose touching the nipple. As the baby roots in response to the stimulus, the head tilts back, the mouth opens, and the lower jaw is planted on the breast.

Note the uncomfortable looking position of the baby's lower arm in **Fig. 88**. When an infant begins to struggle at breast, it could be that some part of his body is twisted or strained. Sometimes a baby suffers minor neck, shoulder or clavicle injury during delivery, which influences how he responds to handling in the early postpartum period. Observe, also, how the mother's arm in **Fig. 88** does not adequately support the baby. The baby's body appears to be falling away. The mother's arm needs to be under the baby, providing sufficient postural support to stabilize the baby's position at breast.

Positioning the infant's arm around the mother's side may be uncomfortable for some newborns. It can be useful, instead, to gently place the baby's lower arm across his chest before rolling him onto his side (**Fig. 89**). This will round the shoulder, placing it in a more comfortable position. Bringing the infant's upper torso into physiologic flexion may reduce the discomfort of torticollis. Note also that the infant in **Fig. 89** has a healing incision on her abdomen and is using a feeding tube device. She suffered a bowel rotation, which was corrected surgically. The baby needed supplementation with pumped milk until she grew stronger. Trapping her lower arm across her chest prevented her from grabbing the feeding tube.

When one arm is brought to the midline of the baby's body, the other hand tends to seek it. Improving physiologic flexion helps state stability and calms some disorganized infants (**Fig. 90**).

Fig. 91 emphasizes that the newborn may be too small to be placed in the crook of the mother's arm at the side of her body. Passive support of the head on the mother's forearm more correctly aligns the baby in front of the nipple. This woman has very long arms. In assisting a woman with comfortable positioning, the LC needs to take into consideration the size of the baby, the size (length, width, and weight) of the woman's breasts, the location of her nipples, the length of her arms, and the length of the mother's torso.

The 6 week-old baby pictured in **Fig. 92** is being breastfed in the cradle position. She has gained 3 pounds (1358 g) above her birth weight and is big enough to be comfortably positioned in the crook of her mother's arm. Careful attention to positioning technique generally is a concern of *early* breastfeeding. As time goes by, each dyad works out their own way of doing things. The hallmark of good positioning is simple: both mother and baby are comfortable, avoiding strain and exertion. Effective breastfeeding allows the newborn to self-regulate intake by efficiently emptying the breast (Daly 1993). The baby will release the breast spontaneously when satiated, and growth will be appropriate (Kent 2007).

The mother in **Fig. 93** is breastfeeding in the cradle position. This mother is using a nursing pillow to support the baby. Her 6 week-old baby needs less postural control and support from her mother than would a newborn. Laying a newborn baby directly on the pillow is generally not a good idea. As the baby sinks into the pillow he may slip off the breast. Sometimes a firm commercial breastfeeding pillow helps, but many pillows are the wrong height and interfere with good positioning. If the mother has a short waist, a pillow may place the baby above the level of the nipple. This forces the mother to lift her breast to the baby, putting strain on her shoulders. Remind the mother of a newborn that her arms support the baby and the pillow supports her arms.

Notice how the mother in **Fig. 93** turns the baby's body in toward her own. Pulling the hips close stabilizes the baby's body. When babies are well-positioned, face-to-face gazing can occur. This facilitates bonding and gives pleasure to both mother and baby.

The mother in **Fig. 94** has slightly over-rotated the body of her infant. Observe how this buries the baby's face so that the mother and baby are not able to see one another. The mother is putting too much pressure on the baby's top shoulder, causing the over-rotation. This will cause the "down" side cheek to back away from the breast. The nipple may emerge from the baby's mouth looking pinched.

Maternal overweight and obesity are associated with poor breastfeeding outcomes (Jevitt 2007). Poor outcomes in this population may result from difficulty in positioning caused by short arms relative to body mass, large breasts, no lap, and issues related to body image (Rassmussen 2006). In order to reduce the risk of early discontinuation of breastfeeding in overweight or obese mothers, the LC must assist with sensitive counseling and teach creative positioning. It is important to choose positions that support both the baby and the breast. If the breast is heavy and the nipple ill-defined, some mothers may use a free hand to shape the breast to help the baby latch (as in **Fig. 96, Fig. 100** and **Fig. 101**).

The football hold is pictured in **Fig. 95**. Note how the baby's flexed hips enable the mother to position the baby's body in a relaxed fashion. If the baby's feet touch the back of the chair, he may reflexively push off, going stiff and arching away. Putting the baby's bottom against the back of the chair may be a solution.

Fig. 96 shows a slight variation of the football hold that is especially useful for preterm babies or hypotonic babies because it gives the mother good control of her baby's body (Tully 1991, Brodribb 1998). Once again, the mother uses active support at the nape of the baby's neck with her hand. She supports the baby's torso with her forearm. Her free hand supports her breast and performs deep breast compression.

It is important when demonstrating the football position to caution the mother against placing her hand on the baby's head and pushing it toward the breast. The mother in **Fig. 97** was instructed to move her hand position and to support the baby at the neck and shoulders as shown in **Fig. 98**. Now she is less likely to hyperflex the baby's head, mashing the baby's nose into the breast and constricting the throat. If the baby's breathing and swallowing are inhibited by the mother's poor positioning technique, breastfeeding turns into a struggle as the baby attempts to communicate discomfort.

A modified cross-cradle position is useful for women with short arms, large breasts, or during engorgement because it helps the mother better support her breast. Note how the mother in **Fig. 99** rests the weight of the breast on her wrist. Her baby's head rests passively in the palm of her hand, but her other arm actively guides the baby and holds him close with support at the nape of the neck and along his torso. When the baby is well positioned, both cheeks will touch the breast and the nose will be clear to breathe.

Fig. 100 shows a mother with large breasts positioning her infant on a table in a modified cross-cradle position. The table stabilizes the baby and the weight of the breast. Using her free hand, the mother shapes and holds the breast in the baby's mouth.

Creative positioning may also assist a baby in a hip brace (See **Fig. 365**). Some babies when first placed in a brace for hip dysplasia do not feed well for a few days until they become accustomed to the restriction of their legs. The LC can teach the mother to use a breastfeeding pillow to help position the baby in a cross-cradle position.

The mother in **Fig. 101** is nursing in the side-lying position. An obvious advantage of side-lying is increased rest for the mother (Milligan 1996). Side-lying also protects the infant's ability to self-attach (Colson 2005). A mother recovering from an episiotomy, a painful perineal tear, or hemorrhoids may find side-lying more comfortable than a seated position. Lang (2002) states that this position may help the woman "who is disabled and cannot take the weight of the baby in her arms." The authors have found side-lying to be another useful feeding position for women with large breasts. The bed supports the weight of the breast. This frees up the mother's hands to guide the baby during latch-on if such help is required.

Hypertonic babies or babies who resist touch also may benefit from a side-lying nursing position. The baby may feel less constrained and more in control -- an important issue if previous breastfeeding experiences have resembled a wrestling match! Infants who previously experienced great difficulty breastfeeding often enjoy being placed in a side-lying position and allowed to re-discover the breast at their own pace. Observing her infant's capacity for self-attachment is an encouraging experience for a mother who feels she is struggling to establish breastfeeding.

Notice that the side-lying mother in **Fig. 101** has oriented the baby slightly below the level of her breast. The baby has to tip his head back to latch, clearing a breathing space for his nose and allowing the mother and baby to look at one another. Note how the mother is using her free hand to guide her breast. She could easily employ deep breast compressions to increase milk intake, if needed (see **Fig. 43**).

The infant's bottom arm may be drawn across the chest, rolling the bottom shoulder and hip toward the mother's body. The "edges" of the mother and baby come together in a "V." If the baby cannot look into his mother's eyes, his head is too close to her armpit, and he should be moved down her torso in the direction of his feet. A rolled-up cloth can be used at the baby's back to keep the baby slightly turned toward the mother.

Fig. 102 shows a 22 month-old toddler nursing to sleep in side-lying position. This older child typically does not require assistance from his mother to latch onto the breast. Moments before this photo was taken, the over-tired toddler began crying. Many mothers who breastfeed beyond infancy find that comfort nursing is an important aspect of calming and caring for their older children. Howard (2004) reported that "Nursing to comfort a crying infant was a highly effective calming method and a strong independent predictor of extended long-term breastfeeding duration." The mother in this photo remarked that she viewed breastfeeding as an essential mothering technique. The ability to comfort her toddler at the breast was even more important to her than the nutritional benefits of breastmilk.

The seated straddle position shown in **Fig. 103** may be helpful for the baby when the mother has a rapid milk ejection. It also may assist infants with clefts of the palate. Some infants with swallowing or breathing disorders may benefit from upright feeding positions that reduce choking. The head must be well-supported at the neck in an extended position to maintain airway patency (Wolf 1992).

The baby in **Fig. 104** has been struggling with his mother's oversupply and forceful milk ejection reflex. Here the mother is reclining in a chair with the baby lying on top of her. The baby is in a prone feeding position, sometimes called "posture feeding." Such positioning is believed to stimulate primitive neonatal reflexes (Colson 2008).

The mother in **Fig. 105** was injured during the repair of her episiotomy after delivery. Sitting was painful for over a year. Her LC (KH) mentioned this mother's problem to Chris Mulford, an IBCLC colleague. Chris had experienced back pain and found that standing and lying were the only positions in which she was comfortable. Chris suggested breastfeeding standing up. The mother was delighted with this suggestion. She wore a nursing pillow wrapped around her waist and rested it on the changing table. The height of this table worked well for her. The story illustrates the creative process that mothers and LCs employ to solve problems.

Fig. 106 illustrates that nipple placement on the breast may vary between mothers. When the nipple is placed on the "downhill slope" of the breast, it can be challenging for the mother to position the baby. Mothers worry when they are unable to see what the baby is doing during latch-on. Some mothers will temporarily tighten the straps on their nursing bras to help raise the breast, tipping the nipple up so it is visible. Other mothers find that all they need to do is lower the level at which they hold the baby. If the baby feels the chin touch the breast and the nipple stroke his nose, most normal babies can latch themselves without the mother needing to see what the baby is doing. The mother in **Fig. 106** demonstrates the technique in **Fig. 107**. In this position, the baby is almost lying flat on his back under the breast.

Breastfeeding texts often refer to ways of holding the breast. **Fig. 108** shows a mother holding her breast with the "scissors" hold. Many books discourage this hold; however, it is frequently seen in fine art depictions of breastfeeding. The scissors hold is clearly effective for this mother, perhaps because she has long fingers. LCs are not obligated to correct mothers if what they are doing works.

Fig. 109 and **Fig. 110** show a modification of the cradle hold that increases maternal control of the infant's body.

This position is especially useful if the mother has short arms. The preterm infant shown in **Fig. 109** lacks good postural control. The LC removed the nursing pillow and showed the mother how to hold the baby more securely. The mother of the baby in **Fig. 110** has been encouraged by the LC to lie back and to support the weight of the baby on her semi-reclined body.

A final word on positioning. It is best to hold the baby at the breast in a way that feels comfortable to the mother and secure to the baby. Remember: the normal baby can latch him or herself on without much assistance. The skill of positioning may not be as instinctive to the mother initially as the skill of latching is to the baby. It helps to reassure mothers that their coordination will improve with practice. As the baby gets older, technique goes by the wayside. **Fig. 111** illustrates that this 5 month-old has her own ideas about breastfeeding!

Visual Images of Latch-on

Latching on is an activity that relates more specifically to the infant drawing the breast into the mouth. Note how the mother in **Fig. 112** has positioned her newborn baby with his chin touching her breast. Observe how the baby uses his hand to grasp and guide the breast.

The mother in **Fig. 113** positions her breast so that baby's mouth is level with the round underside of the breast. The baby's nose is level with the nipple. As the mother's breast gently touches the baby's chin, the infant instinctively gapes and tips back the head (**Fig. 114**). Notice in this photo that the nipple is aimed toward the palate. In **Fig. 115** the baby is drawn in close by the mother with support at the shoulders.

When latched, we see in **Fig. 116** asymmetric attachment to the areola. Notice the nose is tipped away from the breast and the chin tight up against the globe of the breast. This orients the baby's head so that breathing, wide jaw excursions, and unrestricted swallowing are facilitated. The slight extension of the head that permits these activities also enables the baby to look into her mother's eyes. *En face* (face-to-face) gazing provides bonding opportunities.

Sometimes, the LC or the mother makes a breast "sandwich" (Wiessinger 1998) as shown in **Fig. 117** in order to assist a baby who is having difficulty latching -- especially to a flat nipple or to an engorged breast. Some weak infants may need the mother to continue to hold the wedged tissue for the duration of the feed. Other infants may only require such assistance until successfully latched.

Helping parents read the body language of their infant can be useful in reassuring them that their baby is well-latched and taking a good feeding. Note the baby's open eyes, alert affect, and wide gape in **Fig. 118**. After several minutes of robust, rhythmic sucking with few pauses, the baby may briefly rest. Generally, another milk release stimulates another round or 2 of active sucking, after which the baby's eyes may close. Some babies will detach, others will suck until falling asleep. Providing the infant is growing well, the mother should allow the baby to set the pace.

In **Fig. 119** the baby has closed his eyes. His fist is beginning to relax, a sign that Springuel (1994) points to as an indication that the baby is getting full.

In **Fig. 120**, the baby's hand is even more relaxed. The parents may note longer pauses between sucking bursts. Some mothers may be tempted to end the feed at this point. However, this is an important phase of the feeding. As the breast softens, the fat concentration of the milk rises. The baby may be more satiated and "settled" after the feeding if allowed to self-terminate the feed.

Fig. 121 beautifully illustrates a completed breastfeeding. The infant has released the breast and appears totally relaxed, with an open hand resting gently on the mother's breast. Note the round shape of the nipple. The shape demonstrates no evidence of compression injury. After such a feeding, both mother and infant typically appear mutually satisfied with the experience.

Fig. 122 illustrates a baby who is poorly latched to the breast. Her nose is pushed into the breast, her chin rests on her chest, and her view of her mother is inhibited. It may be that the mother's hand, unseen in this photo, is pushing on the back the baby's head. Pressure on the back of the head flexes the neck, inhibiting both breathing and swallowing. The baby may begin to struggle to protect the airway.

The infant pictured in **Fig. 123** has been rolled slightly to the side to allow a view of a poor latch. Note that the infant's chin is too far away from the breast. Poor proximity between the lower jaw and the breast will result in the jaw closing on the shaft of the nipple. This may result in painful breastfeeding and compromised milk transfer. The nipple will emerge from the baby's mouth looking pinched or flattened into a shape resembling an "orthodontic" pacifier or a new tube of lipstick.

The mother in **Fig. 123** has a large areola. She may have been following the advice to "get all the areola into the baby's mouth." Helpers must remember that the mother's view of the baby at breast is limited to the top half of the areola. If the mother is attempting to follow instructions to cover up as much areola as possible, she should be reminded that it is *lower jaw* coverage that matters. Since areolae come in many sizes, telling women to cover the areola is an inappropriate description and may result in incorrect lower jaw positioning.

The poorly gaining infant in **Fig. 124** has a shallow latch on a long nipple. Priority was given to placement of the upper rather than the lower jaw. However, to compound the problem, the nipple may be marginally too long to fit in the baby's mouth without triggering a gag reflex. Notice how the nipple is bent at an angle.

Bending the nipple in a way that constricts the easily compressed milk ducts may obstruct milk flow (Morton 1992, Geddes 2007). The baby in **Fig. 124** closed his eyes almost immediately after latching. Flat or depressed feeding affect early in the feed may indicate poor milk transfer. It is important for the LC to confirm this impression with a test weight. Rather than allow ineffective sucking to proceed indefinitely, a mother in this situation should be encouraged to relatch the baby, and to employ stimulation techniques such as breast compressions to improve milk transfer. Or, she may need to discontinue the breastfeeding session to allow enough time to express milk. Appropriate interventions such as pumping and alternate feeding protect the milk supply and provide milk for supplementation.

When the mother of the baby in **Fig. 124** was taught to draw the baby's entire body in closer, jaw closure occurred over breast tissue, not just on the nipple shaft. Despite the long nipple, this positioning change effectively improved the infant's latch. When optimally latched, the baby took in more milk (confirmed by a test weight). The mother observed changes in the infant's feeding behavior. He opened his eyes and appeared more engaged in the activity. He breastfed with audible swallows. His diaper output increased. Within a few days, he recovered his birth weight and continued to grow well.

The infant in **Fig. 125** is not gaining weight and her mother has cracked nipples. Notice how the baby's upper lip retracts (rolls in). The angle at the corner of her mouth is very narrow - a clue that the latch is part of the problem.

Rolling in the lips can be abrasive to breast tissue and may be a marker for poor oral stability. During feeding, the lips help hold the breast in the mouth to form an effective seal. Normally, the lips should shape to the breast in a relaxed manner, neither too loose (spilling milk), nor too tight.

If a baby is premature, weak, or thin, the lack of sufficient fat pads in the cheeks will decrease ability to maintain the shape of the mouth. Thus, the infant may struggle to hold the breast. The baby may compensate by putting too much pressure on the lips. Decreased or increased lip tone should be noted when evaluating poorly feeding infants (Wolf 1992). Maturation and growth will help resolve many such problems. The mother can assist the baby by supporting the breast so the infant does not have to work so hard to hold the breast in his mouth. Temporary pumping and supplementation may be needed to protect the milk supply and the baby's intake until the infant matures.

The infant in **Fig. 126** is grasping only the nipple. The narrow angle at the corner of the baby's mouth indicates that the baby's jaw compressions will fall on the shaft of the nipple, resulting in pinching. The mother will experience pain, and milk flow will be limited. Note the distance between cheek and chin, and the breast. The cheeks and chin should be in direct contact with the breast.

In **Fig. 127** the nipple appears pinched. **Fig. 128** shows a pinched nipple that resembles the shape of an "orthodontic" pacifier or a new tube of lipstick. When babies grasp only the shaft of the nipple, jaw and tongue compression form a characteristic creased shape. Looking at the nipple as it emerges from the baby's mouth may provide information about the latch.

When an infant is well latched, as is the 24 hour-old baby in **Fig. 129**, the angle at the corners of the mouth will be very wide; this one is 150°. Note how the chin touches the breast, and the nasal passages are clear. Proof of a good latch is verified by lack of pain during the feed. The nipple will emerge from the baby's mouth looking undistorted as in **Fig. 130**. Notice that the baby ends the feed right where she started, with the nose opposite the nipple.

Brodribb W (Editor). *Breastfeeding Management in Australia, 3rd ed.* East Malvern: Merrily Merrily Enterprises, 1998; pp. 52-53, Fig. B 2.5.

Daly S, DiRosso A, Owens R, et al. Degree of breast emptying explains changes in the fat content, but not fatty acid composition, of human milk. *Experimental Physiology* 1993; 78(6):741-0755.

Colson S. Maternal breastfeeding positions: have we got it right? *The Practising Midwife* 2005; 8(11):29-32.

Colson SD, Meek JH, Hawdon JM. Optimal positions for the release of primitive neonatal reflexes stimulating breastfeeding. *Early Human Development* 2008; 84(7):441-449.

Geddes DT. Gross Anatomy of the Human Breast, in *Hale & Hartmann's Textbook of Human Lactation.* Amarillo, TX: Hale Publishing, 2007; pp. 19-34.

Geddes DT, Kent JC, Mitoulas LR, et al. Tongue movement and intra-oral vacuum in breastfeeding infants. *Early Human Development* 2008; 84(7):471-477.

Glass R, Wolf L. Incoordination of sucking, swallowing, and breathing as an etiology for breastfeeding difficulty. *Journal of Human Lactation* 1994; 10(3):185-189.

Glover R. *Follow Me Mum* (video). Perth, Australia, 2000. Contact: reblact@rebeccaglover.com.au

Gunther M. Instinct and the nursing couple. *Lancet* March 15, 1955; 575-578.

Gunther M. Sore nipples, causes and prevention. *Lancet ii* 1945; 590-593.

Howard C, Lanphear N, Lanphear B, et al. Variations in parental comforting practices and breastfeeding duration. Abstract for the 9th Annual Meeting of the Academy of Breastfeeding Medicine, Oct 20-25, 2004, in *ABM News and Views* 2004; 10(S):31-32.

Jacobs LA, Dickinson JE, Hart PD, et al. Normal nipple position in term infants measured on breastfeeding ultrasound. *Journal of Human Lactation* 2007; 23(2):52-59.

Jevitt C, Hernandez I, Groer M. Lactation complicated by overweight and obesity: supporting the mother and newborn. J*ournal of Midwifery and Womens Health* 2007; 52(6):606-613.

Kent JC. How breastfeeding works. *Journal of Midwifery and Womens Health* 2007; 52(6):564-570.

Lang S. *Breastfeeding Special Care Babies, 2nd Ed.* Philadelphia: Bailliere Tindall, 2002; p. 49.

Milligan RA, Flenniken PM, Pugh LC. Positioning intervention to minimize fatigue in breastfeeding women. *Applied Nursing Research* 1996; 9(2):67-70.

Morton J. Ineffective suckling: a possible consequence of obstructive positioning. *Journal of Human Lactation* 1992; 8(2):83-85.

Neifert M, Lawrence R, Seacat J. Nipple confusion: toward a formal definition. *Journal of Pediatrics* 1995; 126(6):S125-129.

Newton N, Newton M. Psychologic aspects of lactation. *New England Journal of Medicine* 1967; 277:1179-88.

Prime D, Geddes D, Hartmann P. Oxytocin: Milk Ejection and Maternal-Infant Well-being, in *Hale & Hartmann's Textbook of Human Lactation*. Amarillo, TX: Hale Publishing, 2007; p. 150.

Ramsay D, Mitoulas L, Kent J, et al. Ultrasound imaging of the sucking mechanics of infant feeding from the breast and an experimental teat. Proceedings of the 12th International Conference of the International Society for Research in Human Milk and Lactation. Sept. 10-14, 2004; Queen's College, Cambridge, UK.

Ramsay DT, Kent JC, Hartmann RA. Anatomy of the lactating human breast redefined with ultrasound imaging. *Journal of Anatomy* 2005; 206(6):525-534.

Rassmussen KM, Lee VE, Ledkovsky TB, et al. A description of lactation counseling practices that are used with obese mothers. *Journal of Human Lactation* 2006; 22(3):322-327.

Redstone F, West J. The importance of postural control for feeding. *Pediatric Nursing* 2004; 30(2):97-100.

Royal College of Midwives. *Successful Breastfeeding, 3rd ed.* London: Churchill Livingstone, 2002.

Savage-King F. *Helping Mothers to Breastfeed*. Nairobi: African Medical and Research Foundation, 1992.

Smilie C. Baby-Led Breastfeeding: The Mother-Baby Dance (video). Los Angeles, CA: Geddes Productions, 2007.

Springuel E. Empowering parents while you educate them about breastfeeding. Conference presentation. The Lactation Consultant in Private Practice Workshop, Philadelphia. PA, 1994.

Tully MR, Overfield M. *Breastfeeding: A Special Relationship* (video). Raleigh, NC: Eagle Video Productions, 1991.

Varendi H, Porter R, Winberg J. Does the newborn baby find the nipple by smell? *Lancet* 1994; 344(8928):989-990.

Wiessinger D. A breastfeeding teaching tool using a sandwich analogy for latch-on. *Journal of Human Lactation* 1998; 14(1):51-56.

Wolf R, Glass L. *Feeding and Swallowing Disorders in Infancy*. Tucson, AZ: Therapy Skill Builders, 1992; pp. 120-21.

Woolridge M. Aetiology of sore nipples. *Midwifery* 1986a; 2(4):172-176.

Woolridge M. The 'anatomy' of infant sucking. *Midwifery* 1986b; 2(4):164-171.

Notes:

Flat and Inverted Nipples

In the 1950's, pioneering lactation physiologist, Mavis Gunther, described women with flat and inverted nipples whose infants became "apathetic" when put to breast. She speculated that baby humans (like other young animals) have an in-born receptivity to certain qualities and patterns of stimuli that evoke responses important to survival. These responses are not merely reflexive; they are behavioral triggers set in motion by certain physical signals. Normal feeding will be interrupted if the baby does not receive these signals. Gunther theorized that babies *expect* a protractile nipple tissue that is sufficiently elastic to pull deeply into the oral cavity. Ultrasound research confirms that normal nipples extend during sucking to within approximately 5 mm of the infant's hard/soft palate junction (Ramsay 2004a, b, Jacobs 2007).

Clinicians have observed that when babies are presented with breast tissue that is problematic to manipulate, it is as if a short-circuit occurs. The baby acts bewildered, shaking his head back and forth, bumping against the breast, or batting at the nipple with his fists. Some babies scream, others simply tune out and fall asleep. The mother may say, "It is as if he cannot figure out how to close his mouth around my breast." She may complain that the baby does not like breastfeeding, her milk, or her.

There may be other reasons why infants may struggle with flat or inverted nipples. Ramsay's ultrasound studies of breast anatomy (2005) identified that nipple ducts are easily compressed and collapse with gentle pressure. When infants encounter flat or inverted nipples, they may exert such high suction trying to draw in the teat that they collapse and occlude milk ducts. The resultant poor milk flow may frustrate the infant, and contribute to increasing levels of engorgement. Engorgement, itself, contributes to further flattening of the nipples, creating a cycle of frustration. To break this cycle, manage both engorgement and excess edema. Several papers explore a technique of massage used to redistribute fluid edema that accumulates close to the nipple as a method of improving nipple protractility (Miller 2004). Cotterman (2004) names this technique Reverse Pressure Softening (RPS).

Cooper (1995) identified 5 infants with severe breastfeeding malnutrition. The mothers of 3 of the 5 infants had inverted nipples. Even in populations of well-educated and highly-motivated mothers, the presence of flat or inverted nipples is associated with sub-optimal breastfeeding behavior on Days 0, 3, and 7, and with resulting delayed onset of lactation (Dewey 2003). The presence of inverted nipples therefore identifies an elevation of risk for serious breastfeeding problems. Infants of mothers with inverted nipples should be closely followed for adequate weight gain, and should receive special assistance until their infants are latching effectively.

Nipple Elasticity and Nipple Confusion

Infants whose mothers have difficult to manipulate breast tissue may react with relief when presented with a bottle teat. Possessing far greater proprioreceptive stimulus than a flat or inverted nipple, a bottle teat elicits the full feeding response. Gunther (1955) called such substitution a "super-sign" and Woolridge (1996) called it a "supernormal stimulus."

Once exposed to the super-sign, the baby may refuse the breast if there has been no improvement in the protractility of the maternal nipple or softening of the breast tissue. In such cases, the breast cannot "compete." The quick, easy milk flow rate of the bottle, combined with the stimulating effect of the artificial teat, overwhelms the signals the baby is receiving from the flat or inverting nipple and partially explains the condition called "nipple confusion." It may also explain why some studies show that many newborns can easily go back and forth between bottle and breast with no apparent difficulty (Cronenwett 1992), and why other experts connect early bottle teat exposure with breastfeeding failure (Newman 1993).

The unexamined, confounding factor in studies of nipple confusion may be the nipple protractility of the mothers involved. If women have erectile nipples with good elasticity, their babies may not be as vulnerable to what is termed nipple confusion. Thus, women with normal nipple elasticity may have less difficulty resuming breast-feeding after their babies have been exposed to bottle teats.

Much debate surrounds the definition and even the existence of what is termed "nipple confusion" (Dowling 2001). Some breastfeeding experts have attempted to clarify the discussion about nipple confusion by proposing a clinical definition (Neifert 1995). They make the point that it is important to distinguish between preference and dysfunction. Many skilled practitioners find that it is not especially difficult to coax babies back to breast who have merely become too familiar with bottles. "Confusion" is not an appropriate term to ascribe to a baby who is functionally incapable of breastfeeding, either temporarily or enduringly.

Flat Nipples

Nipple protractility cannot be visually assessed. The mother or LC must manually compress the tissue behind the nipple. Either the nipple will evert, it will flatten, or collapse inward in a telescoping fashion (see also **Figs. 210** and **211**). Drawing up any part of the areolar tissue between the thumb and forefinger assesses elasticity. Ideally there is some degree of "stretch" to the areolar tissue.

In addition to having larger breasts, excess periareolar adipose tissue may flatten the nipples of obese women (Jevitt 2007). Engorgement also dramatically reduces the elasticity and protractility of the nipple-areolar complex, sometimes creating a temporary flattening.

Hand expression, pumping, reverse pressure softening, and cold compresses help reduce swelling and soften the breast, making it easier for the baby to grasp.

Note: *Any recommendation of the use of cold compresses must take into account cultural beliefs about avoidance of cold in the postpartum period.*

Fig. 131 shows a flat nipple. There is poor definition of the nipple, even when the mother compresses the breast. Large, robust babies suck so effectively that they can often manage a somewhat inelastic nipple. If the baby is weak, small, premature, ill, or compromised in some way, the combination of impaired stamina *and* flat or inverting nipples frequently leads to breastfeeding problems.

In **Fig. 132** a woman pulls back on her breast tissue to create more definition of her nipple. This is a variation of the sandwich technique. Thinning the breast in the same dimension as the corners of the baby's mouth sometimes helps the baby sense the nipple more effectively. If the mother can plant a wedge of breast deeply in the baby's mouth, this action will often trigger sucking (see **Fig. 117**).

Fig. 133 shows a woman shaping her flat nipple into what is colloquially called the "teacup" or inverted nipple hold. Sometimes a mother can wedge enough tissue to help the baby latch. The mother or LC continues to hold the nipple into a pinched-up shape until the baby is sucking well before releasing the hold.

Inverted Nipples

The nipple contains milk ducts, sensory nerve endings and smooth muscle fiber (Lawrence 2005). These tissues are normally capable of elastic stretch, and ultrasonographic photographs taken during breastfeeding show nipple elongation (Smith 1988). Ramsay (2005) observed changes in the length of the nipple relative to the hard/soft palate junction depending upon whether the posterior tongue was in an elevated or dropped position. Ultrasound images suggest that sucking is an active process that moves and expands the nipple. The effect of nipple inversion upon sucking has not been well-studied.

Alexander (1992) estimated that as many as 10 percent of pregnant women have non-protractile nipples. These women may possess nipple tissue that is functionally inadequate to be optimally manipulated by their infants during sucking.

Devices such as breast shells are often suggested to pregnant mothers when flat or inverted nipples are identified. Alexander failed to find any significant value in prenatal therapies to stretch the nipples such as the use of breast shells or Hoffman's exercises. Some LCs report good anecdotal results, but Alexander connected prenatal use of one particular brand of this device with *decreased* incidence of breastfeeding. In this study, the researchers used breast shells with larger openings than those typically used in the US for this purpose. McGeorge (1994) examined the Niplette™ and found some clinical benefits. This device is a commercially developed nipple everter, used to assist women with inverted nipples.

Postpartum nipple protractility appears to increase in response to both sucking and pumping. Over time, many women with flat or inverted nipples report increased elasticity. On rare occasions a women can have a type of congenital nipple inversion that is not remedied by stretching.

Some women have nipples that appear to invert at rest, but that evert well upon compression. Others have apparently protuberant nipples that flatten upon compression (see **Figs. 210** and **211**). If the baby grasps and compresses the areolar tissue and the nipple retracts, the baby may be frustrated and uncertain about how to latch.

Figs. 134, 135, and **136** show an inverted nipple at rest, during compression, and pulled back so the nipple protrudes. This mother was not able to breastfeed her first 2 children, but pumped her milk for many months for them. With the help of an LC, she was able to breastfeed her third child. Women find that nipple protractility changes with more months of breastfeeding or pumping, thus providing more opportunity for the tissues to experience stretch. This information may prove encouraging to affected women.

Dimpled Nipples

The dimpled nipple is a form of nipple inversion in which the tissue inside the fold can become adhered. Variations of nipple configuration can create painful situations for breastfeeding mothers. The woman in **Fig. 137** has just finished pumping her breasts. **Fig. 138** shows the same nipple 2 minutes later when the nipple has resumed its dimpled shape.

In this woman's case, breastfeeding and pumping have pulled the adhered tissue apart for the first time. The adhered skin is very fragile compared to skin that receives a normal amount of light, air, and friction from clothing. When the nipple folds back on itself after breastfeeding or pumping, moisture is often trapped in the dimple, causing maceration and bleeding. After breast-feeding or pumping, it is important to instruct the moth-er to hold the nipple in a position that allows it to air dry and to keep this area very clean to prevent infection. Applications of topical antibiotic and antifungal creams may be used to protect the skin from infection, or to treat infection if it occurs. With repeated exposure to light and air, the tissue can heal.

Using Nipple Shields to Bring the Breast-Refusing Infant to Breast

Since breastfeeding is the natural culmination of the birth process, it is safe to assert that the baby who will not breastfeed is a baby who *cannot* breastfeed. The job of the LC is to determine what barriers prevent the baby from breastfeeding. If the infant cannot overcome the confusion caused by flat or inverting nipples, the LC must consider three issues:

- How is the baby to be fed while nipple remediation takes place?
- How long will it take before the baby can manage the nipples?
- Can the baby be kept at breast until the nipples evert?

Pumping and breastfeeding (if the baby will accept the breast) will usually pull out flat and inverted nipples. This can take a few days, a few weeks, or even months depending on the severity of the nipple inversion and the elasticity of the breast tissue. If the baby is never put to breast during the remediation period, it may become more difficult to transition the baby to the breast. This is true no matter how the baby has been fed in the interim.

The Clinical Rationale for Use of Thin Silicone Shields

A thin silicone nipple shield can be an appropriate clinical tool to assist the breast-refusing baby (Wilson-Clay 1996). The clinical goal of the shield is to supply a degree and quality of oral stimulation not being provided by the

mother's nipples. It also uses a familiar sensation to coax to breast an infant who has already imprinted preferentially on the supernormal stimulus of bottle teats.

Chertok (2006) demonstrated no significant difference in maternal hormonal levels and infant breast milk intake for breastfeeding sessions with and without nipple shields. Therefore, unverified concerns about risks of ultra thin shields must be weighed against evidence suggesting that these shields effectively prevent the abandonment of breastfeeding in some cases.

Fig. 139 illustrates the lack of elasticity in the nipple of a G1 P1 L1 mother with a non-nursing infant (*see note at the end of this chapter*). Her nipple is pictured moments later (**Fig. 144**) after her infant took his first effective breast-feeding at 2 weeks old using a nipple shield. A test weight performed before and after the breastfeeding confirmed that the infant consumed 79 ml. The infant continued to breastfeed with the shield for several weeks, and contin-ued to gain > 1oz/day (30g). The nipples gradually became more elastic, and the mother experienced no diffi-culty in transitioning the baby to direct breastfeeding.

The Clinical Importance of Nipple Shield Design

Antique shields did not fit closely to the breast (see **Fig. 140**). Thick, latex shields sat directly on the breast and were associated with decreased milk transfer and infants who failed to thrive. Shields of these designs should be avoided. Thin silicone shields do not appear to alter suck-ing patterns or significantly change the level of prolactin stimulation (Woolridge 1980, Chertok 2006).

Shield thickness is not the only issue to consider when making a clinical decision about their use as an intervention. If a nipple shield is to be an effective therapeutic tool, the teat height must not be so long that it triggers the infant's gag reflex, or causes jaw closure and tongue compression to fall on the shaft of the teat. Using a too-long nipple shield creates a real risk that the baby will be unable to extract milk effectively, setting up a cascade of events including poor infant growth and decreased milk supply. These considerations relating to nipple shield height may not be fully appreciated unless one considers that the heights of commercially available nipple shields range from 1.9 cm to 6.4 cm (Drazin 1998).

Fig. 141 demonstrates graduating sizes of 3 Medela nipple shields. Sizes pictured are 16 mm, 20 mm, and 24 mm.

The diameter of nipple shields also can vary widely (Frantz 1994). This variability appears to be an attempt by manufacturers to accommodate the wide ranges of human nipple diameters. Several researchers have looked at the variability in size of human nipples. The average nipple diameter appears to be 15-16 mm (Zeimer 1993, Stark 1994, Zeimer 1995, Ramsay 2005). Wilson-Clay and Hoover first presented similar findings on ranges and averages of nipple sizes in the second edition of *The Breastfeeding Atlas* (2002), and expand the discussion in the current edition (see **Ch. 10**). Infants have been observed to have difficulty grasping, sealing off, and manipulating maternal nipples when the nipple diameter is larger than average. Large nipple shields can, themselves, cause similar problems for some babies.

To further complicate any discussion about nipple shields, care must be taken to accurately describe the style as well as the size of the nipple shield being used. Mothers may purchase these devices without appropriate guidance. The nipple shield in **Fig. 140** was purchased at a pharmacy (chemist's shop) in London, UK in 2002. This device has a design similar to antique models of nipple shields, and is not likely to assist with breastfeeding.

It may be that the wide variability in response and outcome reported in shield use is related to inappropriate choices in shields that fail to calculate the effect of the height and base diameter of the shield on the infant's response to its use. In general, practitioners who successfully use nipple shields find they get best results by matching the shield size with the size of the infant's mouth. This often means selecting the shortest available teat with the smallest base diameter. Inevitably, some of the small size shields are not wide enough at the base to accommodate some women's nipples. For women with wide diameter nipples, their breastfeeding problem may be related to the nipple diameter issue *with or without* a shield in place. Issues of "fit" must be factored into clinical observations, choice of equipment, and predictions of outcome.

Applying a Nipple Shield

LCs have devised various ways to apply a nipple shield and use different vocabularies to describe these methods. Some center the shield on the nipple with the "brim" turned up like a sombrero. They then smooth down the brim onto the breast. This helps it stay in place.

Other LCs stretch the part of the shield where the "nipple" joins the "areola." They place the stretched shield over the mother's nipple, release the tension and withdraw their fingers. As the stretched shield returns to its normal shape, it will draw the mother's nipple into the teat cavity before the baby begins to suck. This trick not only helps the shield stay in place better, it also reduces the initial work the baby must exert in order to draw the nipple into the teat cavity.

Some LCs turn all but the top half of the teat portion inside out before placing it over the nipple as demonstrated in **Fig. 142**. Others warm the shield with hot water to make it more pliable.

Fig. 143 shows a newborn infant breastfeeding with a thin silicone nipple shield placed over his mother's nipple. This 6 day-old infant screamed whenever he was put to the breast. He was exclusively bottle-feeding when first evaluated by the LC. His mother was ready to wean. LCs often choose to try a nipple shield in situations when the infant is refusing the breast and weaning is imminent. With the nipple shield mimicking the familiar sensation of the bottle teat, the infant went to breast easily, sucked with good rhythm, swallowed audibly, and perceptibly softened the breast. Test weights confirmed a normal milk intake. Note how the baby's lips are flanged on the breast, suggesting that the baby has a good latch.

Fig. 144 demonstrates how the baby has drawn the mother's nipple into the shield. This woman had flat nipples with poor definition, but her baby was healthy and vigorous. Within a few days of such stretching, nipple elasticity dramatically improved. After the baby had breastfed for a few minutes, and was not as hungry, the mother removed the shield, thus beginning the process of weaning the infant from the shield. When babies are not too hungry, tired or frustrated, they are more willing to latch on without a shield. As this baby grew more confident that he would be able to satisfy his hunger at the breast, he became more patient when latching without the shield. His mother gradually used the shield less and less, and the baby came to trust and love breastfeeding.

Smaller infants or infants with neuromuscular issues (for example, infants with Prader-Willi Syndrome, Down Syndrome, and other genetic disorders) may need to rely on the nipple shield intervention for longer periods.

Preterm infants seem to especially benefit from nipple shields. Meier studied a group of 34 premature babies who averaged 31.9 weeks gestational age. These babies were able to take in 14 ml more milk when at the breast using a nipple shield than when at breast without a nipple shield (Meier 2000). On average they took in approximately 75 percent more milk (3.9 ml without the nipple shield and 18.4 ml with the nipple shield). This represents a statistically and clinically significant increase in intake. The researchers further observed that use of the shield helped correct problems like "slipping off the nipple" and "falling asleep" at breast.

The data from the Meier (2000) study indicate that "for preterm infants who demonstrate insufficient milk intake during breastfeeding, the nipple shield can serve as an effective, temporary milk transfer device without adversely affecting the total duration of breastfeeding." Most of the babies were off the nipple shield in 2 to 3 weeks. Duration of breastfeeding was longer for the babies whose mothers used the nipple shields compared to those who did not.

Fig. 144 is of special interest when discussing the findings of Meier. In this photograph, the nipple remains in an extended position even though the baby has come off the breast. After the first suck, the baby is relieved of the work necessary to keep the nipple elongated. Additionally, the pooled milk in the tip of the shield serves as a reservoir that provides the baby with an encouraging milk reward when nutritive sucking resumes. These observations may identify the shield mechanisms that assist the weak or premature infant to sustain more stable feeding behavior.

Nipple shields are imperfect devices, and some mothers become concerned when the base of the shield curls up and covers the baby's nose. Avent® and Medela® make shields with a cutout space. Some people prefer this design because these nipple shields do not roll over the baby's nose. Others feel the traditional design stays in place better and slips less owing to its greater surface area.

Fig. 145 pictures a 7 day-old infant who is poorly latched to a nipple shield. This baby had latch difficulties in the hospital following a traumatic delivery and little milk transfer was occurring. Note how the baby's mouth is positioned on the shaft of the shield. The baby had lost more than 9 percent of his birth weight, and was still losing weight. This picture and case illustrate the pitfalls of unsupervised nipple shield use. The need for the shield implies that an infant is feeding dysfunctionally. Such infants need close follow-up and their mothers require additional support to ensure good latch.

When repositioned and appropriately latched with the shield in place, test weights showed that the baby consumed 52 ml of milk from the breast in approximately 15 minutes. The LC recommended weight checks every other day until the baby recovered his birth weight, which occurred within 4 days. As the baby regained strength and recovered from the traumatic birth, the mother was able to withdraw the use of the shield. By the middle of the third week after birth, the baby nursed well directly from the breast, and was gaining slightly over one ounce a day (35 g).

Anyone who provides a mother with a nipple shield must also provide follow-up. Positioning and latch should be *directly* assessed to make sure the baby is not sucking only on the shaft of the shield. Many mothers with well established milk supplies find it unnecessary to pump

when they are using a shield. However, until milk transfer is assessed and found to be adequate with the shield in place, the mother should pump after most feedings to insure a robust milk supply. Weight checks provide the information needed to decide whether the baby is able to maintain the milk supply during the period of nipple shield use.

Many clinicians have concluded that keeping the baby at breast with a simple, inexpensive device such as a shield is reasonable when measured against the work of pumping and bottle-feeding and the risks of weaning. While breastfeeding without any paraphernalia is optimal, mothers whose infants are finally brought to breast with nipple shields are usually grateful the tool exists

Note:
Throughout the book, we describe mothers using terms that refer to the number of pregnancies a woman has experienced (gravida), her number of births (para), and her lactation experience (lacta). Thus, G1, P2, L2 designates a woman who has been pregnant once, and given birth to and breastfed twins.

Alexander J, Grant A, Campbell M. Randomised controlled trial of breast shells and Hoffman's exercises for inverted and non-protractile nipples. *British Medical Journal* 1992; 304(6833):1030-1032.

Chertok IR, Schneider J, Blackburn S. A pilot study of maternal and term infant outcomes associated with ultrathin nipple shield use. *Journal of Obstetrics, Gynecologic and Neonatal Nursing* 2006; 35(2):265-172.

Cooper W, Atherton H, Kahana M. Increased incidence of severe breast-feeding malnutrition and hypernatremia in a metropolitan area. *Pediatrics* 1995; 96(5):957-960.

Cotterman K. Reverse pressure softening: a simple tool to prepare areola for easier latching during engorgement. *Journal of Human Lactation* 2004; 20(2):227-237.

Cronenwett L, Stukei T, Kearney M. Single daily bottle use in the early weeks post-partum and breastfeeding outcome. *Pediatrics* 1992; 90(5):760-66.

Dewey K, Nommsen-Rivers L, Heinig M. Risk factors for suboptimal infant breastfeeding behavior, delayed onset of lactation, and excess neonatal weight loss. *Pediatrics* 2003; 112(3):607-619.

Dowling D, Thanattherakul W. Nipple confusion, alternative feeding methods, and breast-feeding supplementation: state of the science. *Newborn and Infant Nursing Reviews* 2001; 1(4):217-223.

Drazin P. Taking nipple shields out of the closet. *Birth Issues* 1998; 7(2):41-47.

Frantz K. *Breastfeeding Product Guide*. Sunland, CA: Geddes Productions, 1994; pp. 45-46.

Gunther M. Instinct and the nursing couple. *Lancet,* March 19, 1955; 575-578.

Jacobs LA, Dickinson JE, Hart PD, et al. Normal nipple position in term infants measured on breastfeeding ultrasound. *Journal of Human Lactation* 2007; 23(1):52-59.

Jevitt C, Hernandez I, Groer M. Lactation complicated by overweight and obesity: supporting the mother and newborn. *Journal of Midwifery Women's Health* 2007; 52(6):606-613.

Lawrence RA, Lawrence RM. *Breastfeeding: A Guide for the Medical Profession, 6th ed.* Philadelphia, PA: Elsevier Mosby, 2005, p. 48.

McGeorge D. The "Niplette:" an instrument for the non-surgical correction of inverted nipples. *British Journal of Plastic Surgery* 1994; 47(1):46-49.

Meier P, Brown L, Hurst N, et al. Nipple shields for preterm infants: effect on milk transfer and duration of breastfeeding. *Journal of Human Lactation* 2000; 16(2):106-114.

Miller V, Riordan J. Treating postpartum breast edema with areolar compression. *Journal of Human Lactation* 2004; 20(2):223-226.

Neifert M, Lawrence R, Seacat J. Nipple confusion: toward a formal definition. *Journal of Pediatrics* 1995; 12(6):125-129.

Newman J. Nipple confusion (letter). *Pediatrics* 1993; 92(2):297.

Ramsay D, Mitoulas L, Kent J, et al. Ultrasound imaging of the effect of frenulotomy on breastfeeding infants with ankyloglossia. Abstract of the 12th International Conference of the International Society for Research in Human Milk and Lactation. Sept. 10-14, 2004a; Queen's College, Cambridge, UK.

Ramsay D, Mitoulas L, Kent J, et al. Ultrasound imaging of the sucking mechanics of infant feeding from the breast and an experimental teat. Abstract of the 12th International Conference of the International Society for Research in Human Milk and Lactation. Sept. 10-14, 2004b; Queen's College, Cambridge, UK.

Ramsay DT, Kent JC, Hartmann RA. Anatomy of the lactating human breast redefined with ultrasound imaging. *Journal of Anatomy* 2005; 206(6):525-534.

Smith W, Erenberg A, Nowak A. Imaging evaluation of the human nipple during breastfeeding. *American Journal of Diseases of Children* 1988; 142(1):76-78.

Stark Y. Human Nipples: Function and Anatomical Variations in Relationship to Breastfeeding. Master's Thesis, Pasadena. CA: Pacific Oaks College, 1994.

Wilson-Clay B. Clinical use of silicone nipple shields. *Journal of Human Lactation* 1996; 12(4):279-285.

Woolridge M, Baum J, Drewett R. Effects of a traditional and of a new nipple shield on sucking patterns and milk flow. *Early Human Development* 1980; 4(4):357-364.

Woolridge MW. Problems of establishing lactation. *Food and Nutrition Bulletin* 1996; 17(4):316-327.

Ziemer M, Cooper D, Pigeon J. Evaluation of a dressing to reduce nipple pain and improve nipple skin condition in breastfeeding women. *Nursing Research* 1995; 44(6):347-351.

Zeimer M, Pigeon J. Skin changes and pain in the nipple during the first week of lactation. *Journal of Obstetric, Gynecological, and Neonatal Nursing* 1993; 22(3):247-256.

Sore Nipples

Many factors and conditions can contribute to sore nipples. Identifying the cause of nipple pain is a critical component of understanding how to relieve it. Experienced lactation consultants have learned the limitations of phone counseling when a mother complains of sore nipples. Visual assessment is crucial because the appearance of the nipple may provide essential clues to the nature of the problem.

The diagram below clarifies the terminology employed to describe the location of nipple trauma:

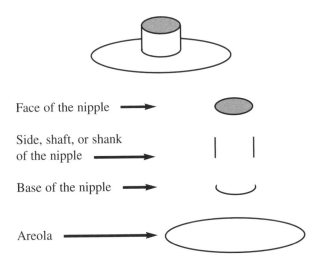

Face of the nipple ⟶

Side, shaft, or shank of the nipple ⟶

Base of the nipple ⟶

Areola ⟶

Early Onset Nipple Pain

Studies of sore nipples during the first 2 weeks postpartum suggest that the height of nipple soreness occurs between Days 3 and 7, with peak levels occurring on Day 3 (*Best Practice* 2003). Some mothers report pain for as long as 6 weeks (Zeimer 1990). Many theories attempt to explain early nipple pain, but breastfeeding supporters seem reluctant to acknowledge how common early nipple pain appears to be. Perhaps breastfeeding activists fear that acknowledgement of early discomfort will discourage women from breastfeeding. However, early onset nipple pain is frequently reported by mothers and has been described in the literature for many years. Women with sore nipples require attention to prevent untimely weaning.

Lactation specialists in the developed world wonder if nipple pain in early lactation occurs in cultures where breastfeeding remains the norm. An IBCLC who formerly practiced in Zimbabwe states, "...My impression is that African (indigenous) mothers experience exactly the same kind and severity of *all* breastfeeding problems as mothers

of other races, including nipple pain and damage" (Morrison 2002).

Gunther (1945) observed that nipple pain occurred in a majority (64 percent) of nursing mothers. In Ziemer's 1990 sample of 100 mothers, 96 reported nipple pain at some point in the study. Foxman, in a personal communication, (March 2002) noted "nearly universal" nipple tenderness during the first week postpartum in a cohort of 946 women in a prospective mastitis study. Additionally, "nipple cracks and sores were reported by more than a third of all participants in the first week postpartum" (Foxman 2002).

Early Postpartum Nipple Sensitivity

Normal phyisological changes might contribute to the phenomenon of early postpartum nipple tenderness. Breast sensitivity increases significantly following birth (Prime 2007). Increased sensitivity provides a benefit by enhancing nipple responsivity to the tactile stimulation necessary to release oxytocin and trigger the milk ejection response. As the milk ejection response becomes better conditioned, enhanced nipple sensitivity may become less critical and thus decline.

Early breast and nipple pain may be associated with other normal hormonal changes. Cox (1999) observed a relationship between nipple growth and prolactin levels, noting that nipple sensitivity at 20 weeks gestation coincides with rising levels of serum prolactin. The dramatic postpartum rise in prolactin levels may also contribute to a similar transient period of increased nipple tenderness. Mothers may find it comforting to learn that early postpartum tenderness will similarly resolve.

During the early postpartum period, many women report pain only when the baby first latches on, lasting about 20 to 30 seconds. Such pain may result from a kind of low load muscle strain as nipple tissue adjusts to stretching. Because unexplained discomfort is more alarming than pain that has an explanation, mothers are reassured when the LC compares nipple stretching discomfort to other familiar activities such as muscle soreness after exercising.

Many LCs will suggest that mothers use the "30 second rule." If the pain subsides once the baby is well latched, the mother can safely ignore it. If discomfort persists, the mother should remove the baby and re-latch. If tissue breakdown occurs, mothers need to know this is a sign they need extra help.

Early postpartum latch discomfort usually resolves within a week or so, and is typically not associated with skin damage. Nipples do not "toughen up;" they will return to normal levels of sensitivity over time. Anticipatory guidance helps the mother view early nipple sensitivity as a temporary inconvenience.

Nipple Pain Resulting from Tissue Damage

Mothers need help distinguishing between common, temporary tenderness and acute pain with resultant nipple damage. Such pain is not considered normal. Nipple pain resulting from trauma may be associated with skin changes that include *erythema* (redness), *edema* (swelling), *fissures* (cracks), blisters, inflamed areas with associated swelling and pain, skin color changes, scabs, peeling, pus, and delayed healing.

Wounds tend to occur on the nipple face, although some (notably those caused by a too-tight pump flange) may occur at the base of the nipple. Some early skin changes on the nipple face appear to be caused by suction damage (Zeimer 1993). A second characteristic wound commonly seen on the nipple face in early breastfeeding is the compression stripe, caused when some aspect of sucking injures the nipple. Woolridge (1986) described suction and compression damage as two *primary* physical causes of nipple pain. *Secondary* causes such as infections or dermatitis may occur once the skin integrity is breached.

Mohrbacher (2004) proposes consistency in describing nipple trauma. She suggests the following staging system:

- **Stage I** -- superficial pain, intact skin (redness, bruising, swelling)
- **Stage II** -- superficial pain, tissue breakdown (abrasion, shallow fissure, compression stripe, blistering)
- **Stage III** -- partial thickness erosion (skin breakdown to the lower layers of the dermis; deep fissure)
- **Stage IV** -- full thickness erosion (full erosion through the dermis)

Suction Lesions

Woolridge explains that when milk flows, suction pressure diminishes. Hence "… if little milk issues from the nipple, or the baby's appetite has not been assuaged after milk flow has ceased, then unrelieved suction will be applied to the nipple surface and this may lead to suction trauma" (Woolridge 1986).

In the first days of breastfeeding, it is possible that the typically low volumes of available colostrum cause some babies to apply unrelieved suction in an attempt to access milk. Certainly, many mothers report that breastfeeding feels more comfortable after their milk comes in. BWC has observed that mothers with chronic low milk supply often complain of sore nipples. Perhaps infants confronted with a low milk supply, engorgement, or blocked ducts exert higher levels of suction, traumatizing the nipples. Similarly, mothers report that *dry pumping* (in the absence of a milk ejection) feels uncomfortable. These observations support those of Woolridge that low milk flow may contribute to nipple pain.

Variant Sucking Dynamics

In spite of apparently normal milk flow, some mothers report on-going nipple pain that fails to resolve. They describe painful or "strong" infant sucking in spite of attentive positioning and careful latch technique. Using ultrasound and pressure transducers, researchers have observed that some infants appear to generate unusually high levels of suction causing significant nipple distortion while breastfeeding (McClellan 2008).

BWC has worked with mothers whose babies and breasts seemed unremarkable except for reports of persistent pain while breastfeeding. Nipple shields helped some of these mothers manage discomfort; others were not assisted by shield use. Pumping with hospital grade breast pumps permitted protection of the milk supply; however, if these mothers breastfed more than a few times a day, their nipple tissue began to break down. Over the course of 3 to 4 months, some of the mothers reported being able to drop pumping sessions and add in more daily breastfeedings without experiencing pain. Some resumed breastfeeding at all feeds while others continued to require some pumping breaks.

It is possible that these cases represent clinical evidence of the phenomenon McClellan reports. Perhaps these babies begin to suck differently over time, or their mothers tolerated the sensation better as nipple sensitivity decreased. Perhaps the babies' mouths grew bigger. When the LC provides information about these variant sucking patterns, some mothers may decide to continue pumping in hopes of eventual improvement or change.

Breast Engorgement and Nipple Pain

Unrelieved engorgement flattens nipples and makes them difficult for the infant to grasp. Geddes (2007) speculates that engorged women may experience transient decrease in milk production owing to increased intra-alveolar pressure that (in animal models) flattens *lactocytes* (milk making cells). The infant may compensate for the harder-to-grasp nipples and try to generate better milk flow by exerting higher levels of negative pressure (see **Ch. 7**).

A Relationship Between Infant Pain, Comfort Sucking, and Nipple Pain?

Sucking is analgesic in infants (Gray 2002). Perhaps infants recovering from birth trauma spend more time sucking or may suck more aggressively in an attempt to regulate state behavior and cope with pain. Because the nipple sensitivity is markedly increased in the first 24 hours postpartum (Geddes 2007), mothers of infants with birth trauma may experience more nipple pain.

Images of Nipple Trauma

Engorged women whose milk flow is inhibited by breast edema may exhibit starburst-shaped lesions on the center of the nipple face. In these cases, the baby appears to have sucked so hard that the stretched, fragile nipple tissue tears. The baby may exert excessive negative pressure because:

- engorgement prevents easy teat formation
- flat nipples are difficult to grasp with normal levels of suction
- engorgement reduces milk production and flow
- nipple pain may inhibit milk release (let-down)

Fig. 146 shows the nipple of a woman 7 days postpartum. Note the inflammation and swelling on the nipple face. The surface of the nipple appears as a collection of vesicles producing Stage I nipple damage. The woman's nipples developed suction lesions on Day 2 prior to hospital discharge. The nipple trauma became more pronounced over time, and the woman developed mastitis that required oral antibiotic treatment. Observe also the venous engorgement visible on the breast.

Fig. 147 shows an engorged breast on Day 4 with a flat nipple and Stage II damage.

Nipple lesions often have a characteristic appearance. The nipple (when viewed in profile) appears distorted into a shape resembling a new tube of lipstick, or an "orthodontic" pacifier. The wounds produced are called "positional stripes." The stripe across the face of the nipple runs parallel to an imaginary moustache on the baby's upper lip as the baby nurses.

The LC and the mother should observe the shape of the nipple immediately after the baby comes off the breast. Distortion of the shape of the nipple is especially traumatic during breast engorgement, because swelling causes the nipple tissue to become more fragile as it stretches and thins. The skin rapidly breaks down, owing to repeated trauma.

Compression lesions may result from shallow latch, behavioral adaptations, anatomic anomalies of the infant's mouth or the mother's nipples, or variant sucking dynamics. For instance, a baby might pull off, or compress or crimp the nipple to slow the milk flow, especially if the mother has a forceful milk ejection reflex. Certain infant anatomical problems may contribute to nipple distortion such as tongue-tie, short tongue, small mouth, receding chin, or high palate. Large or long maternal nipples may prevent a good latch, causing the baby to pinch the nipple.

Fig. 148 shows a pinched nipple seconds after the baby came off the breast. Note the characteristic misshaping of the nipple, producing Stage II trauma.

Fig. 149 shows Stage II trauma on Day 4 postpartum when scabs have formed over the broken skin. The orientation of the "positional stripe" provides information about which position the mother has been using, in this case, the cradle hold. The LC must evaluate the infant for anatomic or behavioral issues that may explain trauma. If not managed, repeated trauma creates the risk of infection and delayed healing.

Deep fissures can appear on the face of the nipple, as in **Figs. 150-151** where Stage III damage is observed. The mother in **Fig. 150** is 4 weeks postpartum. She breastfed 2 older children without difficulty, but her youngest baby was born with a tongue-tie. The mother developed fissures on both nipples that became infected and required antibiotics. The LC explained that taking a break from breastfeeding might speed recovery. Resting on a pump removed the source of the trauma and allowed her nipples to heal. She elected not to seek a frenotomy for the infant, and primarily bottle-fed pumped milk for 4 months and then weaned to formula.

Fig. 151 demonstrates a partial thickness wound where the dermis has been breached to the moist underlying layer. The wound appears to be in the healing phase when new cell proliferation occurs. Note the "beefy red" new capillary bed. This skin is very fragile and prone to re-injury and infection. The mother was told to wean so the fissure would heal. Determined to breastfeed, the woman persevered. The physician was treating the mother's nipples with nystatin for a yeast infection when the LC (KH) saw her.

The LC speculated that rapid milk ejection and oversupply probably contributed to the nipple damage. She explained to the mother that the infant may have been deliberately pinching off the nipple in an attempt to regulate the force of the milk flow. Milk oversupply finally was brought under control at 10 weeks, permitting the infant to discontinue the compensatory sucking behavior. Eliminating nipple trauma and using nystatin cream helped heal the mother's nipples while the baby continued to breastfeed. Perhaps significantly, this family's 2 dogs had fungal skin infections. Animals may serve as a reservoir for human *Candida* infection (Edelmann 2005).

Fig. 152 shows a badly eroded nipple before and during treatment, illustrating Stage III damage. The reddened area and the mother's complaints of severe pain prompted the midwife to prescribe an antibiotic cream and an antifungal cream. Within 5 days, partial regeneration of the tissue can be observed. If a mother with this degree of tissue damage cannot tolerate breastfeeding, an alternate method of milk expression will keep the breasts draining and protect the milk supply while the nipples heal.

Fig. 153 shows a mother with Stage IV nipple damage. She is holding a flat toothpick next to the fissure to help illustrate the depth of the wound which is 7 mm.

Negative Pressure Wound Debridement

Negative pressure therapy is used to treat pressure and diabetic ulcers (Enoch 2003, Kirby 2007). It is possible that both pumping and breastfeeding offer the mother some protection from infection by constant removal of exudate from the wound bed. The effect of pressure debridement on the healing of nipple wounds may be an unexamined issue in breastfeeding. It may help explain why all mothers with nipple fissures do not develop infections in spite of inconsistent wound care practices and constant re-exposure to oral pathogens in the mouths of infants.

Sore Nipple Treatment Controversies

Research has not provided consistent guidance on the most effective way to manage nipple tissue damage. Various methods have been tried, many of them part of cultural traditions, including the use of peppermint water, olive oil, applications of wet tea bags, lanolin, and hydrogel pads, etc. (Riordan 1985, Hewatt 1987, Spangler 1993, Buchko 1994, Pugh 1996, Lavergne 1997, Beauchamp 2005, Sayyah 2007). The apparent efficacy of some of these preparations may stem from unexplored antiseptic and anti-inflammatory effects, or other issues unique to breastfeeding (see above for discussion of negative pressure wound debridement).

Fetherston (1998) supported the use of nipple creams to help heal sore nipples and identified this method of nipple care as a protective factor against development of mastitis. However, she identified wearing a nipple airer (breast shell or tea strainer) as a risk factor for breast infection. She speculated that such devices may become contaminated as a result of poor hygiene or ineffective sterilization practices, or they may indent the areola and cause blockage and bruising. Ramsay (2004) identified that milk ducts "readily collapsed under slight pressure similar to that required to compress a superficial vein on the back of the hand." It may be that devices such as shells, strainers, and even improperly held pump flanges cause blockages by collapsing ducts. Poor breast drainage and nipple fissures are risk factors for mastitis, and care should be taken to avoid behaviors that increase risk of infection.

It is difficult to achieve accurate and consistent comparisons between sore nipple treatment methods (Page 2003). Perhaps different types and degrees of nipple trauma respond to different methods of treatment. Some cases of sore nipples resolve on their own by improving breastfeeding technique and increasing the volume of milk transfer. Women with compromised immune systems however, including those with IgA deficiency may be at high risk for breast infections (Fetherston 2006). Hospital transmission rates of Methicillin Resistant *Staphylococcus aureus* (MRSA) have increased in recent years. Close follow-up of postpartum women with nipple fissures is critical, as MRSA cannot be treated with ordinary antibiotics and is highly contagious (Saiman 2003, Beam 2006).

It is important to base practice on evidence. A comparative study assessed sore nipple treatment in 90 primiparous mothers of term infants (Akkuzu 2000). Three techniques were examined for effectiveness in preventing or reducing nipple pain and cracked nipples in the first 10 days postpartum. Subjects were randomized into 3 groups with one group using applications of warm compresses, one group applying expressed breast milk, and one group using no treatment other than keeping the nipples clean and dry. The warm compress group had the most cracks. The expressed milk group had the fewest complaints of pain and the fastest healing of cracks. On the final day of assessment, the clean and dry group had the fewest cracked nipples. The authors concluded that mothers should be instructed to keep nipples clean and dry following the recommendations of WHO/UNICEF.

Hydrogel Dressings

Hydrogel dressings have been proposed as a treatment for fissured nipples based on moist wound healing theory. There is a difference between surface wetness and the preservation of internal moisture (the basis for moist wound healing theory). Wet breast pads and wet, dirty dressings cause maceration, expose fissures to pathogens, and do not speed healing. Hydrogel dressings that have begun to appear cloudy due to accumulation of fluids may pose an infection risk.

Ziemer examined the use of polyethylene film dressing in a group of 50 Caucasian women. The treatment was used on one breast between feedings, with the opposite breast serving as the control. Use of the occlusive dressing during the first week postpartum appeared to have limited influence on improvement in damaged skin condition; however, use of the dressing did significantly reduce reports of pain during the study period (Zeimer 1995).

Brent (1998) compared use of a hydrogel wound dressing (Elasto-gel™) with lanolin cream and breast shells in a sample of 42 breastfeeding women with sore nipples. She reported significantly more infections in the dressing group, which resulted in early discontinuation of the study. These researchers concluded that lanolin and shells should remain first-line therapy for sore nipples.

Dodd (2003) investigated the use of MaterniMates™ hydrogel dressing. Ameda purchased this product in 2003 and re-named it Comfortgel Hydrogel Pads. Dodd found significantly greater reduction in pain scores in mothers experiencing sore nipples who used these gel pads. The study protocol emphasized maternal handwashing before handling the dressings. Additionally, after removing them, mothers were instructed to wash the dressings with warm water, pat them dry, and advised to place the dressings on a clean surface. After feeding, the mothers were asked to rinse their breasts with warm water and pat themselves dry before re-applying the cleaned dressings. Whenever the hydrogels turned cloudy, the mothers were instructed to discard them and open a new dressing. Using this protocol, no mother using hydrogels experienced infection.

In essence, participants in the Dodd study were following the WHO/UNICEF recommendations (to keep their nipples clean), while receiving the pain reduction benefit associated in several studies with use of hydrogels. This model is worth further consideration. Clearly the emphasis on hygiene is key to the lack of reported infections in this population of hydrogel using women.

Immediate Wound Care for Cracked Nipples

Acute (newly acquired) skin wounds elsewhere on the body are routinely cleansed in order to remove contaminants that could impede healing and cause infection. Generally this process involves use of running water and mild soap (Potter 2001).

It can be difficult to delineate between wounds that are contaminated and those that are infected. *Host factors* (the strength of the maternal immune system) play an important role in the rate of wound healing. Postpartum women have somewhat depressed immune response and increased vulnerability to infection.

Bacteria have the ability to generate a protective coating (a sticky goo called a *biofilm*) over wound colonies. Saliva potently stimulates biofilm production (Hale 2006a). Repeated exposure to infant saliva may make nipple infection harder to eradicate. Biofilms prevent topical medications from penetrating to the wound. Antiseptic measures and gentle *debridement* (wound cleansing) may be helpful in penetrating biofilms in order to eradicate pathogens, promote wound healing, and prevent progression to infection (Ryan 2007).

Since breastfeeding books commonly discourage nipple cleansing, mothers may need clear and specific explanation about why it is important to gently cleanse fissured nipples. Explain that while it is unnecessary to engage in elaborate routines to clean *intact* nipple skin, cracked nipples require the same first aid attention normally followed when taking care of a bite wound on a finger.

Cleanse nipple wounds once a day with warm, soapy water. Following each breastfeeding, mothers should flush the nipple wounds with normal saline solution or tap water (Fernandez 2002). This reduces the likelihood that pathogens from the baby's mouth will re-colonize open nipple fissures. Handle injured nipples with clean hands. Air or gently pat dry before applying expressed milk, purified lanolin, topical antibiotic cream, or a clean hydrogel dressing.

Non-healing Cracked Nipples

The LC may encounter a mother who reports a nipple wound that has been present for days, weeks, or even months in spite of standard care. Enoch (2003) states that *chronic* wounds have several distinctive factors. They fail to heal in a timely, orderly manner, and remain stuck in the inflammation or proliferative phase. The main barriers to healing in chronic wounds appear to be:

- accumulation of *necrotic* (dead) tissue
- pathogen imbalance
- altered exudate levels

Chronic wounds appear to have underlying pathogenic abnormalities that cause constant accumulation of necrotic tissue, prolonging the inflammatory response, and mechanically obstructing the process of healing. The baby's sucking or the pump may continually remove accumulations of necrotic tissue and hide the fact that the wound is manifesting altered exudate levels.

The terms *local infection* and *critical colonization* refer to wounds that will not heal but may not display classic signs of infection (Enoch 2003).

The mix of microorganisms within a wound may also be an issue. The microflora may include fungi as well as bacteria. Giandoni (1994) identified cutaneous candidiasis as a cause of delayed wound healing.

Identifying best practices for the management of cracked nipples awaits more conclusive evidence (Kvist 2007). To prevent infection, the LC focuses on correcting primary sources of nipple trauma, providing appropriate first aid care, and emphasizing ongoing hygiene to speed healing. Close follow-up is required to identify progression to mastitis, which requires medical evaluation and treatment.

Bacterial Nipple Infections

Nipple trauma that does not heal after latch-on and positioning have been corrected may be an important sign of infection. The risk of constant re-exposure to pathogens via contact with the infant's mouth is a factor that may distinguish nipple injury from other types of wounds. *Staphylococcus aureus* (including also MRSA) is carried nasally and may be communicated orally. Nasal carriage can occur in the baby, the mother, or the HCP. This pathogen is associated with mastitis in breastfeeding women (Amir 2006, Kim 2007).

The majority of cracked nipples and breast infections occur during the first 2 weeks postpartum, when pathogens from the hospital environment may be present (Kitajima 2003). Livingstone (1999) states that, "Contaminated wounds are often slow to heal and can lead to widespread infections. *Staphylococcus aureus* ascends lactiferous ducts [causing] infections, mastitis, and breast abscess." Ramsay's ultrasound detection of milk backflow provides a plausible explanation for migration of pathogens into the ductal system (Ramsay 2004).

Mupirocin (Bactroban®) is an excellent preventative topical antibiotic for superficial skin wounds. It is highly active against *staphylococci* and most *streptococci*. There also is evidence to suggest it has anti-candida activity *in vivo* (Nicholas 1999, de Wet 1999). Mupirocin is minimally absorbed topically and is rapidly metabolized when ingested orally, so it is unlikely to produce side effects in infants (Hale 2008b).

It is important to treat cracked nipples promptly and thoroughly with cleansing, drying, and appropriate topical medication to eradicate pathogens. Once nipples become infected, pain is intense, and the appearance of nipple wounds distressing. Systemic antibiotics prevent mastitis when nipples are infected (Livingstone 1999).

Fig. 154 shows an infected, cracked nipple. The appearance of pus indicates the potential for the spread of the infection to underlying tissue and subsequent systemic symptoms. This situation requires both topical and oral antibiotics. It is not appropriate to use hydrogel dressings on infected skin.

Protocols for treating breast infections are reviewed in **Ch. 11**.

Fungal Infection

Two terms refer to fungal infections involving *Candida* species: *candidiasis* and *candidosis*, which are used interchangeably in the literature.

Using accurate assay methods, Hale (2006a) described detection of *Candida albicans* in human milk seeded with yeast cultures. However, using the same assay technique, he was unable to detect *Candida* in milk pumped from women presenting with "classic" symptoms of "ductal" yeast infections, including deep breast pain and burning nipples. Hale's experiment calls into question previous assumptions about whether yeast infections occur within the ducts of the breast.

Yeast infections have been over-identified, resulting in overuse of powerful systemic antifungal medications such as fluconazole. Aggressive over-treatment has also resulted in creating extra work for mothers. Nipple vasospasm, dermatitis, and bacterial infection may be more common than previously believed, and often create symptoms attributed to candidiasis (Livingstone 1996, Huggins 1993, Amir 1993, Anderson 2004, Morino 2007).

Some common "yeast" treatments exert a therapeutic effect upon bacterial infections and dermatitis, adding to the confusion about what is being treated. For instance, topical gentian violet has antiseptic and antibacterial as well as antifungal properties. Oral fluconazole exerts anti-inflammatory activity common to other azole drugs (Gupta 1978). The anti-inflammatory activity is amplified when used in combination with ibuprofen (Arai 2005). Fluconazole also has been demonstrated to exert protective effect against sepsis (Khan 2005).

Full or partial resolution of breast pain following the use of topical and oral "yeast" medications may create a mistaken impression that they have cured a candida infection. Research on deep breast pain suggests that the etiology of deep breast pain is more likely to be bacterial than fungal (Thomassen 1998), and antibiotic therapy more effective in fully eradicating symptoms. Therefore, based on evidence, LCs must reconsider their assumptions with regard to the cluster of symptoms previously attributed to yeast infections of the breast.

Superficial *Candida* Infection of the Nipple

Topical skin infections of *Candida*, particularly *comorbid* infection (combinations of bacterial and fungal organisms) have been identified on the nipple.

Yeast infection of the nipple presents as the onset of pain after early postpartum nipple discomfort has resolved. If untreated, superficial fungal infections may cause skin breakdown. Early nipple skin breakdown in the first few weeks postpartum is more likely to result from sucking trauma or bacterial infection. The late onset of pain and a renewal of nipple tenderness are important signs of superficial fungal infection.

Yeast infection of the nipple generally coincides with the appearance of a fungal infection in the infant's mouth (called *thrush*), or a fungal diaper rash.

Most infants have a white, milky coating on their tongues. Thrush appears as a fuzzy white plaque that spreads to cover the oral mucosa. White on the tongue is not thrush unless it becomes progressively thicker and spreads to other oral surfaces. It is important to realize that other causes may alter the appearance of the infant's oral mucosa. **Fig. 155** shows a white tongue.

Untreated oral candida infection rapidly spreads to the lips (**Fig. 156**) and to the oral mucosa. The infant in **Fig. 157** has fungal lesions on the inside of the cheeks on the buccal pads. The infant in **Fig. 158** has fuzzy white lesions covering much of her mouth.

Oral nystatin is the front line medication to treat infant thrush in the US, and miconazole oral gel outside the US. Maternal treatment involves use of topical ointments or creams containing nystatin, miconazole, mupiricin, or clotrimazole. Breastfeeding can continue and these medications do not have to be washed off the breast. They are re-applied sparingly after each feeding.

Gential violet is an antifungal agent that some doctors recommend as an over-the-counter treatment for thrush, providing care is taken to avoid swallowing. Gentian violet is typically applied to the baby's mouth and the

mother's nipples once a day for 3 to 4 days (**Figs. 159** and **160**). After coating the baby's mouth with gentian violet, place the infant face down on a disposable pad so that excess medication is drooled rather than swallowed. Over-use of gentian violet has been associated with ulceration of the mouth and throat (Utter 1990). Mothers often use purified lanolin to coat the skin around the baby's mouth to prevent the purple dye from staining the baby's face.

Yeast diaper rashes (**Fig 161**) typically do not respond to standard care, but improve when treated with antifungal creams or ointments.

Fig. 162 shows a nipple that is becoming tender and inflamed. Note the accumulations of white material on the nipple surface.

Occasionally, fungal infections are communicated on the hands of another family member, or perhaps from a pet. Good handwashing of at least 15 seconds duration is important in preventing cross-infections. Cross infection should be investigated if yeast infections recur. Treat any family member or pet with symptoms of fungal infection such as athlete's foot, diaper rash, vaginal yeast infection, finger or toenail fungus, jock itch, dandruff, ringworm, etc. Fungal infections can be persistent and take weeks to clear up, especially during hot, humid weather. Fungal infections are particularly difficult to eradicate in people with immunosuppression, especially from HIV/AIDS.

Fungal and Bacterial Infections of the Nipple

Fig. 163 shows an infected nipple that required treatment with antifungal and antibiotic ointment.

Fig. 164 shows extreme tissue breakdown in a woman with a persistent, untreated infection. Her story demonstrates what can occur when only telephone consultation is provided to postpartum mothers. The woman had a *dimpled nipple*, the tip of which folds in on itself, see **Figs. 137** and **138**. With this type of nipple configuration, moisture is retained in the crevice, creating a hospitable environment for bacterial and fungal overgrowth. Unless women are shown how to retract the skin to rinse and air dry the nipple after feeding, the unexposed area can become colonized and infected. The woman had numerous phone contacts with nurses in her pediatrician and obstetrician's offices and with a lay counselor, but no one actually looked at her nipples.

At 5 weeks postpartum, the mother phoned BWC, who insisted on seeing her. By this time, deep fissures had opened on both nipples. There was no obvious evidence of infection, but the cracks had not healed. While very sore, surprisingly, the cracks were not painful enough to keep the mother from breastfeeding or pumping. The LC referred the mother back to the obstetrician for medical treatment with a triple nipple cream that included topical antifungal, antibacterial, and steroid medication. It took almost 2 months of treatment before the nipples healed completely.

Until the fissures closed, the mother continued to be at risk for infection. She was advised to avoid swimming pools, maintain careful skin hygiene, and wear clean cotton brassieres. Shortly before her nipples healed completely, they became exquisitely tender. The LC speculated that after such extensive tissue damage, nerve endings that had been destroyed were now regenerating. The woman maintained lactation throughout the experience and breastfed until her baby was 18 months old.

Allergic Reactions

Any condition that affects the skin elsewhere on the body can also affect the skin of the breasts and nipples. Allergic reactions (*dermatitis*) can occur on the breasts. Postpartum women have an enhanced sensitivity to contact with chemicals, irritants, or allergens (Pray 2000). Dermatitis often is mistaken for fungal infection. Women may phone an LC and complain about weeks of pain from unresolved nipple "yeast" in spite of complicated treatments. A reasonable assumption might be to suspect that something else is the problem. Referral to a dermatologist is appropriate in such circumstances.

Possible Triggers of Allergic Dermatitis on the Breast

- Detergent, soap, shampoos, or spray deodorants
- Creams, ointments, or medications
- Reaction to the material of breast shells, nipple
- shields, or pump flanges
- Introduction of solid foods (exposure via infant saliva)
- Baby on medication or teething gels
- Salivary changes owing to teething
- Previous history of atopic dermatitis in other areas of the body that are prone to maceration

When the mother in **Fig. 165** stopped using the medicated cream she had been applying to her nipples, her allergic reaction resolved.

The mother in **Fig. 166** has hives on her breast from an allergic reaction to topical applications of nystatin, an antifungal drug. She chronically suffered from mild outbreaks of eczema but did not associate the patch that developed

on her areola with her chronic skin condition. After talking with friends, she became convinced that the red skin on her areola was a yeast infection. She requested nystatin to treat it. Her pediatrician called in a prescription without evaluating the breast lesion in person. Over the course of 4 days, the mother treated the baby's mouth with nystatin and applied the drug directly to her nipple. Late on a Friday afternoon, she became worried at the appearance of her breast and visited her obstetrician. The obstetrician had left for the weekend, so the office nurse redirected this woman to BWC.

After taking a history and discovering patches of eczema on the woman's elbows, the LC suspected an allergic reaction to nystatin. The LC consulted with the obstetrician by phone and described what appeared to be hives on the breast. The doctor advised the mother to discontinue applying nystatin and suggested an over-the-counter topical corticosteroid cream to control the itching. She directed the mother to take 2 doses of oral Benadryl® (diphenhydramine) elixir per package directions to control the allergic reaction. Within 12 hours the mother's symptoms cleared, and she required no additional care. This story illustrates the importance of direct examination, and the danger of assuming that every red or itchy patch of skin on the breast indicates yeast infection. Exacerbation of symptoms after medication use begins should prompt evaluation for allergic reaction to the drug.

Eczema

The woman in **Fig. 167** has eczema on her nipple and areola. Note the dry, scaly appearance of the reddened skin. An important question for the LC to ask is, "Do you have similar patches of irritated skin elsewhere on your body?" This question may help determine if the condition is directly related to lactation or involves a pre-existing problem that has been exacerbated by the wet-dry, wet-dry nature of breastfeeding. Eczema also may develop when infants begin to eat solid foods if food residue acts as an allergen on the mother's nipples (Amir 1993). **Ch. 12** also contains a discussion of contact allergic reaction triggered by food.

Eczema is common in people with a family history of hay fever and asthma, and is revealed by skin breakdown behind the knees, on the hands and feet, or on any area where the skin is exposed to stress. Prolonged exposure to hot water, chlorine, and synthetic clothing seems to aggravate eczema. Mothers should be advised to take quick, warm showers, avoid swimming pools, and wear cotton clothes so the breast skin can "breathe."

Often a woman with eczema has an existing relationship with a dermatologist, and may have appropriate topical medications on hand. A call to the doctor determines if the medication is safe for use on the nipples (Huggins 1993). Sometimes skin that is damaged and broken from eczema becomes infected. A combination of a topical antibiotic and a topical steroid is usually effective in this case (Hale and Berens 2002).

Prolonged use of steroids can cause health problems for the baby (Amir 1993). The pediatrician should be informed of ongoing steroid treatment in order to monitor the baby. If breastfeeding the infant is too painful for the mother, pumping protects the milk supply. Friction from the pump flange may further irritate eczematous skin. The mother's own milk or olive oil can be used to lubricate the plastic pump flange.

The woman pictured in **Fig. 167** did not have a previous history of eczema. No factor to explain the sudden onset of eczema was discovered. At 11 months postpartum, she called her midwife to report burning nipple pain and shooting, burning breast pain, and was treated by phone with a prescription topical antifungal for 2 weeks. Her baby was treated with oral nystatin even though the baby showed no signs or symptoms of thrush. When treatment did not resolve her symptoms, the mother was given oral fluconazole for 2 weeks, but her condition did not improve.

The woman called KH to request assistance. KH suggested that the woman ask her midwife for a referral to a dermatologist, who diagnosed eczema and prescribed a steroid cream. Over the next month with this treatment, the eczema gradually improved. The mother continued to breastfeed throughout the treatment.

Paget's Disease of the Nipple

A type of breast cancer called *Paget's disease* resembles nipple eczema (see also **Ch. 12**). Paget's disease of the breast accounts for approximately 2 to 3 percent of breast cancers. Clinical features include bloody nipple discharge, erythema and scaling of the nipple, nipple erosion or ulceration, nipple retraction, and a palpable mass or thickening in the breast with or without nipple changes (Burke 1998). It appears *unilaterally* (on one side) and progresses steadily. When eczema does not resolve with appropriate treatment, further investigation including biopsy may be required. See **Figs. 290-292** for photographs of a nipple biopsy to rule out Paget's disease of the nipple.

Psoriasis

Some women who have struggled with psoriasis most of their lives have had outbreaks on their nipples and areolae that have not significantly impacted breastfeeding. **Fig.**

168 shows *psoriasis* on the nipple and areola. This woman had patches of psoriasis on many parts of her body. These patches were salmon-colored with silvery scales. After the birth of each of her 2 sons, the psoriasis spread to her nipples. Breastfeeding was too painful to continue. When the LC suggested contacting her doctor for a steroid cream, the mother explained that she had been dealing with this condition for many years, and a steroid cream would not be helpful in her care. This mother opted to wean. For many other women with psoriasis, a steroid cream has been found to be effective in resolving the problem.

Poison Ivy

Fig. 169 pictures a woman with poison ivy on her breasts. After the skin is washed, oils from the plant that cause the reaction are gone. Thus, there is no risk to the nursing baby from contact with vesicles on the nipple. However, continued nursing poses some risk of secondary infection of the nipple or of excessive pain. Mothers can pump milk until the lesions heal (Lawrence 2005). Hydrocortisone creams and short-term use of oral corticosteroids are considered safe for breastfeeding mothers who develop poison ivy (Hale and Berens 2002, Hale 2008b).

White Spots on the Nipple

Fig. 170 shows a white spot on the nipple face associated with a painful blockage of the milk duct openings (pores). It may be that a blister has formed over a milk duct opening and milk trapped underneath has calcified forming a "caked duct" (Riordan 2005). A strand of dried milk, the end of which is visible at the nipple pore, plugs the duct, preventing free draining. When a duct opening is obstructed, the resulting backup creates a ropy, tender mass that extends into the breast. Inflammatory response to this retained milk may escalate into mastitis.

It was previously believed that women have 15 to 20 ductal openings in the nipple. Ultrasound anatomy studies identify fewer, with on average 9 patent ductal openings at the surface of the nipple. Thus, obstruction of any of the ductal openings has the capacity to significantly affect the drainage of the breast and may impair lactation (Ramsay 2005).

One mother described her experience with a caked nipple pore as follows: Blocking the pore "...was a small chunk (about the size of a mustard seed) that had a cheese curd consistency. I flicked it with my fingernail and dug in a bit and it came partially out. Then I used sterilized tweezers to grab and pull it the rest of the way out. Milk came shooting out of the pore and gushed for a good minute before slowing to a trickle. After the next feeding my nipple still felt a bit sore with a smaller bump under the skin. After the next feeding the bump was completely gone. No discomfort or swelling left at all."

No one is sure how caked ducts form. It may be that such plugs begin as a milk blister (see **Fig 175**) that, over time, solidifies into a callus, trapping milk behind it. Sometimes the baby can dislodge the plugged material from a milk pore while breastfeeding. Some women must use warm water soaks, lubrication with safe oils, and gentle manipulation behind the plug to squeeze it out.

A physician can open a plugged milk pore with a very sharp, sterile needle. Sometimes milk drains out, but often the material in the duct has dried out and any material that exudes is calcified. Opening the pore may make the nipple sore. Mothers should cleanse the nipple and use a topical antibiotic to prevent infection. Lubrication may prevent formation of another callus.

Some practitioners suggest modifying the diet of a woman who chronically experiences plugged ducts by reducing saturated fats and adding lecithin (Lawrence 2005, Eglash 1998). Lawrence (p. 273) speculates that too much calcium in the diet might cause calcium stones that potentially could block a duct.

Not every white spot on the nipple causes pain, and some may result from issues unconnected with blockages of the ducts. For example, some white spots may be accumulations of dead skin, similar to cradle cap (Lawrence 2005). The mother can lubricate the nipple and gently rub off dry skin. **Fig. 171** illustrates a white spot on the nipple that was not painful. It is asymmetrical and does not appear to cover a ductal opening. The white spot shown in **Fig. 170** appears to be more cystic.

Sometimes a bite from a teething baby produces a ragged tear in the nipple skin. As saliva and milk moisture accumulates under the skin edges, the skin may turn white (similar to a cut on the finger that looks white after bathing). This type of nipple white spot may be associated with pain, but should not be squeezed. The mother should cleanse a bite wound, apply topical antibiotic ointment to prevent infection, and report increasing pain to a physician, as bites are often associated with ascending ductal infection and mastitis.

The appearance of a white spot on the nipple may concern mothers. If the nipple does not hurt and milk flow is not blocked, white spots can be ignored.

Cysts

Sore nipples may have unusual causes. Sometimes the fact that the woman is lactating is coincidental. The woman in **Fig. 172** phoned KH to describe a painful "plugged duct." She stated that "white, stringy" material could be squeezed from the white spot on her nipple, and she was unable to "drain it" thoroughly. When the LC saw the nipple, she discovered that the white spot was on the shaft, not the face of the nipple (as would be the case with a blocked pore). The breast was soft, with no evidence of plugging, and the stringy material more closely resembled a sebaceous secretion than dried milk. These clues led the LC to conclude that the condition was unrelated to lactation and appeared to be a kind of pimple. When the woman consulted a physician the next day, he confirmed the LC's suspicion and identified the problem as a sebaceous cyst. The doctor squeezed out a quantity of the oily matter. Removal of the material brought relief from the pain, and the condition resolved.

Vasospasm

Nipple vasospasm is a constriction of the blood vessels with resultant color changes to the face of the nipple (Anderson 2004). Previous nipple trauma may result in a tendency to experience vasospasm. In describing normal wound healing processes, Enoch (2003) states that "Vasoconstriction...occurs in response to initial injury." Vasospasm is currently recognized as an important source of nipple pain in breastfeeding women, and one that mimics the pain of yeast infection (Morino 2007). **Fig. 173** shows a nipple in the blanching phase of vasospasm.

Cold stress may trigger vasospasm of the nipple. Applying dry, warm compresses immediately after breastfeeding relieves the stabbing, shooting pain described by some mothers. Wet compresses should be avoided as evaporative cooling may trigger resumption of vasospasm. The mother who experiences painful vasospasm should keep her breasts warm and take care not to become chilled.

Lactation consultant, Diana West (personal communication 2005) shares the following: "Some women report that they can stop the vasospasm if they push blood into the nipple. This is done by squeezing the base of the nipple and pushing forward (**Fig. 174**). Restoration of blood flow to the nipple then seems to stop the painful, burning sensation."

The mother experiencing painful nipples resulting from vasospasm should eliminate or reduce her exposure to vasoconstrictors such as nicotine and caffeine (which has a rebound vasoconstrictive effect). She should explore with her prescribing physician how she might reduce her exposure to drugs such as theophylline, terbutaline, epinephrine, norepinephrine, serotonin, prostaglandin, and birth control pills. In Lawlor-Smiths' case studies (1996, 1997) of the phenomenon of vasospasm, each of the 5 women described severe, debilitating nipple pain. Blanching of the nipple occured during and immediately after the feeds, and also between feeds. Exposure to cold precipitated nipple blanching and pain in all patients observed by Lawlor-Smith.

Unexplained pain alarms women. It is helpful to explain that vasospasm, while annoying, is essentially a benign condition that cannot damage the breast. Once the mother understands that relatively simple tricks typically manage her pain, she can stop worrying about it. Some women experience vasospasm of the nipple without significant reports of pain. BWC interviewed one mother who had experienced vasospasm and remarked that it did not cause her pain.

Raynaud's Phenomenon

Raynaud's phenomenon, which includes lack of blood flow to the extremities of the body (such as the toes, fingers, nipples, ears, and nose), is found in approximately 20 percent of women of childbearing age (Anderson 2004). Raynaud's also can cause vasospasm of the nipple (Morino 2007). With Raynaud's syndrome there are typically biphasic or triphasic color changes (Lawlor-Smith 1996, Lawlor-Smith 1998). First the body part turns white. In some instances, it then turns blue. Finally, it reddens. Raynaud's phenomenon has been associated with other medical conditions including lupus erythematosus or rheumatoid arthritis, hypothyroidism, and with certain medications. There is an association (poorly described at present) between breast surgery and Raynaud's (Anderson 2004).

If squeezing the base of the nipple or the use of dry, warm compresses do not significantly relieve pain, a physician may prescribe oral nifedipine (Eglash 1996, Anderson 2004).

Blisters

The woman in **Fig. 175** suddenly developed a blister on her nipple after expressing her milk with a hospital grade electric breast pump. The white material on her nipple is milk. She had been pumping uneventfully for many weeks and was surprised to develop nipple trauma at this time. Blisters can result when a pump is creating excessive negative pressure or when the flange is too small. Using a larger flange size brought relief to this mother. It is possible that nipple tissue becomes more vulnerable to normally safe pressure levels as the result of engorgement. Sometimes the baby may cause a blister when the milk supply is low or blocked by sucking extra hard in an effort to obtain more milk.

Montgomery Glands

Montgomery glands (or tubercules) are scattered over the areolar surface. Great variation exists in the number observed, but the average is 9. These areolar skin glands appear to function as scent organs and play a role in helping the baby find the breast (Schaal 2006). Montgomery glands enlarge during pregnancy and become less noticeable after weaning. They have a small ductal subsystem almost like a miniature mammary system (Lawrence 2005). The small ducts that secrete sebaceous material sometimes merge with the ducts that secrete milk. It is common to see drops of moisture on these pimple-like structures. BWC spoke with a mother who reported that her Montgomery glands significantly enlarged during the engorgement phase and appeared inflamed. They were tender before feedings. The discomfort resolved after feedings when the glands returned to a more normal (less swollen) appearance. She could express drops of milk from her Montgomery glands.

Occasionally a mother will report that one of these ducts gets plugged and may become inflamed (**Fig. 176**). This is typically a self-limiting condition, although gentle manipulation to open the pore with heat and massage may help along with application of a topical antibiotic cream to prevent infection.

The woman in **Fig. 176** called her lactation consultant (KH) complaining of a "plugged duct." The LC talked to her about treating a plugged duct, but as they were concluding their conversation, the mother added an aside, "It has been interesting watching this 'second nipple' grow today." The LC asked the mother to describe this "second nipple," and realized that this description did not sound like a plugged duct. The LC saw the mother in person. Visual assessment confirmed her suspicion that the problem was an infected Montgomery gland.

The LC and the mother used warm soaks and attempted to squeeze the lump without success. The LC instructed the woman to call her obstetrician, who phoned in a prescription for an oral antibiotic. Within hours after starting the antibiotic, the woman felt better. The following day there was a head on the infected area. The woman was able to squeeze out the infected material. She observed white, thickened milk, followed by pus, then blood, and then clear serous fluid. The mother washed the area with warm soapy water, rinsed well, and applied a topical antibiotic cream. The area quickly healed. This woman frequently saw milk coming from her Montgomery glands.

Occasionally an infected Montgomery gland becomes a problem for a woman using a breast pump, especially if the inflammation is located where the breast flange rests. A notch can be cut in the flange if necessary. The cut out area is placed so that the sore area is avoided. This trick is also useful to avoid placing friction or pressure on a sub-areolar abscess while pumping. Be aware that the edges may be sharp and care taken to avoid cutting oneself.

Coincidental Dermatitis

Fig. 177 shows a woman with a raised, red rash on her chin who called an LC because of a red, raised rash on her nipples. The LC pointed out that the rashes looked similar. The mother's dermatologist was consulted about the safety of using the same cream in both locations. He approved the cream for use on her nipples, and the condition cleared. The mother elected to pump her milk for several days until the problem resolved.

Skin Tags

The mother in **Fig. 178** has a *skin tag* on the tip of her nipple. She worried that it might affect breastfeeding or cause nipple pain. In her case it did not. Breastfeeding was slightly more uncomfortable on the affected breast. Occasionally skin tags tear off and bleed owing to the stress of breastfeeding. A dermatologist can easily remove them. While the procedure can be done during lactation, it is probably best performed during pregnancy in order to give the nipple time to heal.

The mother in **Fig. 179** has a skin tag on her large areola, located a distance from the nipple. While this will not directly interfere with breastfeeding, some infants like to manipulate skin tags, causing irritation and potential risk of infection. If a mother chooses not to remove the skin tag from her breast, she may wish to keep it covered to discourage the baby from playing with the tag while feeding.

Proper Removal of The Baby From The Breast

The cause of sore nipples sometimes is simple. Often mothers remove their babies from the breast without first breaking suction. This can be traumatic and can create abrasions on the nipple shaft. **Fig. 180** demonstrates insertion of the mother's finger between the gums (not just between the lips). The baby removed in this manner will gum the mother's finger harmlessly instead of biting the nipple. Poor technique in removing a baby from the breast may be a significant contributing factor and help to explain a mother's complaint of persistent nipple pain.

Biting

Older babies, such as the 5 month-old in **Fig. 181** can present a new set of breastfeeding challenges. Easily distracted by the feeding environment, the baby may tug at the breast while trying to look around, or may bite down as the result of teething discomfort. Mothers should make eye contact and use simple language to tell the baby, "Don't bite!" Repeat the same phrase, especially at times during the feeding when the baby typically bites. If the baby ignores the verbal command, some mothers find it effective to remove the baby from the breast, sit the baby down, repeat the verbal command firmly. Yelling at the baby is discouraged since it may precipitate a *nursing strike* (sudden breast refusal). Babies learn from repetition, and if the mother is consistent in her response, it generally does not take long before the biting problem is resolved. If the baby bites the nipples, breaking the skin, gentle cleansing and application of a safe topical antibiotic ointment will prevent infection in most cases.

Hormonal Changes

Hormonal changes unrelated to breastfeeding may cause pain. Occasionally, a woman who has resumed menstruation will notice nipple tenderness prior to the onset of her period. Changes in breasts and nipples sensitivity may be the first indication of pregnancy, even before a woman misses a period. A woman who becomes pregnant may notice persistent nipple discomfort while breastfeeding. Along with heightened sensitivity, some of this pain may result from diminished milk production and compensatory strong suction by the baby.

Akkuzu G, Taskin L. Impacts of breast-care techniques on prevention of possible postpartum nipple problems. *Professional Care of Mother and Child* 2000; 10(2):38-39, 41.

Amir L. Eczema of the nipple and breast: a case report. *Journal of Human Lactation* 1993; 9(3):173-5.

Amir LH, Garland S, Lumley J. A case-control study of mastitis: nasal carriage of *Staphylococcus aureus*. *BMC Family Practice* 2006; 7:57.

Anderson J, Held N, Wright K. Raynaud's phenomenon of the nipple: a treatable cause of painful breastfeeding. *Pediatrics* 2004; 113(4):e360-e364.

Arai R, Sugita T, Nishikawa A. Reassessment of the *in vitro* synergistic effect of fluconazole with the non-steroidal anti-inflammatory agent ibuprofen against *Candida albicans*. *Mycoses* 2005; 48(1):38-41.

Beauchamp GK, Keast RS, Morel D, et al. Phyto-chemistry:ibuprofen like activity in extra-virgin olive oil. *Nature* 2005; 437(7055):45-46.

Best Practice 2003. The management of nipple pain and/or trauma associated with breastfeeding. 2003; 7(3):1-7.

Beam JW, Buckley B. Community-acquired Methicillin-Resistant *Staphylococcus aureus*: prevalence and risk factors. *Journal of Athletic Training* 2006; 41(3):337-340.

Brent N, Rudy S, Redd B, et al. A clinical trial of wound dressings vs. conventional care. *Archives of Pediatric and Adolescent Medicine* 1998; 152(11):1077-1082.

Buchko BL, Pugh LC, Bishop BA, et al. Comfort measures in breast-feeding primiparous women. *Journal of Obstetric, Gynecologic, and Neonatal Nursing* 1994; 23(1):46-52.

Burke E, Braeuning M, McLelland R, Pisano E, et al. Paget's disease of the breast: a pictorial essay. *Radiographics* 1998; 18(6):1459-1464.

Cox D, Kent J, Casey T, et al. Breast growth and the urinary excretion of lactose during human pregnancy and early lactation: endocrine relationships. *Experimental Physiology* 1999; 84(2):421-434.

de Wet P, Rode H, van Dyk A, et al. Perianal candidosis – a comparative study with mupirocin and nystatin. *International Journal of Dermatology* 1999; 38(8):618-22.

Dodd V, Chalmers C. Comparing the use of hydrogel dressings to lanolin ointment with lactating mothers. *Journal of Obstetric, Gynecologic, and Neonatal Nursing* 2003; 32(4):486-494.

Edelmann A, Kruger M, Schmid J. Genetic relationship between human and animal isolates of *Candida albicans*. *Journal of Clinical Microbiology* 2005; 43(12):6164-6166.

Eglash A. Case report. *ABM News and Views* 1996; 2(1):4.

Eglash A. Delayed milk ejection reflex and plugged ducts: lecithin therapy. *ABM News and Views* 1998; 4(1):4.

Enoch S, Harding K. Wound bed preparation: the science behind the removal of barriers to healing. *Wounds* 2003; 15(7):213-229.

Fernandez R, Griffiths R. Water for wound cleansing. *Cochrane Database of Systematic Reviews* 2002; 4(CD003861). Update: Nov. 2, 2007.

Fetherston C. Risk factors for lactation mastitis. *Journal of Human Lactation* 1998; 14(2):102-109.

Fetherston C, Lai CT, Hartmann PE. Relationships between symptoms and changes in breast physiology during lactation mastitis. *Breastfeeding Medicine* 2006; 1(3):136-145.

Foxman B. Personal communication, March. 19, 2002.

Foxman B, D'Arcy H, Gillespie B, et al. Lactation mastitis: occurrence and medical management among 946 breastfeeding women in the United States. *American Journal of Epidemiology* 2002; 15(2):103-114.

Geddes DT. Gross Anatomy of the Human Breast, in *Hale & Hartmann's Textbook of Human Lactation*, Amarillo, TX: Hale Publishing, 2007, pp. 19-34.

Giandoni M, Grabski W. Cutaneous candidiasis as a cause of delayed surgical wound healing. *Journal of the American Academy of Dermatology* 1994; 30(6):981-984.

Gray L, Miller L, Philipp B, et al. Breastfeeding is analgesic in healthy newborns. *Pediatrics* 2002; 109(4):590-593.

Gunther M. Sore nipples, causes and prevention. *Lancet ii* 1945; 590-593.

Gupta AK, Bhargava KP. Some triazole analogs as anti-inflammatory agents. Pharmazie 1978; 33(7):430-431.

Hale T. Candida infections: all the "NEW" details. Conference Presentation, Hale/Hartmann Human Lactation Research Conference, Richmond, VA, Sept. 28-29, 2006a.

Hale T. *Medications and Mothers' Milk,* 13th ed. Amarillo, TX: Hale Publishing, 2008b; pp. 666, 1124-1126.

Hale T, Berens P. *Clinical Therapy in Breastfeeding Patients,* 2nd ed. Amarillo, TX: Pharmasoft Medical Publishing, 2002; pp. 208-212.

Hewat RJ, Ellis DJ. A comparison of the effectiveness of two methods of nipple care. *Birth* 1987; 14(1):41-45.

Huggins K, Billon S. Twenty cases of persistent sore nipples: collaboration between lactation consultant and dermatologist. *Journal of Human Lactation* 1993; 9(3):155-160.

Khan HA. Effect of fluconazole on phagocytic response of polymor-phonuclear leukocytes in a rat model of acute sepsis. *Mediators of Inflammation* 2005; 1:9-15.

Kim YH, Chang SS, Kim YS, et al. Clinical outcomes in Methicillin-resistant *Staphylococcus aureus*-colonized neonates in the neonatal intensive care unit. *Neonatology* 2007; 91(4):241-247.

Kirby M. Negative pressure wound therapy. *British Journal of Diabetes and Vascular Diseases* 2007; 7(5):230-234.

Kitajima H. Prevention of methicillin-resistant *Staphylococcus aureus* infections in neonates. *Pediatrics International* 2003; 45(2):238-45.

Kvist L, Hall-Lord M, Larsson B. A descriptive study of Swedish women with symptoms of breast inflammation during lactation and their perceptions of the quality of care given at a breastfeeding clinic. *International Breastfeeding Journal* 2007; 2(2).

Lavergne NA. Does application of tea bags to sore nipples while breast-feeding provide effective relief? *Journal of Obstetric, Gynecologic, and Neonatal Nursing* 1997; 26(1):53-58.

Lawlor-Smith LS, Lawlor-Smith CL. Raynaud's phenomenon of the nipple: a preventable cause of breastfeeding failure? *Medical Journal of Australia* 1997; 166(8):448.

Lawlor-Smith L, Lawlor-Smith CL. Nipple vasospasm in the breastfeed-ing woman. *Breastfeeding Review* 1996; 4(1):37-39.

Lawlor-Smith C. Nipple Vasospasm, Conference and annual meeting of the International Lactation Consultants Association, July 15-19, 1998, Boca Raton, Fl, US.

Lawlor-Smith LS, Lawlor-Smith CL. Vasospasm of the nipple -- a mani-festation of Raynaud's phenomenon: case reports. *British Medical Journal* 1997; 314(7081):644-645.

Lawrence RA, Lawrence RM. *Breastfeeding: A Guide for the Medical Profession,* 6th ed. Philadelphia, PA: Elsevier Mosby, 2005; p. 612.

Livingstone V, Stringer J. The treatment of *Staphylococcus aureus* infected sore nipples: a randomized comparative study. *Journal of Human Lactation* 1999; 15(3):241-246.

McClellan H, Geddes D, Kent J, et al. Infants of mothers with persistent nipple pain exert strong sucking vacuums. *Acta Paediatrica* 2008; 97(9):1205-1209.

Mohrbacher N. Nipple pain and trauma: causes and treatments, Conference presentation, North Austin Medical Center, Austin, Texas, 2004.

Morino C, Winn S. Raynaud's phenomenon of the nipples: an elusive diagnosis. *Journal of Human Lactation* 2007; 23(2):191-192.

Morrison P. Lactnet communication, Mar 25, 2002. Used with permission.

Nicholas R, Berry V, Hunter P, et al. The antifungal activity of mupirocin. *Journal of Antimicrobial Chemotherapy* 1999; 43(4):579-582.

Page SM, McKenna DS. Vasospasm of the nipple presenting as painful lactation. *Obstetrics and Gynecology* 2006; 108(3 Part 2):806-808.

Potter P, Perry A. *Fundamentals of Nursing, 5th ed.* Philadelphia: Mosby, 2001; pp. 1597-1599.

Pray W. Consult your pharmacist: dermatitis causes are diverse. *U.S. Pharmacist* 2000; 25(8):14-24.

Prime D, Geddes D, Hartmann P. Oxytocin: Milk Ejection and Maternal-Infant Well-being, in *Hale & Hartmann's Textbook of Human Lactation*, Amarillo, TX: Hale Publishing, 2007; p. 147.

Pugh L, Buchko B, Bishop B, et al. A comparison of topical agents to relieve nipple pain and enhance breastfeeding. *Birth* 1996; 23(2):88-93.

Ramsay D, Kent JC, Hartmann RA, et al. Anatomy of the lactating human breast redefined with ultrasound imaging. *Journal of Anatomy* 2005; 206(6):525-534.

Ramsay D, Kent J, Owens R, et al. Ultrasound imaging of milk ejection in the breast of lactating women. *Pediatrics* 2004; 113(2):361-367.

Riordan J. The effectiveness of topical agents in reducing nipple soreness of breastfeeding mothers. *Journal of Human Lactation* 1985; 1(3):36-41.

Riordan J. *Breastfeeding and Human Lactation,* 3rd ed. Sudbury, MA: Jones and Bartlett, 2005; pp. 249, 261.

Rutala W, White M, Gergen M, et al. Bacterial contamination of keyboards: efficacy and functional impact of disinfectants. *Infection Control Hospital Epidemiology* 2006; 27(4):372-377.

Ryan TJ. Infection following soft tissue injury: its role in wound healing. *Current Opinions in Infectious Disease* 2007; 20(2):124-128.

Saiman L, O'Keefe M, Graham P, et al. Hospital transmission of Community-Acquired Methicillin-Resistant *Staphylococcus aureus* among postpartum women. *Clinical Infectious Diseases* 2003; 37:1313-1319.

Sayyah MM, Rashidi MR, Delazar A, et al. Effect of peppermint water on prevention of nipple cracks in lactating primiparous women: a randomized controlled trial. *International Breastfeeding Journal* 2007; 2:7.

Schaal B, Doucet S, Sagot P, et al. Human breast areolae as scent organs: morphological data and possible involvement in maternal-neonatal coadaptation. *Developmental Psychobiology* 2006; 48:100-110.

Spangler A, Hildebrandt E. The effect of modified lanolin on nipple pain/damage during the first ten days of breastfeeding. *International Journal of Childbirth Educators* 1993; 8(3):15-19.

Thomassen P, Johansson VA, Wassberg C, et al. Breastfeeding, pain and infection. *Gynecologic and Obstetric Investigation* 1998; 46(2):73-74.

Utter A. Case report. *Journal of Human Lactation* 1990; 6(2):178-189.

West D. Personal communication. 2005. Used with permission.

Woolridge M. Aetiology of sore nipples. *Midwifery* 1986; 2(4):173-6.

Ziemer M, Cooper D, Pigeon J. Evaluation of a dressing to reduce nipple pain and improve nipple skin condition in breastfeeding women. *Nursing Research* 1995; 44(6):347-351.

Ziemer M, Paone J, Schupay J, et al. Methods to prevent and manage nipple pain in breastfeeding women. *Western Journal of Nursing Research* 1990; 12(6):732-744.

Ziemer M, Pigeon J. Skin changes and pain in the nipple during the 1st week of lactation. *Journal of Obstetric, Gynecologic, and Neonatal Nursing* 1993; 22(3):247-256.

Unusual Presentations of the Breast and Nipple

Sensitivity, tact, and concern for the client's self-image are important whenever the lactation consultant performs a breast assessment. Women are often self-conscious about their breasts. They need reassurance that variations in the appearance of the breasts and nipples are normal and not necessarily predictors of lactation performance. Occasionally, the LC observes variations that *are* likely to impact lactation. The mother needs honest feedback from the assessment in order to make informed decisions, yet the information should be presented in a supportive manner.

Engorgement in the Tail of Spence

Mammary glandular tissue extends into the *axillary* region (the armpit) and is referred to as the *tail of Spence* (Lawrence 2005). Milk is produced in the tail of Spence and drains through the central ductal system. Women occasionally experience significant and uncomfortable engorgement in this area, often complicated by tight brassieres that cut across ducts and prevent normal drainage. Thus, plugged ducts and mastitis can occur in the tail of Spence.

The woman in **Fig. 182** was worried about the swelling under her arm that occurred on Day 3 postpartum. She was relieved to learn that engorgement in the tail of Spence is not abnormal. Cold compresses and ibuprofen eased her discomfort. Within a few days, the engorgement resolved.

The breast is a vascular organ; it is sensitive to bruising and swelling. When swelling occurs, it impairs blood circulation and lymphatic drainage, contributing to discomfort and interfering with thorough drainage of milk. Pooled fluid accumulating anywhere in the body has the potential to cause problems. As pressure increases and the milk volume exceeds the storage capacity of the breast, milk may leak into interstitial spaces, causing localized inflammation, pain, and the risk of infection. For this reason, it is important for women with axillary breast tissue to avoid constricting clothing and brassieres that might bruise the tissue and interfere with drainage, especially during the earliest phase of lactation when physiologic engorgement is commonly observed.

Accessory Breast and Nipple Tissue

Fig. 183 pictures a woman at one month postpartum with *hypermastia* or *polymastia*: the presence of *accessory* (extra) mammary tissue in the axilla. Accessory tissue is different from mammary tissue that is part of the tail of Spence. Accessory (also referred to as *supernumerary*) ducts, nipples, and glandular tissue can occur anywhere along the *mammary ridge,* the so-called "milk line" that extends down the body from the *axilla* (armpit) to the groin and labia. Accessory tissue may appear in other places on the body, including the thighs and buttocks. Polymastia may not appear until enhanced by sex hormones during puberty or early pregnancy. *Polythelia* (supernumerary nipples) is associated with renal anomalies. Pediatricians generally screen infants who present with accessory nipples for renal and other organ abnormalities. While both polymastia and polythelia can occur sporadically, there appears to be a familial link (Grossl 2000).

Accessory tissue can produce milk (Lawrence 2005). The same conditions that affect the breasts can affect accessory tissue, including engorgement, development of cysts, and cancer.

When mammography is used to study accessory breast tissue, the tissue resembles normal glandular tissue, but is separate from it. It should be recognized as a normal developmental variant. Using radiographic studies to distinguish hypermastia from malignant masses can eliminate the need for unnecessary biopsy (Adler 1987).

Note the side of the breast of the woman in **Fig. 184**. She has accessory breast tissue with no nipple.

The woman pictured in **Fig. 185** has accessory breast tissue in the axilla, but no nipple. Following the delivery of her third baby, this area became engorged on Day 3. The engorgement took several days to resolve. Interestingly, she did not experience this swelling with her first 2 children. Unlike glandular tissue in the tail of Spence that drains into the central ductal system of the breast, accessory breast tissue is a separate system. Because there was no outlet for the milk, the unrelieved pressure resulted in involution and atrophy of the glandular tissue, similar to that which occurs when a woman does not breastfeed. After this localized weaning, the tenderness in her axilla resolved. The woman's primary breasts were unaffected by these events.

The woman in **Fig. 186** has a milk pore located on the milk line. This is an *ectopic* duct with no accessory breast or nipple tissue. As she breastfeeds, a drop of milk appears on the surface of her skin.

Fig. 187 shows a breast in profile with a supernumerary nipple positioned slightly above the *mammary fold* (where the breast meets the rib cage). Some supernumerary nipples have a pronounced appearance, as in **Figs. 187, 188, 189,** and **190,** but they generally have only a rudimentary underlying ductal and glandular structure. Small drops of milk may be visible whenever milk ejection occurs, but such tissue typically does not produce copious amounts of milk. Mothers can be reassured that accessory breast and nipple tissue will not interfere with breastfeeding. Occasionally this tissue develops mastitis and requires medical treatment.

Figs. 189 and **190** show well-developed accessory nipples (photos courtesy of Susan Gehrman). When the doctor who delivered this girl observed them, he told her mother, "Don't let anyone even *think* about doing any cosmetic surgery until after she is fully developed, and then think twice if she is going to breastfeed." This family has a history of accessory nipples, most of which are smaller and resemble "moles." The brother of this girl has an accessory nipple, as do an uncle and a female second cousin. Renal anomalies also run in the family. The woman pictured, however, has no history of renal problems.

At age 19, the young woman pictured in **Figs. 189** and **190** delivered her first child, whom she breastfed for 16 months. Her extra nipples leaked milk at every feeding, and breast tissue was easily palpable below both nipples. She had to place cloths over her extra nipples during feedings to catch the leaking milk. In all other respects, lactation was uneventful. At age 22 she consulted a surgeon to discuss removing the accessory nipples. After the consultation she opted to delay cosmetic surgery until after she completes her family.

Underdeveloped Breast Tissue

The young woman pictured in **Fig. 191** has underdeveloped breasts. Her medical history included infertility that did not respond to treatment. Unable to conceive, she adopted 2 children, and attempted lactation with both. She never made more than a few drops of milk, but was able to coax her infants to breast using both a feeding tube device and a nipple shield. In this way, she enjoyed the experience of breastfeeding. The LC may encounter women whose lack of breast development motivates them to seek surgical implants. Their reduced capacity to lactate relates to the underdevelopment of the breasts, not specifically to the implants.

Figs. 192 and **193** picture women with insufficient breast tissue that affected their ability to produce normal volumes of milk for their infants. Both women required the use of infant formula to help their babies grow.

Fig. 193 shows a woman with underdeveloped breasts. She produced about 8 ounces daily for each of her 2 daughters. She breastfed her first daughter and offered supplements of formula by bottle. She breastfed her second daughter using a supplementer device.

Abnormally Shaped Breasts

Breast development often occurs asymmetrically. Most women have one breast that is slightly larger than the other. Sometimes marked breast asymmetry occurs. Occasionally, both breasts have an unusual cone shape. This may have no significance at all, or it may be a marker of a physical problem that will inhibit full lactation.

Huggins (2000) prospectively studied 34 lactating women with abnormally appearing breasts to explore a possible relationship between breast *hypoplasia* (underdevelopment) and milk production. She found that "the majority of the women with some degree of hypoplasia and with an intra-mammary distance of 1.5 inches (approximately 4 cm) or more produced 50 percent or less of the milk necessary to sustain normal infant growth in the first week postpartum." Many of the women in the study reported no pregnancy-related breast growth or changes. While some of these women experienced gradual increases in milk volume after careful management to maximize their production, 61 percent of the women were unable to produce a full milk supply within the first month. Whenever physical markers such as hypoplastic breasts or a wide span between breasts are observed, it is prudent to monitor the infant's growth rate, and to provide extra assistance to the mother to encourage optimal milk production, which may eventually be experienced.

Good counseling skills are critical when a woman presents with these markers, because they may not always predict difficulty with breastfeeding. The LC must avoid creating anxiety or creating a loss of confidence, as this in itself may create breastfeeding problems. However, because the calibration of lactation occurs early in the process, women with unusual breasts deserve extra attention and extended follow-up to make sure they reach their full lactation potential.

Polycystic Ovary Syndrome

Marasco (2000) researched Polycystic Ovary Syndrome (PCOS), and proposed a connection to insufficient milk supply. Symptoms of PCOS include amenorrhea, infertility, hirsutism, hyperinsulinemia, ovarian cysts, persistent acne, obesity, elevated triglycerides, adult-onset diabetes, and possible pathological interference with breast growth. This pathological interference may affect all 3 phases of lactogenesis. Ovarian cysts emit hormones, generally androgens, such as testosterone, that contribute to hyper-androgenism and hyperinsulinemia. Even subtle changes in a woman's hormonal balance appear to influence breast development, and may create a risk of insufficient milk supply that puts infants at risk for failure to thrive. Women with PCOS are also at significantly higher risk for depression (Hollinrake 2007).

More than 30 years ago, a group of researchers (Balcar 1972) used soft tissue radiography of the breast to diagnose PCOS (then called Stein-Leventhal Syndrome). The researchers found 80 percent agreement between abnormal ovarian findings and abnormal breast develop-ment. "Decreases in [breast] gland parenchyma [even in large breasts] may serve to reveal a hormonal disorder…and may in such cases serve as an easy, simple screening test before a more complicated investigation."

Metformin therapy decreases hyperandrogenism and hyperinsulinemia in women with PCOS, reducing some of the symptoms noted above (Kolodziejczyk 2000). What effect metformin therapy has on improving lactation is unclear. Some practitioners have begun using metformin therapy to increase milk production in women with insulin resistance (Gabbay 2003). Metformin is thought to be compatible with breastfeeding (Hale 2008).

Gestational Ovarian Theca Lutein Cysts

Clinicians have identified women, some of whom have lactated previously, who give birth and do not subsequently become engorged or produce milk. Some of these cases may result from the development of ovarian cysts that emit hormones with the potential to interfere with lactogenesis. Failure to lactate following delivery is an abnormal event, and an endocrinology referral is appropriate (Hoover 2002, Betzold 2004). Gestational ovarian theca lutein cysts are brought on by pregnancy and emit androgens, specifically testosterone, in levels that may temporarily suppress lactation. Levels of suppressive testosterone lessen over a period of 3 to 4 weeks as the cycts resolve. Women are encouraged to continue stimulating their breasts with a breast pump or a baby at the breast with a supplementer in hopes that their milk supply gradually will increase.

Both Hoover (2002) and Betzold (2004) followed women whose initially high testosterone levels prevented lactation. As their testosterone levels declined, most of the women produced milk to satisfy 100 percent of their infants' caloric needs. It therefore seems reasonable to encourage maintenance of breast stimulation for at least 4 weeks in order to optimize the likelihood of developing a full milk supply. One case report describes a mother with a gestational ovarian theca lutein cyst whose milk supply suddenly appeared on day 31 postpartum. She had been stimulating her breasts with a pump since the delivery of the baby during which time she had only been pumping small quantities of milk (Betzold 2004).

Insufficient Glandular Tissue

Women with *insufficient glandular tissue* (Neifert 1985) may not experience breast changes during pregnancy and do not report an engorgement phase postpartum. Palpation reveals only patchy areas of glandular tissue in an otherwise flaccid breast. In spite of good management, these women may be unable to produce an adequate milk supply. The occurence of insufficient glandular development of the breasts is unknown. It is assumed to be rare.

Environmental factors may influence breast development in some populations, especially those who are exposed to agricultural or other chemicals. Precocious puberty, with early breast development has been observed in girls with cumulative exposure to environmental chemicals, especially estrogens. While the breasts of some of the chemically-exposed girls studied seem to contain more adipose tissue, their glandular tissue was often poorly developed or, in some cases, absent (Guillette 2006). Additional studies are required to determined whether chemical exposure exerts wide-spread effects on human female breast development with the potential to disrupt lactation.

Other factors may influence breast development, including a connection between insufficient glandular tissue and thyroid disease. Pringle (1988) found abnormal sexual maturation secondary to primary hypothyroidism. The girls studied had isolated breast development, and absent pubertal growth acceleration. Sharma (2006) reported the development of ovarian cysts in girls with long-standing primary hypothyroidism. Restoration of *euthyroid* state (a balanced state with regard to thyroid levels) was associated with resolution of the ovarian cycts. Such findings suggest a need to exclude hypothyroidism in young girls with ovarian cysts. Given the association between ovarian cysts and abnormal breast development, early treatment of hypothyroidism would perhaps protect optimal breast development and prevent potential lactation deficiency.

In **Fig. 194** the breasts have a tubular ("coke-bottle") shape, and were flaccid for a woman 3 weeks postpartum. Referred by her pediatrician, this mother sought help from an LC because her infant was failing to thrive. Test weights and use of a feeding supplementer during the next week determined that her milk supply was stable at about half of what the infant required. The mother decided to supplement with formula by bottle and continued to breastfeed for several months. Once supplementation began, the baby gained well. The mother, who initially blamed herself, was relieved to know that her baby's poor growth resulted from a physical condition over which she had no control.

Fig. 195 also shows a woman with unusually shaped breasts. Her first baby did not gain well, but her second baby gained normally with exclusive breastfeeding. Her situation points out the risks of making assumptions based solely on appearances.

The glandular tissue of the breast increases with each pregnancy. It appears that lactation itself causes additional maturation of the glands (Cox 1999). Additionally, women may enjoy increased confidence and typically find better social support the second time around. Ingram (2001) followed 22 women who had trouble breastfeeding a first child, and documented significantly more milk production during their second lactations.

Since problems during an initial lactation course may be related to poor management, lack of confidence, or some other *secondary* issue, it is wise to give good support and additional encouragement to women who have experienced difficulties in the past. Ingram concluded that, "Health professionals should encourage women to breastfeed all their children, whatever their experience with their first child."

The woman in **Fig. 196**, who has marked breast asymmetry, sought assistance from an LC when her third child was gaining poorly. Neither of her older children had gained weight well while exclusively breastfeeding. The woman followed all the recommendations that would normally result in improved production without noticeable effect. The LC therefore suspected lactation failure owing to insufficient glandular development.

The nipples and areolae of the woman in **Fig. 197** are located in the forward cone of hypoplastic, tubular breasts. The weight of her 3 week-old baby boy stalled at 5 oz. (142 g) below birth weight. This mother experienced low milk supply problems with her first child. The LC obtained pre- and post-feed weights. An hour of continuous breastfeeding augmented with breast massage produced only 1.8 oz. (53 g) of intake. Visual markers are suggestive of abnormal breast development. The lack of breast changes during pregnancy and the first week postpartum, and the confirmation of low intake by test weights, suggest insufficient glandular tissue as a probable cause for the baby's failure to thrive.

After communicating with the physician, the LC initiated interventions to improve the potential for milk production, and advised supplementation to support the baby's growth. The obstetrician wrote a prescription for the galactagogue, domperidone. The pediatrician concurred that the infant required temporary use of supplemental formula. The baby's suck was too weak initially to make effective use of a feeding tube device. The mother used a bottle to deliver supplemental formula.

Within 4 days, the baby regained birth weight and was sucking strongly enough to begin using a feeding tube at breast. The mother felt that her breasts were fuller and firmer as a result of stimulation from the galactagogue and the extra stimulation provided by post-feed pumping. Her production met the majority of her child's growth needs with breast milk, and she continued to use formula as needed. The obstetrician prescribed domperidone for the first 4 months postpartum because the mother noticed an immediate decrease in production when the drug was not used.

Breast Augmentation

Millions of women have undergone breast augmentation. They can be reassured that implants themselves have not been implicated in causing harm to breastfeeding infants (Berlin 1994).

The United States Food and Drug Administration (FDA) brochure, "Breast Implants Consumer Handbook 2004," is designed to help women make informed choices about implants. The brochure also provides a useful overview for the lactation consultant. Topics covered include different types of implants and risks and benefits of different implant insertion sites, potential risks connected with implants, reporting of serious problems, and breast implant resource groups. Updated in 2006, the entire text of the brochure (along with links to other sites, many with photographs) is available to the public on-line at: www.fda.gov/cdrh/breastimplants/.

No conclusive evidence exists at this time connecting systemic illness with breast implants (Kjoller 2002). The AAP (2001) does not consider implants a contraindication for breastfeeding. However, some studies have associated leaking silicone gel and increased risk of fibromyalgia (Brown 2001). Additionally, implants may complicate visualization by mammography and may interfere with the detection of breast cancer. Patients who have implants removed may have cosmetically undesirable effects such as dimpling or puckering of the breasts. According to the FDA, most breast implants have approximately a 10 year life span. Many women with breast implants experience some local complications such as rupture, discomfort, hardening of the scar tissue that the body forms around the implants, disfigurement, and infections. These conditions may require nonsurgical medical treatments and/or repeat surgeries.

Women's reasons for obtaining implants are varied, and after childbirth many women express regret or embarrassment about their prior decision to seek implants. The LC must consider the psychological state of the mother. Unless the woman is experiencing specific problems related to the implants, the best counseling approach is to reflect her feelings in a supportive manner.

Many women lactate fully after augmentation mammoplasty, and lactation consultants should certainly encourage breastfeeding in this population. However, because the effects of the surgery may impair full milk production in some women, mothers with a history of previous breast surgery need close follow-up. Follow-up of the infant is also important to make sure growth proceeds normally (Hill 2004).

It is crucial to ask women who have had cosmetic surgery about their reasons for seeking augmentation as well as asking about their postoperative recovery. Occasionally, the LC will identify a woman who reports that she failed to develop normal glandular tissue during adolescence. While rare, *amastia* (lack of breast tissue, such as seen in **Figs. 191**, **192**, and **193**) occurs unilaterally or bilaterally, and sometimes results from chest wall underdevelopment (Davis 1996). Amastia constitutes a *primary* problem that prevents lactation and is unrelated to the direct effects of augmentation mammoplasty.

Augmentation Incision Options

Breast implants are inserted through incisions in 4 different locations:

- Under the arm
- Under the breast
- Along the edge of the areola (*periareolar)*
- Through an umbilical incision

Because the surgery is done for cosmetic or reconstructive reasons, minimizing the appearance of the scar is felt to be important. Some surgeons prefer to "hide" the incision scar at the edge of the areola. However, the location of the incision influences future lactation. The implications of locating the incision in this area may not be fully discussed with women of childbearing age. Even if a woman denies interest in lactation, the consequences of areolar incision should be discussed prior to her breast surgery.

The Risks of Periareolar Incisions

In one of the few studies to explore this issue, Neifert (1990) prospectively investigated the effects of breast augmentation surgery on lactation outcome. While *any* previous breast surgery correlated significantly with a 3-fold increase in risk of lactation insufficiency, periareolar incisions were almost 5 times more likely to result in problems. Hurst also found a greater incidence of lactation insufficiency in augmented women compared with non-augmented women and specifically associated the periareolar approach as the most likely cause (Hurst 1996).

Periareolar insertion of the implant is more likely to sever ducts and affect the nerves that supply sensation to the nipple. Ultrasound studies of breast anatomy describe an average of 9 ductal openings on the nipple (Ramsay 2005). Since there are fewer patent ducts than previously believed, interruption of even a few ducts could seriously impact milk production.

Nipple innervation is complex and variable between women, making it surgically challenging to avoid interrupting nerves and impacting nipple sensation (Schlenz 2000, Geddes 2007). The lateral cutaneous branch of the fourth intercostal nerve enters the left breast at 4 o'clock and the 8 o'clock position on the right. Rotating the placement of the surgical incision to avoid damage to the nerve may result in greater postoperative nipple sensation and may be an important way for the surgeon to protect the potential for full lactation (Schlenz 2000).

Fig. 198 shows a woman who has had breast implants that were inserted with a periareolar incision. She sought breast augmentation between her first and second births. The surgeon who performed the mammoplasty "shortened" her nipples for cosmetic effect. The woman's subsequent nipple sensation was poor. Her right nipple was numb, and a large fissure had opened on its face. The LC speculated that the mother could not feel when the baby was poorly latched. Although the woman had experienced a normal lactation with her first child, her second infant failed to thrive. She was committed to the experience of breastfeeding and opted to use a supplemental feeding tube device to offer formula to the baby. Breastfeeding on her left side and pumping the right breast with a hospital-grade electric breast pump allowed the nipple fissure to heal. Her milk supply did not respond to the efforts to improve production.

The mother whose breast is pictured in **Fig. 199** also had implants inserted with a periareolar approach; however, the surgeon took care to preserve her ability to lactate by avoiding bisection of the primary nerves to the nipple. The mother reported good nipple sensation. Observation of a spontaneous milk ejection (the nipple is dripping milk) is evidence of an intact neural pathway. This mother made enough milk to fully feed her own baby and to donate to a local milk bank.

Breast Implant Rupture

The mother pictured in **Fig. 200** is 8 months postpartum and has been breastfeeding her daughter. She experienced a rupture of a silicone implant. Her breast has developed an abscess at the location of the leak. The scar tissue in the mammary fold has become fragile and is red and swollen. The mother had been told by her obstetrician to abruptly wean. The LC provided information about the option of unilateral weaning.

The LC put the mother's doctor in touch with a medical expert on silicone implants in another part of the US. After discussion, a more conservative approach was selected that permitted the mother to pump and discard milk from that breast while taking antibiotics to resolve the infection. She slowly reduced the milk supply in the affected breast, which lessened tension on the fragile scar tissue. The immediate crisis resolved, and the mother continued to breastfeed on her unaffected breast. The mother decided to have the implants removed from both breasts, but elected to postpone surgery until the baby weaned.

Breast Implants and Risk of Mastitis

An uncommon complication of breast augmentation is bilaterally massive engorgement after pregnancy. The key risk factor appears to be development of infection in the postoperative period (following insertion of the implant). The resultant formation of scar tissue blocks the mammary ducts and impedes milk outflow (Acarturk 2005).

Hurst (1996) speculates that pressure exerted by the implant itself might occasionally be detrimental to milk production. Prolonged, increased intramammary pressure may cause atrophy of the alveolar cellular wall, thus diminishing secretion. In some women, implants may thus simulate the same effects caused by unrelieved engorgement. It is also possible that implants contribute to increased risk of mastitis if pressure from the implants interferes with drainage of milk. Theoretically, it is also possible that pressure from poorly drained milk may induce a leak in an implant, causing both milk and the contents of the implant to leak into the interstitial space triggering a heightened immune response. Pro-inflammatory cytokines present in milk are capable of provoking severe inflammatory response (mastitis).

While leaking saline might not be problematic, silicone leakage might exacerbate the inflammatory response (Fetherston 2001).

Breast Reduction

Large, heavy breasts may cause shoulder and spinal problems resulting in poor posture, neck and back pain, headaches, and poor body image. Women who seek surgical relief of these symptoms may not discuss lactation with their surgeons. Surgeons should counsel young women fully on options that influence future breast function.

Before 1984, most reduction mammoplasty was done using a technique that essentially removed the nipple and re-centered it on the smaller breast. Modern surgical techniques (referred to as *pedicle* or central cone procedures) theoretically permit lactation (Marshall 1994). Skin and subcutaneous tissue are lifted off the breast except for a conical base that extends to the nipple-areolar complex, which remains intact (Hagerty 1998). Excess breast tissue is carefully sculpted away in an attempt to preserve nerve and ductal systems. Owing to the intermixture of adipose and glandular tissue (Geddes 2007) this is challenging. However, reports describe positive lactation outcomes for women following reduction mammoplasty using superior, inferior, and horizontal bipedicle techniques (Brzozowski 2000, Kakagia 2005, Cherchel 2007, Cruz 2007). It should be noted that positive outcomes are defined as breastfeeding for a period of 2 weeks. Longer follow-up is needed to fully describe outcomes, especially with regard to infant growth.

Anecdotal reports describe wide variations in lactation performance after breast reduction, from total impairment to full lactation (West 2001). The body is wonderfully resilient, but it is difficult to predict how well the breasts will function after such invasive surgery. Mothers can be encouraged to breastfeed, but the LC has an obligation to monitor and protect the infant's growth.

The woman pictured in **Fig. 201** had very large breasts. She lactated normally with her first 2 children. **Fig. 202** shows the same woman after breast reduction surgery. One pound of tissue was removed from one breast and 1.5 pounds of tissue from the other. Following an unplanned pregnancy several years after the breast reduction, her infant daughter was readmitted to the hospital on Day 5 with dehydration and severe jaundice. While her milk "came in," the severed ducts in her breasts no longer drained to the nipple. Over the next week, she endured painful engorgement, and then abrupt involution. Once the LC determined that only a few drops of milk were expressible by hand or with a pump, a plan was developed that included formula feeding at the breast with a supplementer. The mother opted to bottle-feed when she was out in public.

Other Types of Breast Surgery

The woman whose breast is pictured in **Fig. 203** had a lumpectomy to treat breast cancer. A fine scar from a previous biopsy is visible at the periareolar margin and runs parallel to the lumpectomy scar. The bronze color of the breast results from radiation therapy. Irradiation of the breast generally results in diminished capacity to lactate, although some case reports describe partial lactation following treatment (Higgins 1994).

The 46 year-old woman pictured in **Fig. 204** has recently weaned a 6 year-old child. She discovered a lump, and a benign tumor was removed from her breast. The placement of her biopsy incision is away from the areola minimizing the effect such surgery might have on future lactation. Because of the mother's age, it is unlikely she will have more children. Note the rather deflated appearance of the breast tissue. This is typical immediately following weaning. As fat tissue regenerates to replace the atrophying glandular tissue, breasts typically will regain a more rounded contour. This process may not occur as readily in older women.

Counseling Guidelines Concerning Breast Surgery

- The LC should inquire, as part of her routine intake process, whether a woman has had previous breast trauma or surgery. The woman's reason for seeking surgery should be identified (i.e., whether surgery was sought to cosmetically correct underdeveloped breasts).
- Observe the location of scars. Periareolar scars at 4 o'clock on the woman's left breast and 8 o'clock on the woman's right breast are associated with increased risk of lactation insufficiency.
- Ask whether nipple sensitivity was surgically altered.
- Inform the mother how to assess normal feeding (breasts softer after feeding, listening for swallowing sounds. frequent infant stooling, normal infant weight gain).
- Confirm these impressions by test-weighing on an accurate scale and recommend once-a-week weight checks until lactation is well established.
- Perform hand expression and observe pumping to assess for sprays of milk as opposed to drips and for evidence of milk ejection reflex.
- Counsel about full or partial supplementation and the benefits of partial breastfeeding.
- Allow the mother to verbalize feelings, especially of disappointment. Validate her feeling of loss.

- Support her in exploring other ways to find closeness with the infant, such as carrying the baby in a sling, co-sleeping, co-bathing, etc.

Galactagogues

In cases where early milk production appears impaired, whether because of insufficient glandular tissue or from the effects of surgical interruption, use of a galactagogue during the calibration phase of lactation may maximize milk volume. Metoclopramide (Reglan) and domperidone (Motilium) are reported to increase milk production if prolactin levels are low. Metoclopramide stimulates prolactin and has increased milk production by 66 to 100 percent for some women. Central nervous system side effects such as depression may limit compliance, and some women do not respond to metoclopramide (Hale 2008). Central nervous system symptoms such as depression may prevent the long-term use of metoclopramide. Domperidone has good efficacy and fewer side effects (da Silva 2001, Hale 2008).

Areolar Hair

The mother pictured in **Fig. 205** has hair growing around the edge of her areola. She was concerned about whether the hair would bother her breastfeeding baby, and wondered if she should pluck or shave it. The LC reassured the mother that hair on the areola is common. Shaving the hairs may make them stiff or cause breaks in the skin that make it more vulnerable to infection. Because areolar and nipple tissue will be coming in repeated contact with the pathogens in the baby's mouth and from the mother's hands, keeping the skin healthy and intact is important. Hair removal risks irritating the skin and should be avoided.

Unusual Nipple Configurations

Human nipples come in all sizes and shapes. Sometimes an unusual configuration such as the one pictured in **Fig. 206** may cause prenatal caregivers to become concerned. This woman's midwife referred her for evaluation for potential breastfeeding problems. The LC pointed out that while this nipple seemed too long in the vertical plane for a baby's mouth to encompass, breastfeeding in the cradle hold would position the mouth "sideways," providing plenty of room for the nipple to fit between the corners of the baby's mouth. This proved to be the case. Even though the baby was small, she had no trouble managing her mother's nipples as long as she was positioned carefully.

A woman with double nipples would also position her baby at breast so that both nipples fit comfortably into the baby's mouth. **Fig. 207** shows a double nipple. Note the milk dripping from both nipples.

Pierced Nipple

Fig. 208 shows a pierced nipple. LCs who have worked with women who have removed nipple rings early in their pregnancies report remarkably few problems with breast-feeding. The nipple tissue appears to granulate and to function well during lactation. Perhaps the skill of the piercing artist is a factor, or the size of the ring may be a determinant. There are no published studies that explore this practice, but anecdotal reports describe subsequent lactation.

One of the authors (BWC) worked with 2 women who have breastfed after having worn nipple rings. One woman was followed for 3 months, during which time her infant grew well on exclusive breastfeeding. She had no difficulties with sore nipples or mastitis.

The second mother had minor problems with her right nipple, which had been pierced twice. It became infected the first time it was pierced, and the ring had to be removed while it healed. This nipple appeared to have more scar tissue, and the baby preferred the other breast. However, her child grew well during the 4 weeks the LC followed her case.

Fig. 209 shows a nipple that formerly was pierced. The nipple did not experience full healing (granulation of tissue) after the ring was removed, and it clearly is leaking milk through the incision site in the nipple shaft. This photograph was taken when the baby was 9 months old. Leaking from the incision site did not cause problems for the mother or her baby.

Another woman who breastfed for 2 years reported nipple pain where she had previously worn a nipple ring. She assumed the pain was from scar tissue and nerve injury.

Inverted Nipple

Fig. 210 shows a nipple at rest. As was previously discussed in Ch. 7, it can be difficult to identify nipple inversion by appearance only. Some nipples invert only when compressed. **Fig. 211** shows the same nipple being compressed. This mother's infant manifested extreme frustration when put to the breast. Identification of the nipple inversion helped explain why the infant found it difficult to latch on. A nipple shield was employed as a temporary measure to bring the baby to breast until the nipples became more protractile.

Other Unusual Presentations

The mother in **Fig. 212** required open heart surgery as an adolescent. Following the delivery of her first child, she was distressed by a low milk supply and her infant's poor weight gain. In the absence of other factors to explain her situation, the LC speculated that the invasive surgery interfered with her capacity to fully lactate. There are case reports of women with breast deformity caused by intensive care to treat pneumothorax when they were preterm infants.

In order to spare girls the psychological distress of abnormal breast development, and to protect their option to breastfeed, it is recommended that neonatologists place chest tubes away from the breast tissue in female infants. Skin incisions to drain pneumothorax can be alternatively positioned 4-5 cm inferior to the nipple, and chest drains inserted through the fifth or sixth intercostal space during neonatal treatment (Rainer 2003).

The young mother pictured in **Fig. 213** has just delivered her first child. She had been treated 9 years previously for a condition called *hidradenitis* (inflammation of a sweat gland). Some of her lymph glands were surgically removed. The LC in this case was concerned that the mother might experience difficulty with milk drainage owing to scar tissue in the tail of Spence. In the immediate postpartum period, the mother complained of a plugged duct on this breast, slightly below the scar. The LC suggested careful positioning, frequent breastfeeding to keep the breast soft, and use of cold compresses to reduce swelling. The plugged duct resolved, and the mother continued breastfeeding. There is a case report of a women with postpartum axillary breast engorgement who was mistakenly diagnosed with hidradenitis (Silverberg 2003).

Fig. 214 shows a scar from thyroid surgery. Previous history of thyroid disease has been implicated in abnormal pubertal breast development, and is associated in animal studies with diminished lactation. Generally women in this situation are medically monitored and are prescribed replacement thyroid hormone. If they are euthyroid, lactation should be unaffected. However, the presence of such a scar should prompt the LC to discuss the mother's health history carefully for issues that may impact breastfeeding.

Fig. 215 shows a tattoo on the breast. Tattoos do not impact breastfeeding. Donor milk banks have rules excluding milk donations from women who have acquired tattoos from an unregulated site within 12 months of the time of donation (HMBANA 2008). Many states in the

US now regulate tattoo and other piercing establishments, requiring them to use single-use instruments, dye pots, etc. Tattoos from regulated sites do not restrict milk donation.

Figs. 216 and **217** show the swollen feet and ankles of 2 women both of whom are several days postpartum. Both sought help from an LC because of low milk supply. The mother in **Fig. 217** was 7 days postpartum. Her breasts were flaccid, and her infant was still losing weight. She had been diagnosed shortly before delivery with *Pregnancy Induced Hypertension* (PIH). She experienced swelling in her hands and legs, and complained to the LC of headache. The LC advised her to report all of these symptoms to her obstetrician, who rechecked her blood pressure.

The woman in **Fig. 217** also was experiencing severe edema, although she had no history of hypertension. BWC has observed that when women present with significant edema in their extremities, they often experience significant delays in lactogenesis stage II.

Hall (2002) identified maternal hypertension as a risk factor for weaning in the first week postpartum. Hall does not elaborate on the mechanisms. However, BWC observes that mothers in her practice with dramatic swelling in their limbs (with or without elevated blood pressure) notice increases in milk production in an inverse ratio with the decline in edema. As their feet and ankles return to normal size, their breasts fill with milk. Increased dietary consumption of protein is said to assist, as does keeping the feet elevated, and eating foods with diuretic qualities (such as cucumbers, watermelon) seems to reduce the swelling. It would be interesting to see how administration of a single dose of an oral diuretic medication would affect this phenomenon. This issue deserves more attention, discussion, and systematic clinical investigation.

Acarturk S, Gencel E, Tuncer I. An uncommon complication of secondary augmentation mammoplasty: bilaterally massive engorgement of breasts after pregnancy attributable to post-infection and blockage of mammary ducts. *Aesthetic Plastic Surgery* 2005; 29(4):274-279.

Adler D, Rebner M, Pennes D. Accessory breast tissue in the axilla: mammographic appearance. *Radiology* 1987; 163(3):709-711.

American Academy of Pediatrics (AAP). The transfer of drugs and other chemicals into human milk. *Pediatrics* 2001; 108(3):776-789, p. 777.

Balcar V, Silinova-Malkova E, Matys Z. Soft tissue radiography of the female breast and pelvic pneumoperitoneum in the Stein- Leventhal Syndrome. *Acta Radiologica Diagnosis* 1972; 12(3):353-362.

Berlin C. Silicone breast implants and breastfeeding. *Pediatrics* 1994; 94(4 Pt 1):547-549.

Betzold C, Hoover K, Snyder C. Delayed lactogenesis II: a comparison of four cases. *Journal of Midwifery & Women's Health* 2004; 49(2):132-137.

Brown SL, Pennello G, Berg WA, et al. Silicone gel breast implant rupture, extracapsular silicone, and health status in a population of women. *Journal of Rheumatology* 2001; 28(5):996-1003.

Brozozowski D, Niessen M, Evans HB, et al. Breastfeeding after inferior or pedicle reduction mammaplasty. *Plastic Reconstructive Surgery* 2000; 105(2):530-534.

Cherchel A, Azzam C, DeMey A. Breastfeeding after vertical reduction mammaplasty using a superior pedicle. *Journal of Plastic Reconstructive Aesthetic Surgery* 2007; 60(5):465-470.

Cruz NI, Korchin L. Lactational performance after breast reduction with different pedicles. *Plastic Reconstructive Surgery* 2007; 120(1):35-40.

Cox D, Kent J, Casey R, et al. Breast growth and the urinary excretion of lactose during human pregnancy and early lactation: endocrine relationships. *Experimental Physiology* 1999; 84(2):421-434.

da Silva O, Knoppert D, Angelini M, et al. Effect of domperidone on milk production in mothers of premature newborns: a randomized, double-blind, placebo-controlled trial. *Canadian Medical Association Journal* 2001; 164(1):17-21.

Davis A, Kulig J. Adolescent breast disorders. *Adolescent Health Update: A Clinical Guide for Pediatricians. American Academy of Pediatrics, Section on Adolescent Health* 1996; 9(1):1-8.

Fetherston C. Mastitis and implants. *Lactnet*, April 15, 2001.

Gabbay M, Kelly H. Use of metformin to increase breastmilk production in women with insulin resistance: a case series. *ABM News and Views* 2003; 9(3):20-21.

Geddes DT. Gross Anatomy of the Human Breast, in *Hale & Hartmann's Textbook of Human Lactation*, Amarillo, TX: Hale Publishing, 2007; p. 27.

Grossl N. Supernumerary breast tissue: historical perspectives and clinical features. *Southern Medical Journal* 2000; 93(1):29-32.

Guillette EA, Conard C, Lares F, et al. Altered breast development in young girls from an agricultural environment. *Environmental Health Perspective* 2006; 114(3):471-475.

Hagerty R, Hagerty R. Reduction mammoplasty: central cone technique for maximal preservation of vascular and nerve supply. *Southern Medical Journal* 1989; 82(2):183-185.

Hale T. *Medications and Mothers' Milk* 13th ed. Amarillo, TX: Hale Publishing, 2008; pp. 302-304, 614-615, 633-636.

Hall R, Mercer A, Teasley S, et al. A breast-feeding assessment score to evaluate the risk for cessation of breast-feeding by 7 to 10 days of age. *Journal of Pediatrics* 2002; 141(5):659-64.

Higgins S, Huffy B. Pregnancy and lactation after breast-conserving therapy for early stage breast cancer. *Cancer* 1994; 73(8):2175-2180.

Hill PD, Wilhelm PSA, Aldag JC, et al. Breast augmentation and lactation outcome: a case report. *MCN American Journal of Maternal and Child Nursing* 2004; 29(4):238-242.

Hollinrake E, Abreu A, Maifeld M, et al. Increased risk of depressive disorders in women with polycystic ovary syndrome. *Fertility and Sterility* 2007; 87(6):1369-1376.

Hoover KL, Barbalinardo LH, Platia MP. Delayed lactogenesis II secondary to gestational ovarian theca lutein cysts in two normal singleton pregnancies. *Journal of Human Lactation* 2002; 18(3):264-268.

Huggins K, Petok E, Mireles O. Markers of lactation insufficiency: a study of 34 mothers, in K Auerbach, (ed). *Current Issues in Clinical Lactation 2000*, Sudbury, MA: Jones and Bartlett, 2000; pp. 25-35.

Human Milk Banking Association of North America (HMBANA). *Guidelines for Establishment and Operation of a Donor Human Milk Bank*. Raleigh, NC: Human Milk Banking Association of North America, Inc, 2008; in press.

Hurst N. Lactation after augmentation mammoplasty. *Obstetrics and Gynecology* 1996; 87(1):30-34.

Ingram J, Woolridge M, Greenwood R. Breastfeeding: it is worth trying with the second baby. *Lancet* 2001; 358(9286):986-87.

Kakagia D, Tripsiannis G, Tsoutsos D. Breastfeeding after reduction mammaplasty: a comparison of 3 techniques. *Annals of Plastic Surgery* 2005; 55(4):343-345.

Kjoller K, Friis S, Signorello LB, et al. Health outcomes in offspring of Danish mothers with cosmetic breast implants. *Annals of Plastic Surgery* 2002; 48(3):238-245.

Kolodziejczyk B, Duleba A, Spaczynski R, et al. Metformin therapy decreases hyperandrogenism and hyperinsulinemia in women with polycystic ovary syndrome. *Fertility and Sterility* 2000; 73(6):1149-1154.

Lawrence RA, Lawrence RM. *Breastfeeding: A Guide for the Medical Profession* (6th ed). Philadelphia, PA: Elsevier Mosby, 2005; p. 45.

Marasco L, Marmet C, Shell E. Polycystic ovary syndrome: a connection to insufficient milk supply? *Journal of Human Lactation* 2000; 16(2):143-148.

Marshall D, Callan P, Nicholson W. Breastfeeding after reduction mammoplasty. *British Journal of Plastic Surgery* 1994; 47(3):167-69.

Neifert M, Seacat J, Jobe W. Lactation failure due to insufficient glandular development of the breast. *Pediatrics* 1985; 76(5):823-827.

Neifert M, DeMarzo S, Seacat J, et al. The influence of breast surgery, breast appearance, and pregnancy induced breast changes on lactation sufficiency as measured by infant weight gain. *Birth* 1990; 17(1):31-38.

Pringle P, Stanhope R, Hindmarsh P, et al. Abnormal pubertal development in primary hypothyroidism. *Clinical Endocrinology* 1988; 28(5):479-86.

Rainer C, Gardetto A, Fruhwirth M, et al. Breast deformity in adolescence as a result of pneumothorax drainage during neonatal intensive care. *Pediatrics* 2003; 111(1):80-85.

Ramsay D, Kent JC, Hartmann RA, et al. Anatomy of the lactating human breast redefined with ultrasound imaging. *Journal of Anatomy* 2005; 206(6): 525-534.

Schlenz I, Kuzbari R, Holle J. The sensitivity of the nipple-areola complex: an anatomic study. *Plastic Reconstructive Surgery* 2000; 105(3):905-909.

Sharma Y, Bajpai A, Mittal S, et al. Ovarian cysts in young girls with hypothyroidism: follow-up and effect of treatment. *Journal of Pediatric Endocrinology and Metablolism* 2006; 19(7):895-900.

Silverberg M, Rahman M. Axillary breast tissue mistaken for suppurative hidradenitis: an avoidable error. *Journal of Emergency Medicine* 2003; 25(1):51-55.

West D. *Defining Your Own Success: Breastfeeding After Breast Reduction Surgery*. Schaumburg, IL: La Leche League International, 2001.

Anatomic Variability: An Important Issue in Assessment

Breasts, nipples, and babies come in all sizes and shapes. For the most part, breastfeeding accommodates normal anatomic variability. However, anatomic variations that occur at the extremes of the normal spectrum may be an under-appreciated issue in breastfeeding assessment and management. Problems related to poor "fit" between mother and baby may create substantial barriers in the early days of breastfeeding, especially if the baby lacks strength, size, and stamina. Over time, babies grow. Mothers and babies learn how to compensate for anatomic variations in ways that make breastfeeding easier.

Half a century ago, Mavis Gunther (1955) observed: "If the physical shape of the nipple is the sign stimulus of instinctive activity in feeding, it should be possible from the mother's breast shape to predict the baby's feeding behavior." This provocative statement resulted from her observations that infants of mothers with flat or inverted nipples often were "apathetic" when put to breast. See Ch. 7 and **Figs. 210-211** in Ch. 9. However, other variations in addition to flat and inverted nipples may challenge early breastfeeding. These issues are explored in this chapter.

Dyadic Assessment

Assessing an activity that involves 2 people (a *dyad*) necessitates looking at each individual *and* at how partners interrelate. Infant weight, size, tone, maturation, and physical condition all influence breastfeeding. These issues become critical if there is something challenging about the maternal breast anatomy or the infant's oral anatomy. For example, a robust term infant may be able to latch onto an engorged, non-elastic breast with a large diameter nipple. Mastering such challenges may prove daunting to a baby born at 37 weeks, to a tongue-tied infant, or to an infant recovering from injuries sustained during a traumatic delivery.

An experienced LC evaluates dyadic issues such as size and fit in the development of feeding intervention plans. Careful assessment influences equipment and alternative feeding choices.

Breast Size

Women with large breasts may have body image issues. They may experience consequences of breast size that impact health, contribute to physical discomfort, and affect quality of life (Kerrigan 2001). Pregnancy itself causes additional breast growth. Breast tissue also grows during the postpartum if stimulated by sucking (Cox 1999).

Breast changes associated with pregnancy and lactation may increase the concerns of women with large breasts.

The mother pictured in **Fig. 218** has large breasts and cannot easily see her baby. She may find it somewhat difficult to comfortably position herself for breastfeeding, especially since her arms are short. The side-lying position frees the mother's hands and supports her breast. This prevents the drag from the weight of the breast from tiring the baby. Another helpful position for women with large breasts is to support the breast on a table (see **Fig. 100**).

Areola Size

Areolar tissue is usually elastic and more darkly pigmented than the surrounding skin. Such pigmentation may serve as a visual target that helps the baby locate the nipple. Areolae vary in size, and the range of normal is wide. Areolar diameter tends to decrease with increasing age and to increase with increasing weight (Brown 1999). Ramsay (2005) measured 14 women and found a mean areola radius of 27.8 ± 5.5 mm and 25.6 ± 5.5 mm for the left and right breasts, respectively. A large areola placed far forward in the cone of a hypoplastic breast is described in the plastic surgery literature as a marker for abnormal breast development (Williams 1981). **Ch. 9** reviews abnormal breast development.

Figs. 219, 220, and **221** demonstrate the wide variability in areolar size. The woman in **Fig. 219** has a large areolar circumference. However, her breast demonstrates a full and rounded contour in all 4 quadrants. There is no sign of breast hypoplasia or any tubular appearance. The size of her areola is unlikely to affect lactation. The challenge she may face will be how to interpret the misinformed advice to get "all of the areola into the baby's mouth." Clearly, this would be impossible.

The mother in **Fig. 220** has a small diameter nipple and a small diameter areola. She has recently weaned after breastfeeding her third child for 5 years. The upper quadrants of both of her breasts lack a rounded contour; however, (given her history of successful lactation) this is more likely attributable to recent weaning rather than to breast hypoplasia. The rather "deflated" look of her breast probably results from atrophy of glandular tissue – common after weaning. The shape of the breasts typically will alter as fat tissue in the breast regenerates, especially in younger women. Over time, this woman's breasts assumed a more rounded contour. Her areolar diameter remained about 23 mm in diameter, the size of a US or Canadian quarter, an Australian 1 dollar coin, or a 1 Euro coin.

Nipple Diameter

Areolar size is unlikely to impact breastfeeding except when areolar placement serves as a marker for abnormal breast development. However, some clinicians are becoming increasingly interested in the impact of *nipple* diameter on breastfeeding.

Along with breast and areolar size, nipple size increases during early to mid-pregnancy (Rohn 1989, Cox 1999). While areolar and breast growth are positively related to plasma human placental lactogen (hPL) concentrations, nipple growth appears to be related to prolactin concentrations. BWC and KH have observed women with large nipple diameters during the first week postpartum, who, when seen weeks later, presented with more normal sized nipples. Engorgement of the nipple may occur simultaneously with engorgement of the breast. Tissue edema or high levels of prolactin in the early postpartum may influence nipple size, although these phenomena have not been researched.

Several researchers have measured the female nipple in order to begin to quantify the range of sizes. Zeimer (1993) described a wide range of sizes in a group of 20 breastfeeding women. The average size nipple in her study measured 16 mm in diameter, slightly smaller than a US or Canadian dime, the Euro 1 cent coin, or the Australian 5 cent piece. In Zeimer's 1995 study of 50 women, the average nipple diameter was 15 mm.

Ramsay (2005) measured 14 lactating women and described a mean nipple diameter of 15.7 ± 1.8 mm for the left and 15.8 ± 2.4 mm for the right breast.

For her Master's Thesis, Stark (1994) used calipers and measured nipple diameter in a group of 59 breastfeeding women who ranged from 1 to 36 weeks postpartum. She grouped nipple size into categories and plotted percentages for each size range:

Small: <12 mm at base (14 percent)
Average: 12-15 mm at base (62 percent)
Large: 16-23 mm at base (24 percent)
Extra-Large: >23 mm at base (0 percent)

In the list above, the average size nipple diameter is approximately 15 mm. Stark compared her measurements to those of 86 women with breastfeeding problems who were seen for consultation at the Lactation Institute in Encino, California. She described the following size ranges and percentages in this group of mothers:

Small: <12 mm at base (8 percent)
Average: 12-15 mm at base (47 percent)
Large: 16-23 mm at base (38 percent)
Extra-Large: >23 mm at base (7 percent)

Stark observed that: "In both groups, the larger the nipple [diameter] the more likely it was for the woman to have [latch on] problems."

Using an engineer's circle template, BWC measured the base nipple diameters of 34 breastfeeding clients. She noted that many of the mothers' nipples varied in size between their right and left nipples; thus, 68 nipples were plotted as separate data points. BWC's measurements describe the following nipple sizes and percentages:

Small: <12 mm at base (3 percent)
Medium: 12-15 mm at base (15 percent)
Large: 16-23 mm at base (70 percent)
Extra-Large: >23 mm at base (12 percent)

KH measured the nipples of 100 consecutive women who sought assistance for breastfeeding difficulties. Using a ruler, she measured the diameter of the nipple in millimeters. Reporting only the size of the larger nipple, KH found that the average nipple diameter in this group of clients was 17.5 mm; the average nipple length was 9.5 mm. Sizes and percentages in each categories were:

Small: <12 mm at base (14 percent)
Medium: 12-15 mm at base (17 percent)
Large: 16-23 mm at base (58 percent)
Extra-Large: >23 mm at base (11 percent)

While the sample sizes of the nipple measurement studies described here are small and the measuring tools differed, there is reasonable agreement on the ranges. Larger averages in nipple diameter were seen in private practice settings.

Since women who consult a private practice LC are likely to have breastfeeding problems, it is possible that the data collected by Stark at the Lactation Institute, and by BWC and KH are skewed for women with larger than average nipples. A common observation from all these studies is that women with large nipples have more breastfeeding problems.

One report of 18 babies readmitted to the hospital for dehydration identified one mother with "giant" nipples (Caglar 2006). KH observed that among the mothers she assisted with low milk supplies in 2002, a high percentage had large nipples. Nipple size has seldom been mentioned or identified as an issue in studies of low milk supply or readmission for dehydration, but if nipple size complicates early feeding, it may well be a factor in poor early supply calibration. Clearly, the impact of nipple size on lactation requires additional research.

Measuring Tools

Half a century ago, Gunther (1955) observed that, "For the tissues to be accessible, the nipple must not be too large to enter past the baby's bite, and the tissues when drawn forward must be able to pass the gums." If the nipple diameter is too large, a small baby may experience difficulty latching on. Thus size information is pertinent.

It can be difficult to visualize relative sizes. Comparisons with common items may be useful when teaching. **Fig. 222** shows an engineer's circle template with a pencil eraser (top row), a small diameter nipple (second row) and 2 US coins (bottom row) that represent the sizes of nipple diameters referenced. Standardizing nipple measurement is a desirable research goal. Electronic calipers provide consistent, reliable readings. Owing to their accuracy, BWC and KH propose they be adopted in such research.

Sucking Mechanics and Nipple Size

Ramsay (2004b) used ultrasound and intra-oral pressure transducers connected to a feeding tube device to study infant sucking. She observed that "Negative pressure generated by the infant as the [posterior] tongue moved down resulted in opening of milk ducts in the nipple and milk flow from the breast." In order for maximal suction to be generated, the back of the baby's tongue must first rise as high as it can in order to be able to drop far enough to generate significant amounts of negative pressure.

If an infant (particularly a weak or tongue-tied infant) encounters a large diameter nipple, the size of the nipple may block the tongue from rising high enough, limiting the ability of the baby to generate sufficient suction to remove milk. Variations in nipple diameter, along with anomalies of the tongue, may thus explain some cases of inadequate breastfeeding.

Figs. 223, 224, and **225** show mothers who have large diameter nipples. The mother seen in **Fig. 223** was breastfeeding normally on Day 2 postpartum. On Day 3, she became engorged, and the baby was no longer able to latch on. The hospital nurses remarked to KH that the mother's *nipple* also had become engorged. The photograph shows the size of the mother's engorged

nipple, which is now comparable to the diameter of a US quarter. On Day 4, the engorgement resolved, the nipple returned to normal size, and the baby was once again able to breastfeed. This experience suggests that nipples become engorged, and demonstrates how an increase in nipple diameter may frustrate a breastfeeding baby's latch attempts. More research is needed to observe nipple enlargement in the early postpartum, to record how often it occurs, and to note how long it takes to resolve.

The mother in **Fig. 224** is breastfeeding her third and fourth children, a set of twins. Her nipple, in profile, is long, and as large around as a US quarter. Her large, long nipples have not posed problems for her children; all of them grew normally. Note how pliable the nipple tissue appears, even in the photograph. Perhaps the softness of the nipple tissue allowed the babies to easily compress the nipple against the hard palate, permitting room for the posterior tongue to lift and drop. Perhaps the twins had large enough mouths to easily accommodate nipples of this size.

The woman pictured in **Fig. 225** has an abraded nipple and *erythema* (reddening) of the nipple and areola indicative of mastitis. Note the yellow, crystalized exudate that is characteristic of *S. aureus*. She suffered the same type of nipple damage after the births of each of her infant sons. Neither baby was able to latch on comfortably to her nipple during the newborn period. Her nipple tissue appeared rigid, "meaty," and difficult to compress. Her nipple diameter proved challenging even though both her babies weighed more than 7 pounds (3200 g) at birth.

Because these babies were unable to accommodate the size of her nipples, they sucked in ways that were painful to their mother and caused nipple damage. By about 6 weeks postpartum, each of her babies had grown enough to accommodate their mother's nipples, permitting her to breastfed each child for over 2 years, emphasizing the temporary nature of such "fit" problems. In such cases, the main challenge is to preserve breastfeeding during the time period when the babies cannot latch. Because direct breastfeeding will be delayed until these babies grow into the nipple size, the size of the pump flange must also be examined closely. If a woman with large nipples pumps with a standard size flange, she may feel pain and ducts may be compressed, inhibiting milk flow (Geddes 2007).

Long Nipples

Nipple length varies considerably and may also be an unexplored issue in breastfeeding management. A ruler or caliper can assess nipple length (**Fig. 226**). Remember that the human nipple elongates with suction pressure (Ramsay 2004a). Nipples can extend 2 to 3 times their resting length (Smith 1988).

The primiparous mother in **Fig. 227** has a long nipple (2 cm at rest). She has a large diameter nipple with a bulbous shape (20.6 mm at base and 22.3 mm at the tip). One of her 36 week-old twins is pictured on Day 6 in **Fig. 228**. This twin, who weighed 5 lb 2 oz (2337 g) at birth, lost over 9 percent of his birth weight and had an elevated bilirubin level. He had not stooled in 2 days. The baby is unable to pass the bulbous nipple tip between his gums. While he appears to be breastfeeding, he is actually sleeping with the nipple only halfway in his mouth. Test weights following a feeding revealed no milk intake. The other twin had also lost excessive weight and was similarly unable to latch. These preterm twins were released home from the hospital on Day 3 "exclusively breastfeeding" with no early follow-up planned. They were scheduled to see their pediatrician at 10 days postpartum. Thankfully parental awareness and concern about lack of stooling prompted their worried mother to call an LC. In this case, the large size of the mother's nipples, infant prematurity, and small infant size all should have identified a need for closer follow-up.

After observing the twins' inability to latch onto their mother's breasts, the LC evaluated the mother's pumping technique. The mother had rented a hospital-grade breast pump; however, her pump flange was a standard size and was not a good fit to accommodate either the diameter or the length of her nipples.

Implications of Long, Elastic Nipples

The twins' mother is shown pumping in **Fig. 229**. Note the full extension (4 cm) of her nipple. Neither twin could accommodate the length of this nipple without gagging.

The full extension of her nipples filled the entire chamber of the shaft of the pump flanges, and appeared to affect the suction created by the pump. Almost no milk issued forth during pumping. The LC (BWC) called a pump company engineer to discuss the effect on pumping when a nipple entirely fills the flange shaft.

The engineer explained that in order to create suction, some space must be present between the nipple and the walls and end of the flange chamber. Without space for air movement, insufficient pressure is exerted upon the surface area of the nipple and no milk is withdrawn. LCs should observe pumping for several minutes to identify how nipples fit the flange once they begin to elongate and swell. It is

important to observe for pumping adequacy in cases when the infant is not able to directly breastfeed.

At the time of this case, there were no larger sized flanges available to adapt the kit the mother was using. She could not afford the expense of purchasing another pump kit with a larger flange size, nor did she feel she had the time or energy to try to hand express enough milk for 2 infants. Reluctantly, she weaned her twins to formula.

Fig. 230 pictures a nipple that is narrower at the base than at the tip. Note the shadow of this nipple, which emphasizes a not uncommon "doorknob" shape. The LC should also be aware of different terms to describe variants of nipple shape, such as conical or cylindrical.

Note the size of the nipple pictured in **Fig. 231**, which KH measured as 30 mm in diameter. Compare the size of this nipple to the size of the 2.5 week old twin who weighs 7 lbs 5 oz (3310 g). Both of this woman's twins were unable to breastfeed until they reached about 9 lbs (4075 g). LCs must be educated about how to counsel the mother with a fit problem. The infant's milk intake and the milk supply must be protected in such cases until the infant grows.

BWC has taken oral measurements of 98 infants ranging from 35 gestational weeks of age to 3 months. Wearing a non-latex glove or finger cot, BWC allowed babies to draw her finger into their mouths until it reached a depth that triggered sucking. For most infants this depth is near the juncture of the hard and soft palates. BWC made an ink mark on her finger where lip closure occurred (**Fig. 232**), and measured this length with a ruler. The range extended from 1.9 cm to 3.2 cm (**Fig. 233**). The shallower "oral reaches" were associated with the smaller infants, and the longer reaches with larger babies. Infant size (weight), rather than age or head circumference, seems to be the key predictor of longer oral "reach."

Perhaps when small babies with a short oral reach encounter a long maternal nipple, repeated triggering of the gag reflex occurs, contributing to development of feeding aversion. Further, a short reach may cause babies to grasp only the shaft of the nipple, creating nipple pain. Thus, having a short oral length may elevate lactation risk.

Since oral reach seems most related to the infant's size, mothers can be reassured that growth will often resolve the problem. It is useful to point to the dental literature, which describes rapid forward growth of the mandible in the first few months after birth. This growth alters the size of the baby's mouth so that it will eventually accommodate the mother's nipple. Both BWC and KH have worked with many infants who initially were not able to breastfeed owing to "fit" problems, and who ultimately breastfed well once they grew.

It is unnecessary to measure all mothers and infants. However, some mothers will benefit from the explanation that a fit problem is complicating lactation.

Implications of Size Variability on Equipment Choice

Two of the manufacturers of clinical grade breast pumps provide equipment that accommodates variations in nipple size. The LC must ensure that women who are using pumps have correctly fitting flanges.

Fig. 234 illustrates the difference between the openings in the Medela® 24 mm and Personal Fit™ 30 mm flanges. Other Personal Fit™ flanges measure 27 mm and 36 mm. A 40 mm glass flange is also available.

Fig. 235 shows Ameda Custom Breast Flanges™. The Standard Ameda flange size is 25 mm. The Custom Breast Flange with the inset is 28.5 mm and without the inset 30.5 mm. Specialty sizes also include 32.5 and 36 mm flanges.

Figs. 236 and **237** demonstrate the consequences of pumping with a pump flange that is too small. The mother in **Fig. 236** was given a standard size pump kit in the hospital. Observe how the nipple is wedged tightly into the flange opening, creating a strangulation effect that inhibits milk outflow. The woman's breasts remained full and lumpy following pumping, and her pumped volumes were low for a woman 6 days postpartum. At the time of the LC's home visit, the nipples were increasingly sore. In **Fig. 237**, note the cracks that have opened at the base of the nipples, resulting from friction trauma caused by the poorly fitted flanges. The infant was ill and unable to breast-feed, so the poor flange fit jeopardized this woman's milk supply and her infant's growth. It also increased the risk of mastitis. These are unacceptable consequences of incomplete evaluation.

The mother in **Fig. 238**, delivered her second term infant at home. She suffered a substantial blood loss following delivery of an unexpected second placenta. Methergine was administered to control her bleeding. The woman had relatively flat nipples with a large base diameter (approximately 24 mm). She experienced low milk production with her first child. Because the new baby was sleepy and could not latch well to the mother's large, flat nipples, and owing to past milk supply problems, the midwife suggested pumping to help bring in the milk. After 24 hours of pumping, both nipples were swollen and abraded. The LC was consulted on Day 4, and

began to systematically address all the red flags for increased lactation risk. She informed the parents that milk production might remain low until the mother recovered from the metabolic stress of excessive blood loss and the exposure to methergine.

Frustrated by hunger and the large nipples, the baby of the mother seen in **Fig. 238** began rejecting the breast. Effective pumping would prove critical to this case. The LC provided larger pump flanges and wrote down careful pumping instructions. The mother reported greater comfort during pumping with the larger flanges, and thus was able to tolerate increased pumping frequency. At a follow-up visit 2.5 weeks postpartum, the mother's milk supply was still inadequate for the baby's needs. The LC speculated that the woman needed more recovery time from her blood loss. Also, given her history of previous milk supply problems, the LC was concerned that this mother might have a primary milk production insufficiency.

Both BWC and KH consider that more research is needed to investigate the variable responses of the human nipple to pumping. The authors have observed that nipples frequently appear to swell during pumping. Pre- and post-pumping measurements taken with a circle template reveal that nipple size can increase 3 to 4 mm. **Figs. 239** and **240** graphically demonstrate this phenomenon. The mother's pre-pumping nipple size is 20.64 mm. After pumping, her nipple size swells to 23.81 mm. Using coin comparisons, her nipples enlarged from the size of a US nickel to the size of a US quarter. Thus, if a mother has nipples that are 20 mm in diameter or larger, she should use a larger size pump flange if she needs to pump her breasts.

Meier (2004) also examined flange fit in a group of women exclusively pumping for preterm infants, and observed that most mothers required larger flanges. She comments: "...about half of the 35 mothers who served as subjects in the research initially required either the 27 or 30 mm (Medela) shield in order to achieve optimal, pain-free nipple and areolar movement during milk expression. As lactation progressed, 77 percent or slightly over three quarters of the mothers eventually found they needed these larger shields."

Fig. 241 shows the 40 mm Medela® blown glass flange. While expensive, the glass flange provides another option when mothers have unusually large nipples that exceed even the capacity of the 36 mm plastic flanges. KH provided a 40 mm flange for a hospital LC whose patient had an extra large nipple that was not accommodated by using the plastic flanges stocked in the hospital. The hospital LC watched the mother pump with the glass flange and observed milk spraying from a duct opening located on the areola. The mother commented that a firm area of her breast softened and became comfortable. Had it not been for the wider opening of this large flange, that section of the woman's breast would not have been drained.

Fig. 242 pictures a woman with PCOS. This woman has a wide span between her breasts, conical, hypoplastic breast shape, and extremely large diameter nipples. She is shown pumping with a large plastic flange in **Fig. 243**. Her nipples fit tightly even in the larger flange. She is a good candidate for the 36 mm plastic or the 40 mm glass flange.

Both authors have been asked how to determine the appropriate flange size. There needs to be space around the base of the nipple, and we have found that the woman herself is the best judge of which size fits.

Routine lubrication of the nipples or the pump flange is unnecessary and should be suggested only if the mother complains of discomfort. **Fig. 244** shows a woman lubricating her nipples with olive oil prior to pumping. In addition to its lubricating properties, olive oil contains oleocanthal, a natural anti-inflammatory compound that has a chemical profile similar to that of ibuprofen (Beauchamp 2005). Edible oils are safe for the baby.

Fig. 245 demonstrates the consequences of a poor flange fit. Note the abrasions on the nipple face caused by using a 24 mm flange on a nipple with a resting diameter of 29 mm. Note the periareolar scars from previous breast reduction surgery.

Variability in Pacifiers and Teats

Pacifiers, nipple shields, and bottle teats come in a variety of sizes (**Fig. 246**). Some sizes and shapes may be more or less useful in meeting a specific therapeutic goal. For example, NNS may exercise a baby's weak tongue by giving the baby opportunities to move the tongue and jaw at times other than feedings.

Bottle teats come in various sizes and shapes (**Fig. 247**), factors that influence milk flow rate (Matthew 1990). Additionally, they are made of different materials, some of which may expose the infant to the risk of chemical ingestion. All of these elements impact feeding. It is important to chose the most effective size bottle teat or nipple shield when using these devices therapeutically.

Beauchamp GK, Keast RS, Morel D, et al. Phytochemistry: ibuprofen-like activity in extra-virgin olive oil. *Nature* 2005; 437(7055):45-46.

Brown T, Ringrose C, Hyland R, et al. A method of assessing female-breast morphometry and its clinical application. *British Journal of Plastic Surgery* 1999; 52(5):355-359.

Caglar MK, Ozer I, Altugan FS. Risk factors for excessive weight loss and hypernatremia in exclusively breastfed infants. *Brazilian Journal of Medicical and Biological Research* 2006; 39(4):539-544.

Cox D, Kent J, Casey T, et al. Breast growth and the urinary excretion of lactose during human pregnancy and early lactation: endocrine relationships. *Experimental Physiology* 1999; 84(2):421-434.

Geddes DT. Gross Anatomy of the Human Breast, in *Hale & Hartmann's Textbook of Human Lactation*, Amarillo, TX: Hale Publishing, 2007; p. 29.

Gunther M. Instinct and the nursing couple. *Lancet* March 15, 1955; 576-578.

Kerrigan C, Collins E, Striplin D, et al. The health burden of breast hypertrophy. *Plastic Reconstructive Surgery* 2001; 108(6):1591-1599.

Matthew OP. Determinants of milk flow through nipple units. Role of hole size and nipple thickness. *American Journal of Diseases of Children* 1990; 144(2):222-224.

Meier P, Motyhowski J, Zuleger J. Choosing a correctly-fitted breastshield for milk expression. *Medela Messenger* 2004; 21(1):8-9.

Ramsay D, Langton D, Gollow I. Ultrasound imaging of the effect of frenulotomy on breastfeeding infants with ankyloglossia. Abstract of the proceedings of the 12th International Conference of the International Society for Research in Human Milk and Lactation, Sept. 10-14, 2004a; Queen's College, Cambridge, UK.

Ramsay D, Mitoulas L, Kent J, et al. Ultrasound imaging of the sucking mechanics of the breastfeeding infant. Abstract of the proceedings of the 12th International Conference of the International Society for Research in Human Milk and Lactation: Sept. 10-14, 2004b; Queen's College, Cambridge, UK.

Ramsay D, Kent J, Hartmann R, et al. Anatomy of the lactating human breast redefined with ultrasound imaging. *Journal of Anatomy* 2005; 206(6); 525-534.

Rohn R. Nipple (papilla) development in girls: III. the effect of pregnancy. *Journal of Adolescent Health Care* 1989; 19(1):39-40.

Smith W, Erenberg A, Nowak A. Imaging evaluation of the human nipple during breastfeeding. *American Journal of Diseases of Children* 1988; 142(1):76-78.

Stark Y. Human Nipples: Function and Anatomical Variations in Relationship to Breastfeeding. Master's Thesis. Pasadena, CA: Pacific Oaks College, 1994.

Williams G, Hoffmann S. Mammoplasty for tubular breasts. *Aesthetic Plastic Surgery* 1981; 5(1):51-56.

Ziemer M, Pigeon J. Skin changes and pain in the nipple during the 1st week of lactation. *Journal of Obstetric, Gynecologic, and Neonatal Nursing* 1993; 22(3):247-256.

Zeimer M, Cooper D, Pigeon J. Evaluation of a dressing to reduce nipple pain and improve nipple skin condition in breastfeeding women. *Nursing Research* 1995; 44(6):347-351.

Engorgement, Oversupply, and Mastitis

Fullness of both breasts appears to be a normal event in the first several weeks postpartum. Newton (1951) suggested that failure of the breasts to manifest some sign of fullness during this time is a marker for risk of lactation difficulty. However, at the other end of the spectrum, intense, unrelieved engorgement is a marker for inflammatory conditions of varying severity. Regular breast emptying is the first line of defense against inflammatory breast disorders, and failure to remove milk has consequences in terms of breast health and maintenance of milk production. Down regulation of milk supply occurs when a protein called feedback inhibitor of lactation (FIL) accumulates in the breast and interferes with calibration of the milk supply (Daly 1996). Prolonged, unrelieved engorgement may therefore result in diminished milk production that may prove impossible to reverse.

Engorgement

Several theories explain the phenomenon of breast engorgement. The delivery of the placenta alters the maternal hormonal milieu, triggering the onset of copious milk production, typically by 72 hours postpartum. The breasts react to this hormone change with temporary lymphatic edema indicated as swelling. Because of the swelling, some babies experience difficulty latching onto the distended nipple and areolar tissue. Pathologic engorgement may result when the non-latching baby cannot assist the mother in draining colostrum and milk.

Another theory holds that retained milk causes the alveoli to distend. This distention presses against the surrounding milk ducts, prevents the outflow of milk, and creates inflammatory swelling.

Fetherston (2001) describes one aspect of the inflammatory process that occurs during engorgement or periods of milk stasis. Whenever milk flow is blocked, normally tight seals between cells in the ducts become leaky. Protein components from milk and blood begin to seep into the space between these cells. Leaked substances, particularly pro-inflammatory cytokines in the milk, may provoke a host defense reaction, causing systemic responses, such as fever and flu-like symptoms. These symptoms may occur with or without actual infection of the breast. Such inflammatory symptoms are associated with decreased milk production in cattle, and low milk supply is often observed in mothers who suffer from any form of mastitis. Thus, milk stasis and inflammation may initiate a chain of events that ultimately culminates in poor lactation outcome.

It is important for the LC to understand the relationship between prolonged engorgement and down regulation of milk supply owing to the mechanism of FIL. Some women may be more sensitive to inhibitory factors, explaining why one mother may easily recover full production after early inhibition, and why another does not. Removing milk from the breast helps reduce engorgement and swelling. Milk production is endangered when postpartum engorgement is inappropriately or ineffectively managed.

Patterns of Breast Engorgement in the First Two Weeks Postpartum

Because it appears to be normal for mothers to experience some degree of breast engorgement during the postpartum period, the LC must understand how to prevent severe engorgement and how to manage such engorgement when it occurs. Timely care reduces the likelihood that prolonged engorgement and milk stasis will result in down regulation of the milk supply. Unfortunately, engorgement has been poorly studied, and inconsistent advice is often provided to new mothers.

Moon (1989) identified variables that closely correlated with breast engorgement:

- delayed initiation of breastfeeding
- infrequent feeds
- time-limited feeds
- late maturation of milk (i.e., the shift from colostrum to milk)
- supplementary feeds (usually without replacement pumping)

Hill (1994) and Humenick (1994) observed 4 distinct patterns of postpartum breast engorgement:

- Some mothers have *one* experience of very firm, tender breasts followed by a decline in symptoms.
- Some mothers have *multiple peaks* of engorgement before symptoms decline.
- Some mothers have *intense engorgement that persists* for 2 weeks or longer.
- Some mothers experience only *slight breast changes.*

Hill and Humenick thus conclude that the experience of engorgement is not the same for each mother. Not only did 4 distinct patterns emerge, but their research identifies variations in the time to peak engorgement as well. Some mothers became engorged as early as Day 2. Others reached peak levels between Days 9 and 14. During the first 2 weeks some women only experienced firmness with slight tenderness for one day and others had 9 days of very firm, very tender breast engorgement. The LC should avoid describing only one pattern of engorgement. Mothers who experience a variant pattern may otherwise become alarmed.

Breastfeeding Outcome and Patterns of Early Engorgement

Hill and Humenick assert that there is some *predictive value* offered by assessing a woman's pattern of post-partum breast engorgement. Women with profound and persistent engorgement appeared to be at greater risk for problems related to oversupply. Similarly, women who reported only low levels of engorgement were more likely to report low milk supply concerns. The former were more uncomfortable and discouraged about their experience of breastfeeding. The latter reported the highest percentage of early weaning owing to perceived insufficient milk supply.

Hill (1994) also observed that previous breastfeeding appeared to be a more critical variable than was parity in predicting engorgement. "...second time breastfeeding mothers appeared to experience breast engorgement sooner after delivery and at higher levels than did first time breastfeeding mothers, regardless of delivery method." Further, "Growth of the mammary glands *during* lactation may not be a rare phenomenon" (Cox 1999). Previous lactation may stimulate (along with pregnancy-related growth) the amount of functional glandular tissue present, increasing the likelihood of higher levels of early milk production with each lactation.

Pathologic Engorgement

The mother in **Fig. 248** is 3 days postpartum. She is experiencing pathologic breast engorgement that appears to be obstructing milk removal. Her breasts are so swollen that the baby cannot latch. Note the taut appearance of the areolar tissue. When a balloon is over-inflated, it is necessary to let off some of the air pressure before enough of the balloon tissue can be drawn up to tie a knot. Similarly, some of the swelling present in a pathologically engorged breast must be reduced before the baby can draw in enough of the breast tissue for a good latch.

Mothers in such cases used to be cautioned against expressing milk from engorged breasts owing to concerns that milk production would then be over-stimulated. Such fears appear to be unfounded. Thoroughly softening the breasts can sometimes resolve pathologic engorgement.

Fig. 249 shows a woman on Day 8 postpartum. The LC explained to the woman that her breast fullness might continue for another week. Pumping helped soften the woman's breasts to enable her baby to latch.

The woman in **Fig. 250** is engorged on Day 6 postpartum. She has large, dimpled nipples and her infant is unable to latch onto her breasts. Use of a hospital-grade electric breast pump or hand expression can help soften engorged breasts. Careful assessment of nipple diameter is always important in such cases. A poorly sized pump flange may restrict the ability of the pump to adequately drain the breast.

Treatment of Engorgement

A Cochrane Review (Snowden 2001) compared the effectiveness of interventions commonly suggested to relieve engorgement symptoms. It found that cabbage extract and placebo cream were equally effective, suggesting that massage may have been the factor that alleviated symptoms rather than an actual effect of cabbage leaves. Utrasound treatment and placebo were equally effective, suggesting that either radiant heat or massage may have alleviated symptoms. Oxytocin and cold packs had no demonstrable effect on the symptoms of engorgement. The only treatments that significantly improved the total symptoms of engorgement compared to placebo were the use of anti-inflammatory medications. More research is needed to assess the effectiveness of various treatments and to explore the use of non-steroidal anti-inflammatory drugs, such as ibuprofen, in the management of engorgement (Berens 2007).

Breast Massage and Acupuncture

Massage therapists trained in a technique called manual lymphatic drainage may assist mothers experiencing severe breast engorgement. Gentle massage along the lymph drainage pathways may improve lymph flow. Reduced lymphatic congestion may lessen swelling and improve milk flow. BWC has referred several clients to a manual lymphatic drainage therapist when nothing else seemed to relieve their pathologic engorgement. Three women who sought manual lymphatic drainage massage all reported improvement of symptoms, including reduced discomfort and better subsequent milk yields during breast pumping.

Kvist (2007) randomized 205 lactating mothers with inflammatory breast symptoms to 3 groups in order to test the hypothesis that acupuncture hastens recovery. Acupuncture treatment, along with standard care to correct positioning and latch, was less expensive and more effective than the use of oxytocin spray in this sample of women. It is important to note that antibiotic therapy was required to treat 15 percent of the women in the study whose engorgement was connected with mastitis.

Reverse Pressure Softening/Areolar Massage

Postpartum women commonly retain fluids and often experience generalized peripheral edema that affects their hands and feet. Such edema may cause distention of the nipple and areola as well, and may collapse ducts, reducing milk outflow. Miller (2004) and Cotterman (2004) described similar techniques that Cotterman named Reverse Pressure Softening (RPS). Both techniques appear to temporarily shift nipple and areolar edema, permitting better milk outflow.

The LC or mother places her fingers or thumbs at the base of the nipple and presses into the breast tissue, holding for one minute. If effective, nipple elasticity improves, which assists the infant in drawing in more tissue. Because pumping may pull excess interstitial fluid toward the nipple and areola, shifting edema away from the areola with RPS also may help the mother pump more effectively.

Fig. 251 (courtesy of Colette Acker, BS, IBCLC) shows a mother performing reverse pressure softening.

BWC encountered a mother with extreme engorgement who was unable to remove any milk from her right breast. She instructed the mother to take her prescribed dose of ibuprofen, and waited 15 minutes for the anti-inflammatory and pain relief aspects of the medication to take effect, and then BWC performed RPS. Afterwards, the mother was able to pump 18 ml of milk from her previously impacted breast. The milk flow stopped after several minutes of pumping, and it became necessary to repeat the technique, which facilitated removal of another 10 ml of milk.

At this point, using a nipple shield helped the baby latch to the now somewhat softened breast. The baby's sucking stimulated a milk ejection (observed on the other breast). Test weights confirmed infant intake of 12 ml of milk with the shield in place. After the baby stopped feeding, the mother pumped another 15 ml.

Removing a total of 55 ml of milk significantly helped relieve the mother's pain. The mother was advised to repeat the process demonstrated at 2 hour intervals, and to continue taking ibuprofen as described in her post-discharge orders. By the next day, the mother was able to pump 90 ml from her previously impacted breast. The baby was latching more consistently with the shield. As the breasts softened over the next few days, the baby was able to latch without using the shield.

The Risks of Inadequate Management of Engorgement

The risks of inadequate management of prolonged engorgement are illustrated in **Fig. 252.** The mother has unusually flaccid breasts for Day 12 postpartum. Her milk supply is decreased and her baby has not regained his birth weight. She described an intensely painful engorgement phase characterized by full, tight breasts. Believing that it would make her engorgement worse, she did not remove milk from her breasts. Although she put the baby to breast frequently, he was unable to latch well to her tight breast tissue, and mostly slept at the breast. Because milk was not being regularly removed, down regulation of her supply occured. The situation on Day 12 mimics that of a woman who never initiated lactation, and whose milk supply has been allowed to dry up. The woman never regained a full milk supply in spite of an aggressive regimen of pumping and the use of a galactagogue.

Peu d'orange

Figs. 253 and **254** show 2 women with *peu d'orange* (orange peel skin). Pitting edema may occur during severe engorgement or mastitis and is an important symptom of inflammatory breast cancer. The marks on the breast made by the seams of a bra in **Fig. 253** also reveal high levels of edema.

Oversupply

Some mothers appear to make more milk than others, creating as many potential lactation difficulties as under supply (Wilson-Clay 2006). A singleton baby, while thriving, may become overwhelmed by excessive milk volume. The baby may choke, pull away, feed frequently, act colicky, and have explosive, watery bowel movements. The mother may become confused by the negative feed-back from her baby and may conclude that the baby is hungry or is allergic to something in her diet. Some mothers go to extraordinary lengths to avoid certain food groups in an effort to resolve the baby's behavior. The baby's aversive behaviors may escalate to the level of a nursing strike.

Livingstone (1996) describes oversupply as maternal and infant *hyperlactation syndrome*. It is important to appreciate the dyadic emphasis. The mother is at increased risk for developing milk stasis-related disorders such as plugged ducts, mastitis, and abscess. Owing to chronic over-consumption of foremilk, or owing to rapid milk flow rates and gulping, some infants may suffer from digestive disorders (and even respiratory problems if milk is chronically aspirated). The infant may present with some of the symptoms of gastroesophageal reflux disease (GERD). Both members, mother and baby, become deprived of opportunities for pleasurable feedings, thus affecting the interpersonal relationship.

Unless the mother is planning to return to work or school, the management plan should focus on decreasing the rate of milk synthesis. Skillful counseling is required because it is not always obvious to a mother that milk oversupply, is the problem, especially if she has previously interpreted the baby's fussing as a sign of hunger. Consequently, it is difficult for some mothers to trust the LC's advice to reduce milk production. Taking test weights can assist. Weights often reveal that the baby is, indeed, taking in large volumes of milk during very short breastfeeding episodes. Such information helps the mother see that her baby is complaining about too much, not too little, milk.

Reducing Oversupply by Block Feeding

One method to reduce milk oversupply involves changing the pattern of breast usage. Instead of using both breasts, the mother only uses one breast at a feeding. For some women, reduction in supply can be achieved by offering only one breast for a feeding period that extends over several hours. This is called *block feeding*. Many women notice down regulation of supply within a few days of initiating this feeding pattern. Some women with oversupply need to breastfeed from the same breast for as long as 3, 4, 5 or even as long as 6 hours in order to sufficiently reduce their milk production. Excessive pressure in the unused breast can be partially relieved by hand expression or pumping, but the unused breast should not be emptied. Because of local feedback control mechanisms for lactation, the presence of residual milk retained in the breast triggers a gradual reduction in production. In time, the woman's body will make less milk.

In an adaptation of block feeding, van Veldhuizen-Staas (2007) begins the treatment by completely emptying both engorged breasts with a pump, and then breastfeeding the baby. The baby thus gets a feed of cream rich milk from both of the "emptied" breasts. The day is then divided into blocks of time, during which the baby feeds *ad lib,* but only from one breast during the block. The duration of the blocks may gradually be increased from 4, 6, 8, or even 12 hours. Some mothers will require only one thorough mechanical drainage of the breasts at the start; others may require occasional repetition to drain "milk lakes." However, mothers must avoid over stimulation.

Mothers with oversupply need help interpreting the babies' behavior during the down-regulatory period. At the first feed in a block, the infant may spend only a few minutes at the breast gulping down foremilk. The LC teaches the mother to view this as the first "course," not the entire meal. Reassure the mother not to expect the baby to stay on the breast too long. She can allow the baby to come back to the same breast several times over the course of the blocked time period to access the creamier hindmilk.

Consuming a more appropriate balance between fore and hindmilk tends to reduce the baby's watery, explosive stools. A thickening in the consistency of the baby's bowel movements may be the first sign that block feeding is working. As the milk supply normalizes, feedings become calmer and more pleasant for baby and mother, and evening colic may diminish. Sometimes the baby will begin asking for both breasts at some feedings, although the LC counsels the mother to make sure that the baby significantly softens the first breast before switching sides.

Oversupply and the Working Mother or Student

Women with oversupply who plan to return to work or school may wish to approach managing oversupply in a different way. They may wish to maintain some degree of overproduction to protect against possible reduction of milk supply later owing to the extra stress and fatigue that working mothers often experience. These mothers can be advised to briefly pump to soften their breasts prior to breastfeeding. This reduces engorgement and makes it easier for the baby to latch. It also reduces milk spraying that contributes to gulping and possible infant digestive distress. Mothers can freeze their extra milk for later use or donate it to a milk bank.

Pharmacologic Management of Milk Oversupply

Medically supervised pharmacologic treatment may be required to manage milk oversupply that fails to respond to block feeding. Pseudoephedrine is a drug that is usually contraindicated in breastfeeding women owing to its effect in reducing milk production (Hale 2008). Aljazaf (2003) reported that following a single 60 mg dose, the 24-hour milk production of 8 lactating women was reduced by 24 percent. Hale (2008) states that at the 60 mg daily dose, which is a fourth of the normal dose recommended for decongestant relief, "The calculated dose that would be absorbed by the infant was still very low."

Working with supervising HCPs, BWC has observed that one 60 mg of pseudoephedrine daily has helped decrease milk production when mechanical measures have failed. Sometimes it seems most effective to administer the entire

60 mg dose at bedtime to control overnight engorgement. In other cases, spreading the dosage throughout the day provides the greatest relief of symptoms. One mother in BWC's practice reported symptoms of jitteriness that resolved when she discontinued the therapy. In other cases BWC found that using pseudoephedrine effectively reduced maternal hyperlactation symptoms with few maternal side-effects. Pseudoephedrine should be avoided in women with hypertension. Therapies involving drugs must always be supervised by a health care provider.

Estrogen has been observed to reduce lactation in women (King 2007). Some physicians recommend a brief course of oral estrogen once daily for 4 to 7 days in order to regulate extreme oversupply when other methods have failed (Jain 2001, Lawrence 2005). The woman may experience an episode of bleeding afterwards, interrupting lactation amenorrhea and disrupting the contraceptive protection of breastfeeding. Women should be directed to employ contraceptive precautions once menstruation begins. Estrogen hormonal therapy is not advised for anyone with a clotting disorder, nor is it suitable for an immobilized person. It should be used with great care and probably not during the first 3 weeks postpartum (Jain 2001). BWC has worked with women for whom this therapy was effective.

Rapid Milk Ejection Reflex

The milk ejection reflex can be triggered by nipple stimulation or thoughts of the baby. Some women appear to have unusually forceful milk ejection reflexes. This phenomenon is sometimes seen in conjunction with (but may appear independently from) milk oversupply.

Note the milk squirting from the mother's nipple in **Fig. 255**. Rapidly ejecting milk may cause the baby to choke or pull off the breast, and gulping may contribute to symptoms of colic. Some babies appear quite distressed and get anxious at feeding times. As in oversupply cases, the mother may misinterpret her baby's response. She may think the baby is fussing because there is not enough milk when actually the baby is complaining about being overwhelmed by the forceful milk spray.

Choosing a special breastfeeding position may help the baby to manage a forceful milk ejection. Some infants will cope better when breastfed in an upright position or in side-lying. Some mothers lie flat and place the baby *prone* (face down) as in **Fig. 256** or semi-prone as in **Fig. 104**.

Mothers with forceful milk ejections may wish to manually stimulate a milk ejection. They can catch the forceful milk spray with a towel, wait a few moments, and then put the baby to the breast. Occasionally, a nipple shield may be used briefly, at the start of the feed, when the milk ejection is most forceful. The shield acts as a mechanical barrier blocking the milk spray so that it does not choke the baby. When the force of the spray lessens, the mother removes the shield and the baby finishes breastfeeding without it. Employing a nipple shield is useful if the baby has been rejecting the breast in favor of a more consistent or controllable milk flow rate from a bottle.

The Role of the LC in Managing Lactation Mastitis

Plugged ducts and mastitis represent worsening problems along the milk stasis spectrum. When a mother suffers from inflammatory breast disorders, the LC works with the woman's health care providers to help her recover. Further, the LC works to ease the symptoms, discover the factors that have contributed to the current crisis, and help the mother learn how to prevent recurrence. To do this, the LC must have a thorough understanding of inflammatory breast conditions.

The LC must also appreciate that some cases of mastitis can be stubborn to eradicate. Eglash (2007) describes a mother first seen at 5 weeks postpartum who experienced early cracked nipples and one episode of acute mastitis. The woman continued to complain of chronic deep breast pain, which resolved only after several months and numerous courses of different oral antibiotic medications.

Some women who experience chronic mastitis have difficulty obtaining adequate medical attention. Because breastfeeding continues to be viewed by some as a "lifestyle choice," mothers who complain of lingering breast pain often encounter pressure from family members and HCPs to wean instead of receiving help to resolve the problem. Women have told BWC that they were sure if their pain had been located in any other part of the body than the breast, it would have been taken more seriously.

Sadly, women are vulnerable to persuasion when others tell them that breastfeeding has become "inconvenient." In such cases, the LC may advocate for the baby's right to be breastfed and for the mother's right to a full medical assessment and adequate treatment. It may be necessary to help locate professional resources and references in order to assist the HCP in treating the mother, especially if the HCP appears unfamiliar with current guidelines for treatment. A useful source for physician information for treating lactation mastitis is the Academy of Breastfeeding Medicine's Protocol # 4 (ABM 2008). See the references for a web link to this protocol.

Mastitis

Mastitis is a frequently cited reason for early weaning (Fetherston 1998, Snowden 2001). Michie (2003) identified mastitis as a major cause of both early weaning and reduction in milk production. Michie also commented that "...by altering the cellular composition of milk and local defenses within the breast itself, mastitis is a powerful risk factor promoting vertical transmission of infections." During mastitis, activated dendritic cells may be identified in the milk, which may more readily carry virus particles to the infant. This fact has obvious implications in the transmission of HIV, increasing the risk of vertical transmission from mother to infant via breastfeeding (Hansen 2004).

Fetherston (2006) describes increased breast permeability, reduced milk synthesis, and rising concentrations of immune components with increasing severity of breast and systemic symptoms. Such changes, while still not fully explained by current theories, appear to be temporary. Remarkably, human breasts appear to fully recover within about one week after resolution of the symptoms of mastitis.

Better prevention, early identification, and appropriate treatment of mastitis is critical to prevent untimely weaning, protect infant growth, and reduce the risk of transmission of viral disease to infants.

Definitions and Incidence of Mastitis

Controversy exists over the definition of mastitis. Medical texts have tended to define mastitis narrowly as an infectious process of the breast. More recently, experts have begun to understand mastitis as a condition occuring along a spectrum. It ranges from subclinical mastitis and non-infectious inflammation to infectious processes, including breast abscess. (Foxman 1994, Inch 1995, Michie 2003, Amir 2007).

Identifying the incidence of mastitis has been challenging because available studies vary widely in their methodology, diagnosis, and duration. Most studies focus on the early weeks postpartum, the time when mastitis is most common.

In Foxman's (2002) prospective study, 9.5 percent of breastfeeding women reported mastitis during the first 12 weeks of lactation. Amir (2007) examined data from 2 studies and found rates of mastitis of 17 percent with most episodes occurring in the first 4 weeks postpartum. Amir concluded that improved management of nipple damage could potentially reduce the risk of developing mastitis.

Riordan (1990) and Fetherston (1998) found much higher incidence rates for mastitis in separate studies that looked at the incidence over longer time periods. Riordan speculated that because many women self-treat, the true incidence of mastitis may be under-reported and under-appreciated. Mohrbacher (2003) and Riordan (2005) report the incidence of lactation mastitis as approximately 27 percent.

Riordan (1990) retrospectively studied a group of women about their experience with mastitis over the full duration of lactation, rather than focusing only on the first few months postpartum. She found rates of mastitis as high as 33 percent. Some of the women in her study lactated for 60 months. While incidence of mastitis was highest during the early months of lactation, a third of the women recalled developing mastitis after 6 months. Nearly a fourth of them developed mastitis after one year.

The mothers in Riordan's study (1990) ranked the factors they perceived to increase the risk for developing mastitis:

- fatigue
- stress
- plugged (blocked) ducts
- changes in number of feedings
- engorgement/milk stasis
- an infection in another family member
- breast trauma

Fetherston's (1998) prospectively sought to identify predictive factors associated with occurrence of mastitis in a group of Australian women. She found a 27 percent rate of mastitis in the first 3 months postpartum and proposed a broader definition of lactation mastitis as an "*inflammation of breast tissue*...[that] affects different tissues and structures of the breast." Fetherston notes that symptoms vary among individuals, and whether infective or non-infective in origin, symptoms can be equally debilitating. Grouping risk factors into common themes, Fetherston's 1998 study identified 5 factors as most predictive of development of mastitis:

- blocked ducts
- stress
- latch difficulties
- tight, restrictive bras
- nipple pain during a feeding

Maternal stress is not noted as a predictive factor for development of mastitis in primiparous mothers, but *was* predictive in multiparous women (Fetherston 2001). Perhaps women with more children to care for feel more tired and stressed. Previous history of mastitis appears also to be a risk factor. Perhaps mastitis creates internal breast changes or scar tissue formation (such as is noted in dairy cattle). It is also possible that anatomic anomalies contribute to increased risk of mastitis in some women (i.e., ducts blocked by previous surgery, cysts, or tumors, etc).

Foxman (2002) also identified mastitis risk factors similar to Fetherston's:

- previous mastitis history
- breast and nipple pain
- cracks in the nipple

Subclinical Mastitis

Subclinical mastitis is a condition well known in the dairy industry. While it may occur without obvious symptoms, milk production can be impaired. Although low grade or subclinical mastitis is not discussed in most breastfeeding books, it can be detected in women by an increase in a number of specific chemical markers. These include elevations in selected components that may help to protect the nursing infant from developing clinical illness while feeding on mastitic milk (Buescher 2001).

Subclinical mastitis may be connected with milk stasis that triggers inflammatory host responses. Milk stasis may occur owing to a number of reasons, including poor feed frequency, ineffective infant feeding, and incomplete breast emptying. Whenever inflammatory breast changes occur, milk flow becomes further obstructed by swelling. The mother begins to feel aches and other flu-like symptoms. The chemical markers in her milk will be similar to those noted during pregnancy, the colostral phase, engorgement, and during weaning (Rand 2001).

These chemical changes in the milk appear to reveal the presence of a true inflammatory process that may occur in the mammary glands without the classic, full blown symptoms of mastitis, such as fever. Researchers have also identified chemical changes in the milk that initiate inflammatory stimuli in the gut of young infants. Such changes affect infant gut permeability, increasing the risk of infant susceptibility to infection (Hansen 2004).

Studies of women with subclinical and chronic low-grade mastitis have identified high concentrations of immunological factors and elevated sodium and potassium in the milk of HIV-infected mothers (Semba 1999, Kasonka 2006). These milk changes were associated with a higher HIV load in milk and higher mother-to-child transmission of HIV. The impact of improved postpartum health care,

particularly management of maternal infection, on the prevalence of subclinical mastitis requires investigation.

Filteau (1999) linked subclinical mastitis in women to poor infant growth. This may be secondary to impaired milk production since milk supply generally decreases during mastitis. The same study noted that maternal dietary supplementation with vitamin E rich sunflower oil was helpful in reducing subclinical mastitis.

Clearly, more studies are needed to fully identify the true incidence of subclinical mastitis. HCPs must discover ways to assist mothers with subclinical mastitis whose symptoms (mainly low milk supply and low grade breast pain) may be overlooked or dismissed.

Other conditions must be ruled out when evaluating and assessing a mother's report of breast pain. Episodic breast pain coincidental with lactation is also observed among women experiencing vasospasm of the nipple (Page 2006). The pain may radiate deep in the breast and may occur without obvious signs of infection. Identification of nipple blanching confirms this phenomenon. Vasospasm is treated with palliative use of heat and, medically with nifedipine therapy.

A Link Between Milk Oversupply and Risk of Mastitis

In her analysis of the mechanisms involved in mastitis, Fetherston (2001) observed that obstruction of milk flow works against the natural flushing mechanisms of the lactating breast. She further speculates that frequent breast drainage may ease intramammary pressure and reduce inflammatory symptoms.

The flushing mechanism of the breast may be hampered when the rate of milk production is too high and retained milk contributes to chronic breast engorgement (Amir 2000). Vogel (1999) also concluded that mastitis "may be a marker of an ample milk supply." Some mothers appear to produce more milk than one infant can comfortably consume. Milk oversupply needs time to down regulate, and perhaps some women are more prone to mastitis in the interim. Both BWC and KH have observed that mothers in their practices who have been copious milk producers tended to have more episodes of both plugged ducts and mastitis, and have required assistance to diminish milk production.

A Link Between Cracked Nipples and Mastitis

There is a link between cracked nipples and mastitis (Fetherston 2001, Amir 2007). When nipples become cracked in the hospital environment, *nosocomial* (hospital acquired) organisms can ascend into the breast and cause infections. Women may be particularly vulnerable if bacterial colonization of the breasts occurs via cracked nipples during the engorgement phase of lactation, when milk stasis is common and the let down reflex is not well-conditioned. The protective flushing mechanism of the breats may not be as functional as it will be when breastfeeding is more established.

Livingstone (1999) also observed a strong association between cracked, infected nipples and mastitis. After 5 to 7 days of treatment, 12 to 35 percent of the women she observed with infected nipples who were not being treated with systemic antibiotics developed mastitis.

Anatomic ultrasound studies lend support to Livingstone's hypothesis that pathogens introduced through nipple cracks can ascend ducts, causing infection of the breast. Ramsay (2004) observed that "...milk is not stored in the larger ducts close to the nipple but flows back into the smaller collecting ducts and ductules, a phenomenon we have observed as a reversal in flow of the echogenic fat globules within the duct." Thus, mothers with superficial nipple skin damage must be carefully managed in order to prevent infection of the ductal openings with progression to mastitis.

Other Risk Factors for Lactation Mastitis

The literature on mastitis contains references to less common risk factors. When the lactation consultant assesses a mother, it is important to consider that occasionally these issues may be relevant:

- poor maternal health, especially a history of anemia (Minchin 1998)
- reliance upon an ineffective breast pump
- injury to the breast resulting from strenuous exercise or trauma (Fetherston 1997)
- structural abnormalities of the breast such as ductal anomalies, previous breast surgery, breast cancer, cysts, abscesses (Meguid 1995, Dahlbeck 1995, Olsen 1990)
- use of and poor cleaning of nipple shields (Fetherston 1998, Noble 1997)
- smoking (Furlong 1994)
- maternal IgA immunodeficiency (Fetherston 2001)

Treatment of Mastitis

When a mother experiences symptoms of mastitis, it is appropriate for the LC to advise the mother to notify her health care provider. Unless the LC is also a physician,

midwife, or a nurse practitioner, the LC should report to the mother's HCP. Her report should *describe symptoms* observed rather than presenting a diagnosis.

The Royal College of Midwives' (2002) recommendations regarding mastitis state: "...it might be appropriate to delay antibiotic therapy for 12-24 hours, whilst taking corrective measures [to reduce inflammation and promote thorough breast emptying]. If however, there was no improvement during this time, a broad-spectrum antibiotic would be necessary...If it is not possible to provide close professional supervision and support for a mother with mastitis, prophylactic antibiotics will be needed from the outset."

Some HCPs will wish to see the mother; others may phone in a prescription for a drug such as dicloxacillin that is generally effective against *S. aureus*. The ABM (2008) mastitis protocol (citing the WHO publication on mastitis) states that if there is no positive response to antibiotics within 2 days, if the mastitis recurs, if it is hospital-acquired mastitis, or if the mastitis is severe or unusual, breast milk cultures and sensitivity testing should be undertaken.

Once the HCP has been notified of the mother's symptoms, the LC endeavors to alleviate inflammatory symptoms. The HCP may suggest ibuprofen, and cold therapy may be employed as a mechanism of pain relief (if it is culturally acceptable). Flushing the breast (ideally by breastfeeding) is imperative. Mothers may need to use a hospital grade electric pump if breastfeeding is too painful. Gentle reverse pressure softening can be employed (if the mother can tolerate it) to help reduce edema around the nipple that may be hindering milk outflow.

Rest is critical to recovery. Woman with mastitis should be instructed to remain in bed for 2 days. They should be encouraged to take all medication as prescribed (including pain medication if indicated), to eat well, and to drink extra fluids. Breastfeeding should continue. Removing residual milk on the affected side with a pump after breast-feeding helps to keep the breast flushed and to resolve symptoms more quickly.

Mothers pumping for a sick or premature baby should be directed to discard the milk from the mastitic breast until their symptoms resolve (Neifert 1999, Behari 2004). Sometimes babies will refuse to breastfeed from a mastitic breast, probably owing to the salty taste resulting from high levels of sodium and chloride present in milk during mastitis (Newton 1997b). In cases of breast refusal, the mother breast-feeds on the unaffected side and pumps the affected side.

Nasal carriage of *Staphylococcus aureus* is a major risk factor for invasive *S. aureus* disease (Peacock 2003). Amir (2006) identified significantly more infants of mothers with mastitis as nasal carriers of *S. aureus*.

If the infant has been colonized in the hospital setting, mouth-to-nipple contact potentially reintroduces bacterial exposure with each breastfeeding. *Staph* infections may also appear as pustules in the infant's diaper area (Fortunov 2006). Because bacterial contamination of open nipple wounds contributes to the development of mastitis, nipple cleansing and maternal hand-washing after diaper changes are important measures to prevent mastitis so long as cracked nipples are present.

Wound specialists advise flushing open wounds with tap water or normal saline solution. BWC and KH encourage mothers with cracked nipples to rinse their nipples after feeding or pumping. Mothers are also encouraged to clean nipples once daily with mild soap and water. Topical antiseptics or antibiotics may prevent infection.

Nipple cleansing or topical antibiotics are measures that are advised only for short-term first aid until nipples heal. It is unnecessary to engage in special cleansing or topical applications if the nipple skin is healthy. Overuse of soap may cause dry skin or alter the scent of the nipple.

Prescription mupirocin (Bactroban®) has both antifungal and antibacterial properties. It may be applied sparingly to cracked nipples to prevent superficial infection of the wounds. Once infection occurs, systemic antibiotics are generally required.

If cracked nipples result from mechanical trauma, the LC must assess the positioning and latch, evaluate any "fit" issues, and assess the infant's oral anatomy and suck. Assessment and correction of problems will help prevent recurrences of nipple trauma and reduce the risk that the breast will become re-infected.

Images of Mastitis

The left breast of the woman in **Fig. 257** is inflamed on Day 4 postpartum. She complain to the LC on the telephone that her breast felt painfully hot and swollen. When the LC visited, she observed *erythema* (redness) that extended from the nipple to the chest wall (from 4 o'clock to 12 o'clock). The mother's milk flow was blocked and breastfeeding was too painful for her to attempt. The mother reported headache and body aches but no fever; however, she had been taking acetaminophen, which may have masked febrile symptoms.

The mother in **Fig. 258** also was taking acetaminophen and was afebrile. Mastitis typically is unilateral, but *bilateral mastitis* can occur (**Figs. 258** and **259**). Bilateral pathological engorgement may present similarly, but *Streptococcus* infection should be ruled out when bilateral mastitis occurs.

Amir (1999) performed an audit of women treated for mastitis in an emergency room and found that almost 40 percent of the women were afebrile. Only 27 percent ran temperatures of 38.5°C (101°F) or higher. She also noted that some mothers were taking anti-pyretic medications that masked symptoms. Mastitic women without fever should be asked whether they have taken a medication that may be altering their symptoms. Based on this audit, Amir remarks, "…the evidence for the presence of a fever of 38.5°C in women with mastitis needs to be reexamined." Other practitioners have observed mastitis and even abscess without the symptom of fever. Some individuals may only develop fever late in the course of an infection. Therefore, breast *pain* must be considered as an important diagnostic indicator of mastitis.

Milk Cultures

Studies have examined the colony counts of bacteria in expressed milk as a way to definitively diagnose breast infection (Osterman 2000, Thomsen 1983). However, Fetherston points out that this technique, borrowed from bovine science, has limitations when trying to diagnose mastitis in humans. The human breast has a different structure from the udder, in which all lobes drain into a common reservoir. Love (2000) states that, in humans, it is more anatomically correct to think of "…not a breast but 6 to 9 ductal systems."

Because each of these ductal systems is separate from the others, researchers suspect that it may be possible to get confusing results when performing bacteriologic testing. Unless the milk is captured solely from the infected ductal system, mixing of milk from other, healthy lobes may dilute the bacterial colonies obtained from infected lobes. Thus, a colony count may not provide much information. In practice colony counts are seldom done owing to cost and the time it takes to get the culture results. However, milk cultures are useful, to identify the type of pathogens growing in the breast. Identification aids in selection of appropriate antibiotic therapy.

Some practitioners obtain cultures of the mother's milk or of the baby's nose and throat to identify pathogens (Wust 1995) to help in the selection of an antibiotic. These cultures are typically performed when a woman fails to respond to standard treatment with frontline antibiotics.

Risk of Candidiasis Following
Antibiotic Therapy for Mastitis

Secondary candida infection may occur following antibiotic use. Overgrowth of yeast on the nipple surface may be preventable by gentle rinsing of the nipples with clean water following each breastfeeding. Yeast spores may be washed off intact skin, as is demonstrated by the fact that mothers with excellent hygiene sometimes can avoid nipple infection even when their infant has a diagnosed case of thrush. LCs recommend anticipatory guidance to assist women in identifying and obtaining treatment for topical fungal infections that may occur following the use of oral antibiotics.

Both authors have encountered women with chronic breast pain (and probably mastitis) who refused antibiotic treatment owing to an almost phobic fear of secondary yeast infection. In some cases, these women will continue to self-treat what they are convinced is a fungal infection, They may drastically modify their diets and incur exhausting extra laundry and housekeeping duties. Many are willing to repeat numerous courses of powerful systemic antifungal medications in spite of experiencing no real relief of symptoms. The LC must help these women explore the possibility that they do not have a fungal infection, and probably require treatment for bacterial mastitis.

Sharing research evidence may assist the LC in convincing mothers to explore alternatives to repeating treatment for "yeast." Thomassen (1998) studied 3 groups of women: 20 with deep breast pain in one breast, 20 with superficial skin infection of the nipple, and 20 healthy women with respect to the growth of bacteria and fungi. *C. albicans* was found twice as often in the milk of women with superficial lesions as compared to those with deep breast pain. Bacteria were more likely to be found on the nipple and in the milk of those complaining of deep breast pain. "Thus, *if* the deep breast pain syndrome is caused by microbes, this study points to a pathogenic role of bacteria rather than fungi." Persistent, chronic, unilateral deep breast pain should be treated with antibiotics. If signs and symptoms of candidiasis of the nipple occur, topical anti-fungal medication can be prescribed by the HCP (see Ch. 8 for additional information).

Breast Abscess

Mastitis occurs along a spectrum of severity. Failure to resolve symptoms successfully at any stage often results in progression toward more serious disease. Delayed or inadequate treatment of mastitis can result in the development of breast abscesses.

Breast abscesses are pus-filled cysts that develop as a complication of mastitis. A US report puts the incidence of breast abscess as high as 11 percent (Foxman 2002). Incidence seems to vary significantly by country. Amir (2004) cites an occurrence rate of breast abscess in Australia as approximately 3 percent. In a Swedish study, Kvist (2005) examined data for all singleton births from 1987 to 2000 and identified a rate of occurrence of breast abscess of 0.1 percent.

Abscesses are more common in primiparous women, in women older than 30, and in those who give birth post-maturely (Ulitzsch 2004, Kvist 2005). The risk of developing an abscess is increased if abrupt weaning occurs during inflammatory or infectious mastitis, if the wrong antibiotic therapy is chosen to treat a breast infection, if necessary antibiotic therapy is delayed, or if a woman fails to complete the full course of antibiotics.

Aspiration of Breast Abscesses

Abscesses constitute a medical emergency and require prompt medical treatment. Performing mammograms on women with mastitis is painful and breast changes caused by inflammation of the breast may result in increased radiographic density that can obscure focal lesions (Ulitzsch 2004). Ultrasound is a useful tool to rule out inflammatory masses that occur without evidence of focal pus (i.e., when no cyst has formed). If an abscess *is* present, ultrasound can be used to define the area of the abscess and to guide the aspiration needle or catheter to the abscess for drainage (O'Hara 1996, Hayes 1991, Ulitzsch 2004).

Aspiration of material allows culture and sensitivity tests to determine the proper drug therapy to specifically treat the infection. Aspiration and irrigation of the abscess with sterile saline permits withdrawal of the purulent material from the cyst, allowing some abscesses to be treated without incision and drainage (Dixon 1988). For large abscesses (typically those in excess of 3 cm), catheter drains may be placed for several days, allowing for continuous drainage and irrigation (see **Fig. 265**). Such drains may prevent the need for surgical incision (Karstrup 1993, Ulitzsch 2004).

Christensen (2005) studied the results of ultrasound-guided drainage of 151 patients who had *puerperal* (occurring after childbirth) and non-puerperal breast abcesses. Their abscesses were drained by needle or catheter under local anesthesia, and the women were treated with oral antibiotics. Of the women with puerperal abscesses, 97 percent recovered after the first round of ultrasound-guided drainage. Only one required subsequent surgical excision of the abscess cavity or of a fistula. This study supports the use of the aspiration technique as a less invasive treatment than traditional surgery while providing a high rate of success.

Surgical Treatment of Breast Abscess

Recovery can be slow when incision and drainage are used to remove a cyst or abscess from a lactating breast. It is not unusual for the wound to take 4 to 6 weeks to heal. The incision must be kept open and draining so that the wound can fill in and granulate properly from the inside. If the external wound heals over too quickly, fistulas may form under the surface, leading to further complications. The open incision will leak milk during the time the internal healing is occurring. Leaking milk, while messy, may be beneficial, because the milk contains human growth factors, anti-inflammatory factors, and immune factors that bathe the wound and may prevent infection. However, the appearance of the open wound is alarming to women and their families. Leaking may be especially noticeable when the woman experiences a milk ejection. A clean disposable diaper held over the open incision works well to catch leaking milk and to wick the moisture away from the skin. Keeping the skin dry may help to prevent maceration and skin breakdown.

Types of Abscesses

Intramammary unilocular abscesses occur as a solitary locus of infected material deep in the tissue of the breast. Some 65 percent of abscesses are *multilocular* and have a high rate of recurrence (Olsen 1990).

Abscesses can occur close to the surface of the breast near the nipple (*subareolar abscesses*). These often "ripen" as a boil does, are easier to excise, and have a more favorable prognosis. The woman pictured in **Fig. 260** is 6 weeks postpartum. Seen from the side, the shape of a ripening abscess is apparent. Note the *induration* (pulling in) of the nipple. Induration of breast tissue is an important symptom of serious disease and should be reported to a physician.

The woman pictured in **Fig. 261** has an abscess that is *ripening* (coming to a head). She had been self-treating for what she thought was a plugged duct for 3.5 weeks. Since she did not report a fever, the doctor's staff did not take her other symptoms seriously. Because of the risks associated with untreated breast disorders, unexplained breast masses that do not resolve within 3 days should always be examined by a HCP.

The mother pictured in **Fig. 262** developed a subareolar abscess in the 3 o'clock position on her right breast at 3 weeks postpartum. She had an oversupply problem and poorly managed engorgement. She began experiencing mastitis by the end of Week 2, but delayed seeking medical treatment for her symptoms. She sought emergency room care with a walnut-sized breast mass that was identified as an abscess. It was incised and drained. The mother is shown at one month postpartum with an iodine wick that promotes drainage and prevents the surface of the wound from closing before internal healing is complete. The wound is leaking blood and milk. Normally the mother wore a dressing over the wound, but the large dressing seemed to distract the baby during feedings. The mother learned to hold a small piece of sterile gauze over the wound while breastfeeding (**Fig. 263**).

This mother was advised by her doctor to pump the affected breast and to discard the milk; however, the pump flange was difficult to position so that it did not rub against the wound. Further, the mother was unable to soften her breast by pumping. She found that the baby's sucking brought more relief. While some mothers might be too distressed to breastfeed and would prefer to rely on the pump to keep the breast drained, this mother preferred to breastfeed. Because an ill or premature infant might become sick if exposed to the high levels of pathogens in the milk of a mother with breast abscess, the infant should be medically monitored for illness. The infant in this case did not suffer any ill consequences of breastfeeding from the affected breast.

Because of their location, periareolar abscesses create both breastfeeding and pumping challenges. From the standpoint of lactation, surgical incision should be placed as far as possible from the nipple in order to facilitate breastfeeding and pumping. Locating the incision radially, so that it runs along, rather than across the ducts, may be less likely to damage the ductal system.

Fig. 264 shows the same mother's breast at 7 weeks postpartum. The wound closed, and the mother continued to breastfeed uneventfully.

Case Study of MRSA-related Abscess Treated Initially with Percutaneous Drainage

A 36 year-old P1 G1 L1 mother (pictured in **Fig. 265**) gave birth to a healthy male infant at 38 weeks. Both nipples became cracked in the hospital. Treatment with hydrogel dressings and lanolin failed to result in healing the nipples, and the cracks had persisted for 7 weeks. The left breast produced 3 times as much milk as the right. Engorgement may have contributed to poor flushing. The pathogens that were preventing nipple healing may thus have had ample opportunity to ascend into the interior of the breast.

At 4 weeks postpartum the mother experienced an afebrile episode of plugged ducts in the left breast. Her physician called in a prescription for a 7-day course of cephalexin (500 mg twice a day). Owing to infant colic symptoms, the mother discontinued the medication on Day 5 of therapy. Symptoms recurred in the same breast 2 weeks later. Although the mother remained afebrile, she insisted on evaluation. Her HCP prescribed dicloxacillin (250 mg 4 times a day), which failed to resolve her symptoms. It should be noted that according to ABM protocols, the types and doses of antibiotic treatment this mother received were delayed, inadequate, and incomplete. Inadequate antibiotic therapy is a risk factor for abscess. Additionally, the mother was primiparous and older than 30, both issues identified in the literature as risk factors for breast abscess.

By Week 7 a red, swollen area developed at approximately 3 o'clock on the upper, outer quadrant of the left breast. A radiologist performed ultrasound investigation, which revealed a cluster of abscesses. As seen in the photo, a percutaneous drain was inserted to drain fluid from the abscess. Methicillin-resistant *Staphylococcus aureus* (MRSA) was isolated from material aspirated and the mother was immediately admitted to the hospital for incision and drainage of the abscess and intravenous vancomycin therapy. The mother requested emergency weaning advice, but owing to difficulty establishing the infant on formula, she opted to reverse the weaning and continued to lactate on the unaffected breast.

This case (Wilson-Clay 2008) demonstrates how serious infection can occur as the result of non-healing cracked nipples. The absence of fever resulted in treatment delays. Persistant low-grade breast pain was the primary symptom. It failed to sufficiently alarm the HCP and the mother did not receive timely, appropriate care. With the increasing prevalence of drug-resistant pathogens, timely, adequate evaluation of soft tissue infection in postpartum women is critical. MRSA must be ruled out when mastitis fails to resolve with front line drug therapy.

Case Study of Multilocular Breast Abscesses in a Breastfeeding Mother

The 26 year-old primiparous woman in **Fig. 266** has 2 abscesses shown in the healing phase following surgical excision. She visited her physician on Day 21 postpartum to report a pea-size lump in her right breast above the edge of her areola at 12 o'clock. She had no fever, but the area was tender. The doctor identified a plugged duct and recommended application of hot packs and more frequent breastfeeding. The mother had returned to graduate school at 2 weeks postpartum, and she was experiencing

elevated levels of stress and fatigue as the result. She also had a copious milk supply with a prolonged engorgement phase. Her baby was unable to remove enough milk to prevent breast engorgement, and her busy school schedule interfered with adequate time for pumping.

By Friday of the same week, the mother called BWC to report that the lump in her breast had grown to the size of an egg. The woman still reported no febrile symptoms; however, BWC was alarmed by the reported size of the mass. The obstetrician was notified, and the mother was immediately referred to a surgeon. Using ultrasound, the surgeon located a subareolar abscess, and aspirated it for relief of pressure and to culture for drug sensitivity. When the mother asked about her lack of febrile symptoms, the surgeon stated that approximately 25 percent of the women he treated for breast abscess were afebrile.

Fine needle aspiration did not resolve this mother's abscess, nor did oral antibiotics. Incision and drainage were performed 2 days later. Multilocular abscesses were discovered. Drainage tubes removed purulent material. The mother pumped her breasts post-surgically to relieve engorgement, and decided to wean as a result of her emotional trauma.

Slow Weaning on a Breast Pump

The LC devised a slow weaning plan to protect the healing breasts from the stress of engorgement. The mother expressed milk with a breast pump, and gradually reduced the number of minutes spent during each pumping session and the number of daily pumping sessions.

For example, on Day 1, the mother dropped one feeding. She pumped for 12 minutes at all the rest of her regular feeding times. The baby received bottles of pumped milk until it became necessary to use formula. The mother followed this schedule for several days until her breasts felt comfortable at the reduced level of milk production. She then reduced the duration of pumping at each session to 10 minutes, holding at this level for a few days until her milk production stabilized. Next, she dropped another scheduled pumping session. She continued in this manner, alternating between dropping minutes of pumping and dropping entire pumping sessions until milk production ceased. Whenever she became uncomfortable during the weaning process, she was instructed to use the pump briefly to relieve built up milk pressure. Because of her history of abscesses and the milk overproduction issues, an extremely slow and careful weaning was necessary to protect her.

The LC recommended the mother hold her dressings in place using a sports bra. Wearing such a bra also helped to stabilize the mother's breast so that motion would not stress the healing incisions. The soft cotton-lycra bra material allowed the breasts to "breathe," while providing support.

Fig. 267 shows the same mother 6 months after the original surgery. She returned to the breast surgeon when she discovered another mass in her breast. Ultrasound detected a *galactocele*, a sterile, milk-filled cyst. The surgeon reopened the upper incision (covered in the photo) and removed the cyst. In the photo, the mother points to the other original surgical site located at the areolar edge.

Subsequent Lactation Following
Surgery for Breast Abscess

The mother pictured in **Figs. 266** and **267** became pregnant again when her oldest child was only 11 months old. Her surgically-affected breast appeared still to be healing, with reddened, keloid scar tissue that stretched and remained tender to the touch throughout her pregnancy. Her son was born at term, 20 months after the original abscesses were treated. The mother again experienced a copious milk supply. She was counseled to rest and to guard against excessive fatigue and engorgement.

Her nipples became cracked and she complained of a plugged duct in her right breast, although in a different location from the previous abscess sites. The breast surgeon was immediately consulted and placed the woman on prophylactic antibiotics. The mass in her breast persisted. She did not experience fever, but her right breast became increasingly tender, especially over the locations of the old scars. The surgeon detected another galactocele; however, he said that since it was not growing, no immediate action or any surgical intervention was required to excise it. Galactoceles are often left alone providing they are not growing rapidly, are not painful, and do not obstruct or impair lactation.

The mother in this case study experienced 4 episodes of mastitis over the next 6 months; 2 in each breast. When she introduced solid foods to the baby at 6 months, her copious milk oversupply began to resolve. Once production lessened, her baby was able to keep the breasts comfortably drained. She experienced no additional episodes of breast inflammation, and breast-fed her son until he was almost 2 years old.

When this woman's third child was delivered, the surgeon and the LC discussed her situation and suggested the use of prophylactic benadryl during the engorgement phase to see if the drying effect of this medication would help reduce the woman's milk supply and prevent mastitis. The

mother was instructed to take the medication at bedtime. Her baby slept 4 to 5 hours overnight, and her breasts often became painfully engorged by morning. Oral Benadryl appeared to be effective in managing the woman's milk oversupply in the early weeks of lactation, and she avoided developing mastitis. However, because benadryl causes drowsiness, subsequently published research suggests that pseudoephedrine would confer the same benefit without the risk of sleepiness (Aljazaf 2003). If seen today, BWC would refer this mother for consideration of estrogen therapy to reduce milk production owing to her increased risk of breast abscess formation.

Abscess Drainage Tubes

Fig. 268 shows drainage tubes being used to drain pus from an abscess in the breast of a woman who was breast-feeding twins. The mother had recently returned to a part time job. Perhaps extra fatigue and incomplete breast emptying resulted in mastitis with subsequent abscess development. The woman initially had 3 drains, but one had fallen out at the time of the photograph.

Clumps in the Milk

In dairy herds, visible changes in the milk often signal the onset of mastitis. Clots or clumps of cellular debris (pus) in the milk alert the farmer to early stage illness in the animal (Milner 1996). Infected milk in cattle has higher amounts of free fatty acids, suggesting that it is susceptible to spontaneous and induced *lipolysis* (the breakdown of fat). Clumps in a woman's milk may be evidence of a similar mechanism in humans.

Some women report that milk pumped during bouts of mastitis contains congealed globules of material. A mother with mastitis at 3 weeks postpartum has pumped milk from the affected breast and poured the milk through a tea strainer (**Fig. 269**). The clumping is clearly visible. If infection affects the chemical composition of milk, it may be more likely to coagulate (Newton 1997a). Women can be reassured that the clumps will go away. No research reports suggest that mothers should withhold their milk from their infants during mastitis (AAP 2006) unless the baby is in the intensive care unit for illness or prematurity (Neifert 1999, Behari 2004).

The American Academy of Pediatrics (2006) considers the presence of a breast abscess as a contraindication to breastfeeding, and advises mothers not to feed milk from a breast still draining pus owing to the number of pathogens the infant might consume. The mother with a healing abscess in **Fig. 263** is breastfeeding her baby. The pus has been drained, and she is taking antibiotics to protect against infection. The abscess is draining serous fluid, blood, and occasionally, milk. The ABM Protocol #4 supports this mother's actions; however, owing to concerns about emerging pathogens, such as MRSA, increased caution is required in abscess cases. Behari (2004) reported that MRSA-infected breast milk contributes to increased morbidity and mortality in babies in special care nurseries, consequently, milk from a mastitic breast is discarded.

Case Study of a Mother with Methicillin-resistant *Staphylococcus Aureus*

KH consulted with a G1 P1 L1 mother at 4 weeks postpartum who requested a consultation for pain in her right breast.

Sept. 3. Two days before the initial LC visit, the woman's breast surgeon drained a cyst using needle aspiration at 9:00 AM. By mid-afternoon, the mother experienced sharp, shooting pains in that breast. The breast became engorged, and the baby refused it. By late afternoon, the mother began taking ibuprofen for pain. She used a pump to relieve the fullness, and observed blood-stained milk. In the middle of the night the woman began to feel ill. She experienced chills and fever of 103.5°F. She contacted her doctor and began treatment with dicloxacillin at about 5:00 AM. She noticed that her pumped milk had turned yellow.

Sept. 5. When the mother phoned the LC 2 days after the aspiration procedure, she was concerned about blisters that had begun to form on the face of her right nipple. She told the LC that her right breast remained full and firm. She could not get her baby to latch on, and could no longer express any milk. She had been on antibiotics for 40 hours with only minimal improvement.

That evening, the LC made a home visit to evaluate the mother's situation. The mother's entire right breast was red and hot (**Fig. 270**), and her temperature was 102°F in spite of antibiotic therapy. The mother pumped for 2 hours and only obtained 2 ounces (57 g) from her right breast. The pumping had not succeeded in softening the area around the areola, although the breast was somewhat softened toward the chest wall. Milk dripped, rather than squirted, during pumping, suggesting that the flow was blocked. The milk was bright yellow (**Fig. 271**). The LC was concerned about the possibility of subareolar abscesses. She urged the mother to call the doctor immediately to report her symptoms.

Sept. 6. Because the next day was a holiday the mother ignored the LC's advice and chose not to "bother" the doctor. She kept trying to soften the breast during the

night, but was only able to extract an additional ounce (28 g) of milk from her right breast. The LC made a follow-up phone call in the morning. The mother's temperature was still elevated. When she learned that the mother had not reported her symptoms to the doctor, the LC explained that in her opinion the mother's situation constituted an emergency. The mother agreed to phone the physician, who insisted she be immediately evaluated. After examining her, the doctor admitted the woman to the hospital and began antibiotic treatment with intravenous (IV) levofloxacin (Levaquin®). The baby was allowed to accompany her to the hospital.

Sept. 7. Ultrasound revealed no abscesses and suggested a diagnosis of *cellulitis* (mastitis of the interlobular connective tissue). The mother was now pumping orange milk (**Fig. 272**).

Sept. 9. After 3 days of IV antibiotic, the mother still had fever and her condition had not improved. The family was advised to discontinue feeding her milk to the baby due to concerns about prolonged infant exposure to levofloxacin.

Sept. 10. On Day 7 of the infection, cultures indicated that the breast infection was caused by methicillin-resistant *S. aureus* (MRSA). IV vancomycin therapy was immediately begun. After this antibiotic therapy was initiated, the mother slowly began to improve.

Sept. 13. Within 3 days after beginning vancomycin therapy, the mother began breastfeeding again on the unaffected breast. The mother had maintained her milk supply through the crisis by pumping at 3 hour intervals. She was able to pump close to 24 ounces in 24 hours. This volume of milk is considered to constitute a full supply. The milk pumped from the affected breast had clumps of debris in it the size of large coins. After her week-long hospitalization, the mother was discharged home still receiving IV vancomycin.

Sept. 15. The LC made a home visit to take photos. The breast looked more inflamed than it had appeared at the initial visit (**Fig. 273**). The mother was pumping red milk (**Fig. 274**). The area of the breast where infection had destroyed the connective tissue layer is evident in **Fig. 275**. Milk can be seen leaking though the broken skin at the site of the original needle aspiration. The mother used disposable diapers to absorb the leaking milk. **Fig. 276** shows a plug of congealed milk being pulled through a hole at the aspiration site on the breast. The woman's expressed milk still contained clots of congealed material (**Fig. 277**).

Oct. 5. Almost a month later, IV antibiotic therapy was terminated. The mother had been pumping and discarding milk from her mastitic breast during this time. For the next few weeks, the mother continued to pump her healing breast and fed the pumped milk to the baby by bottle.

Oct. 20. In **Fig. 278** the mother is shown feeding the baby from the unaffected breast. For 25 days from the night of the consult, the baby received some formula supplements, but continued breastfeeding from the left breast. Over time, the milk supply increased in the left breast. Within one month the baby's milk needs were entirely satisfied by the healthy breast. The appearance of the breast was much improved, although milk can still be observed leaking from the wound in **Fig. 279**. Around this time, the baby resumed feeding from the affected breast with no ill effects observed.

Nov. 12. The mother saw the doctor for the last time. The broken skin on her right breast had healed and she was no longer leaking milk from the wound. A month later, the mother returned to full-time employment.

Fig. 280 shows the completely healed breast shortly before the baby's first birthday. The mother breastfed this child for 2.5 years, weaning midway through her next pregnancy.

Unanswered questions remain pertaining to this case. Where did the woman acquire this virulent infection? MRSA may be acquired during the hospital stay via cracked nipples. Saiman (2003) described the cases of 8 postpartum women who developed skin and soft tissue infections with MRSA with a mean time after delivery of 23 days. The pathogen, in this case, may have entered the woman's breast at the time of the aspiration procedure. Her husband was a physician. It is also possible he may have unwittingly carried the infection home on his clothes or skin.

Follow-up is an important part of an LC's care plan. This case graphically illustrates the wisdom of close follow-up. Fortunately, KH recognized that this mother's condition was worsening. Her persistence was critical in assuring that the mother followed through in reporting her symptoms to a doctor. Sometimes the LC encounters situations that require immediate medical attention. In such cases, the LC should contact the HCP by phone for guidance. This case also documents the length of treatment sometimes required for full resolution of symptoms. Such experiences are traumatic for the whole family, and the LC provides important emotional support to her client during this time. Sharing case details can often reassure families that this sort of thing has happened to other women and that the problem will eventually resolve.

Inflammatory Breast Conditions and Maternal Depression

BWC has observed clinically that most of the women she has worked with who have suffered from prolonged breast inflammation also appeared to be struggling with some degree of mental depression. These mothers typically appeared to feel as overwhelmed emotionally as they did physically. It may be that illness of any kind triggers some degree of depression; however, BWC routinely provides anticipatory guidance about managing transient symptoms of depression whenever mastitis occurs. This guidance may consist of simple reassurance that mood will lift as soon as she begins to recover. It also involves the advice to rest, eat a nutritious diet, and to seek help with baby care and housework. The family's support must be enlisted. The LC should also discuss with her client and the family the importance of talking to the HCP if depression worsens.

A connection may exist between inflammation in the body and alterations in the brain that affect mood. In fact, Kendall-Tackett (2007) identifies inflammation as the *key* risk factor for depression. She explains that proinflammatory cytokine elevation is part of normal host defense; however, the chemical changes that result exert an effect upon the brain, including the increased release of cortisol, a stress hormone. Kendell-Tacket suggests that in order to prevent postpartum depression, care providers and families should reduce maternal stress and carefully treat inflammatory conditions to protect maternal mood.

Lactation Mastitis and the Baby-friendly Hospital Initiative

A cross-sectional Brazilian study identified a lower prevalence of lactation mastitis in women who delivered in hospitals certified as Baby-Friendly (Vieira 2006). Consequently, the LC should advocate for policy implementations that facilitate more comprehensive care for postpartum women in order to ensure successful initiation of lactation. Mastitis constitutes an important source of physical and mental distress and cost for women and their families. Additionally, premature weaning resulting from mastitis puts infants at risk. More research is required to identify how to prevent mastitis. Optimal protocols for the management of inflammatory conditions of lactation need to be more widely disseminated among medical care providers. Lactation consultants must be better trained to be vigilant with follow-up to make sure problems resolve in a timely and expected manner. They should not fail to advocate for appropriate medical care for clients when necessary.

Academy of Breastfeeding Medicine (ABM) Protocol Committee. Protocol # 4: Mastitis. *Breastfeeding Medicine* 2008; 3(3):177-180. http://www.bfmed.org/ace-files/mastitisprotocol4.pdf Accessed Oct, 2008.

Aljazaf K, Hale T, Ilett K, et al. Pseudoephedrine: effects on milk production in women and estimation of infant exposure via breastmilk. *British Journal of Clinical Pharmacology* 2003; 56(1):18-24.

American Academy of Pediatrics (AAP). Committee on Infectious Diseases. *2006 Red Book: Report of the Committee on Infectious Diseases,* 27th ed. Elk Grove Village, IL: American Academy of Pediatrics, 2006.

Amir L. Mastitis: are we overprescribing antibiotics? *Current Therapeutics* April 2000; 24-28.

Amir LH, Forster D, McLachlan H, et al. Incidence of breast abscess in lactating women: report from an Australian cohort. *BJOG: International Journal of Obstetrics and Gynaecology* 2004; 111(12):1378-1381.

Amir LH, Forster DA, Lumley J, et al. A descriptive study of mastitis in Australian breastfeeding women: incidence and determinants. *BMC Public Health* 2007; 7(147):62.

Amir L, Harris H, Andriske L. An audit of mastitis in the emergency department. *Journal of Human Lactation* 1999; 15(3):221-224.

Amir LH, Garland SM, Lumley J. A case-control study of mastitis: nasal carriage of *Staphylococcus aureus. BMC Family Practice* 2006; 7:57.

Behari P, Englund J, Alcasid G, et al. Transmission of methicillin-resistant *Staphylococcus aureus* to preterm infants through breast milk. *Infection Control and Hospital Epidemiology* 2004; 25(9):778-780.

Berens P. Management of Lactation in the Puerperium, in *Hale & Hartmann's Textbook of Human Lactation*. Amarillo, TX: Hale Publishing, 2007; p. 363.

Buescher ES, Hiar PS. Human milk anti-inflammatory component contents during acute mastitis. *Cellular Immunology* 2001; 210:87-95.

Christensen A, Al-Suliman N, Nielsen K, et al. Ultrasound-guided drainage of breast abscesses: results in 151 patients. *British Journal of Radiology* 2005; 78(927):186-188.

Cotterman KJ. Reverse pressure softening: a simple tool to prepare areola for easier latching during engorgement. *Journal of Human Lactation* 2004; 20(2):227-237.

Cox D, Kent J, Casey T, et al. Breast growth and the urinary excretion of lactose during human pregnancy and early lactation: endocrine relationships. *Experimental Physiology* 1999; 84(2):421-434.

Dahlbeck S, Donnelly J, Theriault R. Differentiating inflammatory breast cancer from acute mastitis. *American Family Physician* 1995; 52(3):929-934.

Daly S, Kent J, Owens R, et al. Frequency and degree of milk removal and the short-term control of human milk synthesis. *Experimental Physiology* 1996; 81(5):861-875.

Dixon J. Repeated aspiration of breast abscess in lactating women. *British Medical Journal* 1988; 297(6662):1517-18.

Eglash A, Proctor R. A breastfeeding mother with chronic breast pain. *Breastfeeding Medicine* 2007; 2(2):99-104.

Fetherston C. Management of lactation mastitis in a Western Australian cohort. *Breastfeeding Review* 1997; 5(2):13-19.

Fetherston C. Risk factors for lactation mastitis. *Journal of Human Lactation* 1998; 14(2):101-109.

Fetherston C. Mastitis in lactating women: physiology or pathology? *Breastfeeding Review* 2001; 9(1):5-12.

Fetherston CM, Lai CT, Hartmann PE. Relationships between symptoms and changes in breast physiology during lactation mastitis. *Breastfeeding Medicine* 2006; 1(3):136-145.

Filteau S, Rice A, Ball J, et al. Breast milk immune factors in Bangladeshi women supplemented postpartum with retinol or beta-carotene. *American Journal of Clinical Nutrition* 1999; 69(5):953-958.

Fortunov RM, Hulten KG, Hammerman WA, et al. Community-acquired *Staphylococcus aureus* infections in term and near-term previously healthy neonates. *Pediatrics* 2006; 118(3):874-881.

Foxman B, Schwartz K, Looman S. Breastfeeding practices and lactation mastitis. *Social Science Medicine* 1994; 38(5):755-761.

Foxman B, D'Arcy H, Gillespie B, et al. Lactation mastitis: occurrence and medical management among 946 breastfeeding women in the United States. *American Journal of Epidemiology* 2002; 155(2):103-114.

Furlong A, al-Nakib L, Knox W, et al. Periductal inflammation and cigarette smoke. *Journal of the American College of Surgeons* 1994; 179(4):417-420.

Hale T. *Medications and Mothers' Milk,* 13th ed. Amarillo, TX: Hale Publishing, 2008; pp. 805-806, 1101.

Hansen L. *Immunobiology of Human Milk.* Amarillo, Texas: Pharmasoft Publishing, 2004; pp. 196-203.

Hayes R, Michell M, Nunnerley HB. Acute inflammation of the breast–the role of breast ultrasound in diagnosis and management. *Clinical Radiology* 1991; 44(4):253-256.

Hill P, Humenick S. The occurrence of breast engorgement. *Journal of Human Lactation* 1994; 10(2):79-86.

Humenick S, Hill P. Breast engorgement: patterns and selected outcomes. *Journal of Human Lactation* 1994; 10(2):87-93.

Inch S, Fisher C. Mastitis: infection or inflammation? *The Practitioner* 1995; 239(1553):472-476.

Jain E. Personal correspondence, 2001.

Karstrup S, Nolsoe C, Brabrand K, et al. Ultrasonically guided percutaneous drainage of breast abscesses. *Acta Radiologica* 1990; 31(2):157-159.

Karstrup S. Acute puerperal breast abscesses: US-guided drainage. *Radiology* 1993; 188(3):807-809.

Kasonka L, Makasa M, Marshall T, et al. Risk factors for subclinical mastitis among HIV-infected and uninfected women in Lusake, Zambia. *Paediatric Perinatology and Epidemiology* 2006; 20(5):379-391.

Kendall-Tackett K. A new paradigm for depression in new mothers: the central role of inflammation and how breastfeeding and anti-inflammatory treatments protect maternal mental health. *International Breastfeeding Journal* 2007; 2:6.

King J. Contraception and lactation. *Journal of Midwifery and Womens Health* 2007; 52(6):614-620.

Kvist LJ, Hall-Lord ML, Rydhstroem H. A randomised-controlled trial in Sweden of acupuncture and care interventions for the relief of inflammatory symptoms of the breast during lactation. *Midwifery* 2007; 23(2):184-195.

Kvist LJ, Rydhstroem H. Factors related to breast abscess after delivery: a population-based study. *British Journal of Obstetrics and Gynecology* 2005; 112(8):1070-1074.

Lawrence RA, Lawrence RM. *Breastfeeding: A Guide for the Medical Profession, 6th ed.*. Philadelphia, PA: Elsevier Mosby, 2005; pp. 575, 579.

Livingstone V. Too much of a good thing. Maternal and infant hyperlactation syndromes. *Canadian Family Physician* 1996; 42:89-99.

Livingstone V, Stinger LJ. The treatment of *Staphylococcus aureus* infected sore nipples: a randomized comparative study. *Journal of Human Lactation* 1999; 15(3):241-246.

Love S. Dr. *Susan Love's Breast Book,* 3rd ed. Cambridge, MA: Persues Publishing, 2000; p. 11.

Meguid M, Oler A, Numann P, et al. Pathogenesis-based treatment of recurring subareolar breast abscesses. *Surgery* 1995; 118(4):775-82.

Michie C, Lockie F, Lynn W. The challenge of mastitis. *Archives of Disease in Childhood* 2003; 88(9):818-821.

Miller V, Riordan J. Treating postpartum breast edema with areolar compression. *Journal of Human Lactation* 2004; 20(2):223-226.

Milner P, Page K, Walton A. Detection of clinical mastitis by changes in electrical conductivity of foremilk before visible changes in milk. *Journal of Dairy Science* 1996; 79(1):83-6.

Minchin M. *Breastfeeding Matters, 4th ed.* Victoria, Australia: Alma Press, 1998; p. 152.

Mohrbacher N, Stock J. *The Breastfeeding Answer Book, 3rd ed.* Shaumburg, IL: La Leche League International, 2003; p. 500.

Moon J, Humenick S. Breast engorgement: contributing variables and variables amenable to nursing intervention. *Journal of Obstetric, Gynecologic and Neonatal Nursing* 1989; 18(4):309-315.

Neifert M. Clinical aspects of lactation: promoting breastfeeding success, in CL Wagner, DM Purohit (eds). *Clinics in Perinatology: Clinical Aspects of Human Milk and Lactation.* 1999; 26(2):281-306.

Newton E. Personal communication; 1997a.

Newton E. *Mastitis: Cause, Diagnosis, Treatment.* Schaumburg, IL: La Leche League, Int., 1997b; p. 4.

Newton M, Newton N. Postpartum engorgement of the breast. *American Journal of Obstetrics & Gynecology* 1951; 61(3):664-667.

Noble R, Bovey A. Therapeutic teat use for babies who breastfeed poorly. *Breastfeeding Review* 1997; 5(2):37-42.

O'Hara R, Dexter S, Fox J. Conservative management of infective mastitis and breast abscesses after ultrasonographic assessment. *British Journal of Surgery* 1996; 83(10):1413-1414.

Olsen CG, Gordon RE. Breast disorders in nursing mothers. *American Family Physician* 1990; 41(5):1509-1516.

Osterman K, Rahm U. Lactation mastitis: bacterial cultivation of breast milk, symptoms, treatment, and outcome. *Journal of Human Lactation* 2000; 16(4):297-302.

Page SM, McKenna DS. Vasospasm of the nipple presenting as painful lactation. *Obstetrics and Gynecology* 2006; 108(3 Pt 2):806-808.

Peacock SJ, Justice A, Griffiths D. Determinants of acquisition and carriage of *Staphylococcus aureus* in infancy. *Journal of Clinical Microbiology* 2003; 41(12):5718-5725.

Ramsay D, Kent J, Owens R, et al. Ultrasound imaging of milk ejection in the breast of lactating women. *Pediatrics* 2004; 113(2):361-367.

Rand S, Kolberg A. Neonatal hypernatremic dehydration secondary to lactation failure. *Journal of the American Board of Family Practice* 2001; 14(2):155-158.

Riordan J. *Breastfeeding and Human Lactation, 3rd ed.* Boston, MA: Jones and Bartlett Publishers, 2005; pp. 250-255.

Riordan JM, Nichols FH. A descriptive study of lactation mastitis in long-term breastfeeding women. *Journal of Human Lactation* 1990; 6(2):53-58.

Royal College of Midwives. *Successful Breastfeeding, 3rd ed,* London: Churchill Livingstone, 2002; pp. 105-110.

Saiman L, O'Keefe M, Graham P, et al. Hospital transmission of community-acquired methicillin-resistant *Staphylococcus aureus* among postpartum women. *Clinical Infectious Diseases* 2003; 37(10):1313-1319.

Semba R, Newton K, Taha T, et al. Mastitis and immunological factors in breast milk of human imunodeficiency virus-infected women. *Journal of Human Lactation* 1999; 15(4):301-306.

Snowden H, Renfrew M, Woolridge M. Treatments for breast engorgement during lactation *Cochrane Database System Review 2001;* (2): CD00046.

Thomassen P, Johansson V, Wassberg C, et al. Breast-feeding, pain and infection. *Gynecologic and Obstetric Investigation* 1998; 46(2):73-74.

Thomsen A, Hansen K, Moller B. Leukocyte counts and microbiologic cultivation in the diagnosis of puerperal mastitis. *American Journal of Obstetrics and Gynecology* 1983; 146(8):938-941.

Ulitzsch D, Nyman M, Carlson R. Breast abscess in lactating women: US-guided treatment. *Radiology* 2004; 232(3):904-909.

van Veldhuizen-Staas C. Overabundant milk supply: an alternate way to intervene by full drainage and block feeding. *International Breastfeeding Journal* 2007; 2:11.

Vieira GO, Silva LR, Mendes CM, et al. Lactational mastitis and Baby-Friendly Hospital Initiative, Feira de Santana, Bahia, Brazil. *Cad Suade Publica* 2006; 22(6):1193-1200. (in Portuguese, abstract in English)

Vogel A, Hutchison L, Mitchell E. Mastitis in the first year postpartum. *Birth* 1999; 26(4):218-225.

Wilson-Clay B. Milk Oversupply. *Journal of Human Lactation* 2006; 22(2):218-220.

Wilson-Clay B. Case report of Methicillin-resistant *Staphylococcus aureus* (MRSA) mastitis with abscess formation in a breastfeeding woman. *Journal of Human Lactation* 2008; 25(3):326-329.

Wust J, Rutsch M, Stocker S. *Streptococcus pneumoniaeas:* an agent of mastitis (letter). *European Journal of Clinical Microbiology and Infectious Diseases* 1995; 14(2):156-157.

Notes:

Breast Cancer: Issues For Lactation

Epidemiological evidence suggesting that prolonged breast-feeding protects against breast cancer has accumulated in recent years (Chang-Claud 2000, Zheng 2000, Kim 2007, Shema 2007). Studies show a decreasing risk of breast cancer with increasing number of months of breastfeeding. The mechanisms of this protective effect are not fully understood.

Perhaps lactation has a flushing effect on debris that accumulates in the ducts of the breast (Helewa 2002). The yellow color of colostrum derives from the presence of carotenoid fat globules. Djuric (2005) studied nipple aspirate fluid taken from women who had never lactated and women who lactated only for short periods, compared to nipple fluid aspirated from women who lactated 6 months or more. Carotenoid and tocopherol levels were significantly higher in nipple aspirate fluid from women who lactated for 6 months or more. Carotenoids and tocopherols are thought to be protective against breast cancer. Carotenoids may dilute and help expel substances stored in the non-lactating gland such as DDT, PCB, and other environmental contaminants (Patton 1990).

Fully breastfeeding women also enjoy extended periods of lactation related amenorrhea. Perhaps a lifetime reduction in number of months of breast exposure to hormones that potentiate the growth of cancer cells explains the protective effect of breatfeeding.

At one point, it was thought that a woman's intake of dietary fat might increase her risk of developing breast cancer, and that increasing dietary fiber might reduce it. Studies do not support this theory (Rohan 1988, Willett 1992). However, diet in *early childhood* may affect the risk of developing breast cancer later in life.

Freudenheim (1994) observed that having been breast-fed is associated with a decrease in breast cancer. Martin (2005) performed a meta-analysis on a large cohort of cancer patients and identified a significantly reduced risk of premenopausal breast cancer in women who had been breastfed.

A number of countries have noted increasing rates of breast cancer in their populations as rates of breastfeeding incidence and duration have fallen (Shema 2007, Kim 2007). Because having been breastfed as a child and breastfeeding each appear to be independently protective, the choice to breastfeed may be one of the few proactive measures that can be undertaken to lower a woman's lifetime risk of developing breast cancer. In fact, the

evidence for a protective effect of breastfeeding is now sufficiently well-established to motivate changes in cancer prevention policy recommendations. In 2002, the Collaborative Group on Hormonal Factors in Breast Cancer concluded that "The longer women breastfeed the more they are protected against breast cancer. The lack of or the short lifetime duration of breastfeeding typical of women in developed countries makes a major contribution to the high incidence of breast cancer in these countries." Such statements have resulted in specific recommendations to women urging exclusive breastfeeding for 6 months, and the continuation of breastfeeding after the introduction of solids as a cancer prevention strategy (WCRF 2007).

Families should also be aware that radiation exposure to breast tissue during childhood, experienced, for example, during diagnostic scans, may affect breast development and impact lactation later in life. Whenever possible, breast tissue should be shielded, even in young children (Coursey 2008).

The protective effect of breastfeeding does not alter the fact that it is still possible for an individual woman to develop breast cancer during pregnancy or lactation. Individuals who have been breastfed may still develop breast cancer. The incidence of breast cancer in young women has risen, and because many women now delay child-bearing, pregnancy following treatment for breast cancer is more common (Dow 1994). Owing to these demographic factors, more women will develop breast cancer during pregnancy and lactation. The LC must be aware of the symptoms that require evaluation to rule out breast cancer.

Breast Cancer During Pregnancy and Lactation

Breast cancer is the second leading cause of cancer deaths among American women. The American Cancer Society in 2007 reported that about 178,000 women are diagnosed with breast cancer each year in the US. Of these, 25 percent develop tumors in their child bearing years (Camune 2007). The incidence of breast cancers occurring in pregnant or lactating women is felt to be 2 to 3 per 1,000 (Steyskall 1996).

Unfortunately, diagnosis and treatment are often delayed in pregnant and lactating women. The reasons for this are complex and include both lack of awareness, health care provider distraction, and psychological denial. As with other types of cancer, early identification provides the best chance of survival.

Prenatal care should include serial breast examinations, and women should continue monthly breast self-examinations during lactation. It is normal for lactating breasts to feel lumpy, and plugged ducts and mastitis are not unusual events. However, a discrete lump that is different from surrounding breast tissue may be a sign of breast cancer (Lind 2004). Breast exams increase the woman's familiarity with changes in her own breasts, alert her to masses that do not resolve with standard treatment, and alert her to masses that recur persistently in the same area of the breast. A physician should evaluate such masses.

Health care providers may be distracted by conditions such as pregnancy and lactation, dismissing or ignoring symptoms that would, in a nonlactating woman, trigger prompt evaluation. Misdiagnosis of carcinoma of the breast is the most frequent cause of malpractice litigation in the United States. The willingness to seek a second opinion has saved many lives.

Private practice lactation consultants may encounter situations where a woman presents with suspicious findings (Petok 1995). It is important for LCs to know the warning signs for breast cancer in order to refer women for prompt medical evaluation.

Red Flags and Warning Signs for Breast Cancer

The following warning signs require prompt referral to the woman's primary care provider:

- Skin color changes on the breast, especially in the absence of fever (Dahlbeck 1995, Cristofanilli 2003)
- Skin texture chances, *peu d'orange* (pitting),
- **Figs. 253** and **254**, edema, *indurations,* **Fig. 289**.
- Masses, especially fixed, irregular shaped lumps
- Copious, spontaneous, clear or bloody nipple discharge (typically unilateral)
- Mastitis that occurs repeatedly in the same area and does not resolve with conservative treatment (i.e., with appropriate drugs and management)

Diagnostic Tests and Lactation

It is possible to perform diagnostic tests on pregnant and lactating women without weaning, although mammograms are more difficult to interpret owing to the density of the pregnant and lactating breast. Ductal lavage is a technique to achieve non-invasive access to breast tissue. It involves duct cannulation and endoscopy. The duct is washed, and the flushed tissue is examined for breast cancer and precancerous changes (Love 1996). However, whether the ductal lavage technique is diagnostically useful during lactation is unknown.

Ultrasound (**Fig 281**) is a safe diagnostic technique that can be used during pregnancy and lactation. It is painless and useful in distinguishing between cystic (fluid-filled) and solid masses (Freund 2000, Lind 2004).

Galactoceles are a type of cyst that can form in the breast during lactation. The material aspirated from such a cyst is milk. Abscesses are another type of cystic lesion, and the aspirate will include purulent material (pus). Needle biopsy can be performed to examine cells aspirated from masses that have been identified by ultrasound. Ch. 11 contains a full discussion of types of abscesses.

Tumors are solid (rather than cystic) masses. Many types of tumors (such as fibrocysts) are benign. A breast biopsy is the most definitive type of diagnostic measure used to identify the nature of a mass and to rule out cancer. Because it is a surgical procedure, it is the most invasive diagnostic tool. While it is often necessary, biopsy poses a certain degree of risk to current or future lactation owing to incision and removal of tissue (Osuch 1998). Such risk, however, must be evaluated in terms of its potential for saving the mother's life.

Inflammatory Breast Cancer

Inflammatory breast cancer is a particularly aggressive form of cancer with a high mortality rate. Early diagnosis is critical. However, diagnosis of this type of breast cancer may be delayed because it shares important symptoms with mastitis: pain, tenderness and firmness of the breast. While a woman with inflammatory breast cancer typically experiences no fever, the breast becomes warm, red, heavy and edematous, often presenting with peu d'orange pitting. The area of redness is generally large, often covering the whole breast. The nipple appears flattened and *indurated* (retracted). Nipple skin may become crusted (Dahlbeck 1995). Inflammatory breast cancer may occur during pregnancy and lactation, and can be difficult to detect with mammography. Examination of malignant cells accessed by fine needle or excision biopsy confirms the diagnosis.

African American women have a higher incidence of inflammatory breast cancer than do Caucasians and other ethnic groups (Cristofanilli 2003).

Women and clinicians may be distracted by the presence of pregnancy and lactation, attributing important signs of breast cancer instead to plugged ducts or to mastitis. It is important to remember that if appropriate antibiotic therapy does not result in marked improvement within 2 days, or if symptoms recur in the same area of the breast, further evaluation is required to rule out other disease, including breast cancer.

Breastfeeding after Treatment for Breast Cancer

Breastfeeding is discontinued during chemotherapy for breast cancer because the drugs used are toxic and may harm a breastfeeding baby. Additionally, it is felt that the mother needs to conserve metabolic energy toward her survival.

Some women become infertile as the result of chemotherapy, and experience chemical menopause. Others succeed in becoming pregnant after treatment and can breastfeed. No survival disadvantage has been identified by subsequent pregnancy or lactation (Dow 1994, Kasum 2006, Camune 2007). There is no contraindication for breastfeeding after treatment for breast cancer (Danforth 1991). Lactation usually proceeds normally in the unaffected breast. In the treated breast, functional lactation is possible, but generally milk production is significantly diminished in the majority of patients (Moran 2005).

Some women elect to preserve part of the affected breast by choosing lumpectomy rather than mastectomy. Radiation therapy and the damage to the structures of the breast caused by invasive surgery may render the breast incapable of lactation. Partial lactation has occurred in some cases, resulting in some ability to lactate on the treated breast (Higgins 1994).

David (1985) reports a case of a 36 year-old woman who had a "poorly differentiated infiltrating ductal carcinoma in the right tail of Spence area." The mass was excised and her nodes were unaffected. She received radiation therapy, and became pregnant a year later. Her treated breast did not enlarge as much as the untreated left breast during the pregnancy, but following the birth the treated breast did lactate. The milk was slightly thicker, and it produced about half the amount of milk that the left breast produced.

BWC worked with a woman who breastfed unilaterally following treatment for breast cancer with lumpectomy. The lumpectomized breast became engorged following the birth of the baby. The mother observed spontaneous leaking. Because the woman elected not to stimulate that breast, it soon involuted. She breastfed her child uneventfully on the unaffected breast.

Lumpectomy

The 48 year-old woman shown in **Fig. 282** has a radial incision over the location of a lumpectomy. She had breastfed her children. A history of having breastfed does not justify complacency regarding the development of lumps in the breast. Interestingly, a faint scar from an earlier biopsy is visible, running exactly parallel to the lumpectomy scar, at the areolar edge. This earlier biopsy revealed a benign tumor. For a younger woman, with more childbearing years ahead of her, a radial rather than a circumferential incision might lessen the impact of such invasive surgery.

The same woman is pictured in **Fig. 283** during radiation therapy. Note the bronzed appearance of the skin. Approximately 90 percent of patients treated with radiation therapy will develop some degree of radiation-induced dermatitis (Harper 2004) that can produce significant discomfort and limit daily activity. Previously, soap and water washing of irradiated skin was discouraged owing to concern that a drying effect of soap would exacerbate radiation dermatitis. When systematically evaluated, however, moist *desquamation* (shedding of skin) developed in 33 percent of those who did not wash the skin as compared with 14 percent of those who washed with soap and water. Roy (2001) hypothesized that washing may reduce moist desquamation by removing skin microbes that act as inflammatory stimuli at the basal layer of the skin. The study concluded that washing the skin does not increase skin toxicity.

Fig. 284 shows the scar from an axillary biopsy taken to discern whether cancer has spread to the lymph nodes. The presence or absence of spread to the nodes defines the *stage* of the cancer. Staging is a way to conceptualize each case of breast cancer so that appropriate treatment can be selected. Stage 1 is a tumor with no affected lymph nodes. Stage 2 is a small tumor with positive lymph nodes, or a larger tumor with positive or negative nodes, or a large tumor with negative nodes. Stage 3 is a large tumor with positive lymph nodes, or a tumor with "grave signs." Stage 4 is a tumor that has obvious metastasis (Love 2000).

The woman in **Fig. 285** was treated 8 years prior for breast cancer with lumpectomy, radiation therapy, and chemotherapy. Her left breast did not experience any changes during pregnancy or postpartum. She planned to breastfeed using her right breast. It is interesting to note the size difference in her breasts from the increase in breast development during pregnancy.

Breastfeeding after Mastectomy

A 32 year-old woman is pictured in **Fig. 286**. She had 3 children at the time that she was diagnosed with breast cancer. Her affected breast was removed, and she was told that she would experience chemical menopause. She and her family were shocked when she became pregnant 4 years later. She described herself to the LC as having been "traumatized by my medical treatment." She had a home birth supported by a midwife, and 2 weeks later, requested to see the LC because of a cracked nipple on her remaining breast. Her baby was gaining well, and judging from the orientation of the wound, the main issue appeared to be a routine positioning and latch-on problem.

The mother was instructed to gently cleanse the wound in order to prevent nipple infection and mastitis and to pump the breast to give the nipple a chance to heal. The midwife prescribed mupirocin to prevent infection. The baby was bottle-fed pumped milk for 5 days until the wound healed. An experienced breastfeeding mother who was determined to succeed, this woman was not worried about subsequent breast refusal. As expected, the baby easily transitioned back to breastfeeding, and uneventful lactation proceeded.

The 28 year-old woman in **Fig. 287** is shown breastfeeding her 18 day-old third child following mastectomy for breast cancer. The woman's husband had discovered a lump in her left breast the previous summer. The mother was breastfeeding their 2 year-old son at the time. Because the mother was deaf, the father phoned BWC to describe the persistent mass in the breast. BWC recommended medical evaluation. A breast surgeon performed a needle biopsy and detected cancerous cells in the aspirate. The surgeon recommended immediate weaning and mastectomy to remove the breast and axillary lymph nodes.

BWC assisted with an emergency weaning and took photos of the process. In **Fig. 288** faint bruising appears over the location of the biopsy at 8 o'clock on the left breast. On Day 3 of the weaning (**Fig. 289**), engorgement has lessened to the extent that it is possible to perceive an induration on the underside of the breast where the tumor is located.

Chemotherapy and radiation treatment followed the mastectomy. During radiation treatment, the woman became pregnant, and her healthy daughter was born at term. Breastfeeding continued uneventfully for 5 months, during which time the baby grew normally feeding only from one breast. Gradual weaning was begun at this point to allow the mother's physicians to perform diagnostic tests in response to elevated tumor markers in her blood. Sadly, 5 years after these photos were taken, the young mother died of breast cancer.

Biopsy to Rule Out Paget's Disease of the Nipple

The 32 year-old mother whose nipple is pictured in **Figs. 290-292** nursed her first child uneventfully for 15 months. After the birth of her second child, she developed an eruption on her left nipple that continued essentially unabated for 5 months. The LC observed an oozing, crusty left nipple on Day 7 postpartum. The right nipple

was also cracked and irritated. The LC adjusted the mother's positioning, and antibiotics were begun within 24 hours because the mother had developed febrile symptoms. After a week on antibiotics, the mother developed the symptoms of what she suspected was a yeast infection. At 6 weeks postpartum, after constant medical treatment, the nipples appeared to be healing. However, because the nipples were still slightly inflamed, the mother consulted the first of 4 dermatologists. The first dermatologist advised the mother to apply a hydro-gel after each feeding, which immediately worsened her symptoms, especially on the left nipple.

Over the next months, the mother consulted 3 other dermatologists and continued contact with her obstetrician and her LC. The mother was treated for yeast infection, staph infection, and contact irritant dermatitis with Diflucan, Loprox, Ketoconazole, Zithromax, Locoid ointment, Elocon cream and Vaseline. Cultures from her milk and the baby's mouth and nose all showed normal flora. For a period of 3 months, the mother exclusively pumped, feeding the baby by bottle. While her nipples improved during the time she pumped, they never healed completely and worsened as soon as she resumed any breastfeeding.

At 6 months, the left nipple again appeared erythematous and edematous. A fourth dermatologist advised a punch biopsy to rule out *Paget's disease* (a type of cancer of the nipple that resembles eczema and is also referred to as erosive adenomatosis.) In **Fig. 290,** the dermatologist injects Lidocaine into the nipple to numb it. A numbing cream was applied previously to the nipple to reduce the sting of the injection.

In **Fig. 291** a small punch tool is used to remove a core of tissue (seen being removed in **Fig. 292**) that was sent to a lab for analysis. The sample indicated that there was no evidence of disease. In fact, there was no conclusive evidence even of a contact or irritant dermatitis. In short, nothing was discovered to explain this woman's chronic nipple irritation.

The dermatologist sutured the wound made by the biopsy. BWC expressed concern about the stitches, fearing they would interfere with breastfeeding. The mother phoned BWC several hours later to report that clots of blood had appeared in her pumped milk. Her breast was not draining well and felt engorged. In contrast to pumping, the baby was able to soften the breast, but the knot in the stiff sutures dug a deeper hole in her nipple each time the baby nursed. Additionally, her bra was rubbing on the sutures and this irritated the wound. The mother called the doctor who instructed her to remove the sutures. The doctor advised her to keep packing the hole in her nipple with mupirocin. However, within 24 hours, the mother's breast was bright red. She was diagnosed with mastitis and was treated with oral antibiotics. Once she began the oral antibiotics, healing proceeded uneventfully.

Several studies have discussed the development of atopic dermatitis, a chronic inflammatory skin disease, where colonization of skin with *S. aureus* is known to produce toxins with superantigen activity. Perhaps sensitization occurred early in the course of this mother's situation. At the time of the biopsy, her results showed only a dilated vasculature, a very non-specific finding; however, the LC was uncertain whether tests for superantigen activity were performed.

Although the mother in this case stated that she had no food allergies, she consumed large amounts of dairy products which she felt constituted the mainstay of her diet. BWC had advised a dairy elimination very early in the case, but the mother only abstained from dairy for about a week. During the biopsy, the LC and dermatologist discussed the possibility of a relationship between diet and the woman's sore nipples. After this discussion, the mother removed dairy products for several weeks and felt that it did make some difference. As time went on, the baby exhibited signs of atopic disease. He developed eczema and constipation around 6 months, and his mother had to remove dairy from his diet entirely by the time he reached toddlerhood.

Reaction from exposure to dairy protein in the mother's diet could have provoked salivary changes irritating to the nipple. It was interesting, however, that the nipple condition never totally resolved, even when the baby was not breastfeeding directly for long periods of time. The woman continued to breastfeed past the baby's second birthday. Her nipples, however, remained vulnerable, and breastfeeding was never comfortable for her. BWC stayed in contact with this woman, and 10 years later the woman reported no breast or nipple complications from her experience.

BWC is generally reluctant to advise dairy restriction; however, she observed another client whose sore nipples cleared up (after all other suggestions failed to bring results) when dairy protein was taken out of the woman's diet. Dairy elimination was trialed on the premise that a sensitive baby might experience salivary changes in reaction to exposure of the offending protein through the milk, and that these changes might irritate the nipple. A 3 week dairy elimination resulted in healed nipples. At the time, the supervising physician felt the improvement was merely coincidental; however, the mother was so relieved

to have no more nipple pain that she remained on the dairy-free diet.

It became clear that her baby was allergic to dairy protein when, at age 5 months, the father gave the baby a taste of ice cream from a spoon. A drop of ice cream also spilled on the baby's cheek. Within an hour, the baby was taken to the emergency room with symptoms of anaphylactic shock. The cheek was scalded where the ice cream touched it.

Extreme reactivity to minute quantities of allergen by skin contact is not unique. Another 5 cases are reported in the literature. One involved a 3 month-old male who later proved to have multiple food allergies. He developed localized skin irritation when his mother kissed him after eating cereal with milk (Tan 2001). In all 5 cases, reactions occurred while the children were being breastfed (exclusively in 4 and mixed feeding in one). A connection between food allergy and sore nipples deserves more investigation, and while it is important to rule out breast cancer (especially Paget's disease of the nipple), there may be alternate etiologies involved when nipples fail to heal.

Complex cases remind LCs that multiple causes exist for breast lumps and skin conditions of the nipples. Rarely are they cancer, but the LC has an ethical responsibility to not overlook suspicious symptoms that require further investigation by a qualified physician.

Note: Dr. Susan Love, author of *The Breast Book*, has launched an initiative to create a large pool of research subjects to help better understand the nature of breast cancer. To become involved and sign up, go to www.armyofwomen.org.

Camune B, Gabzdyl E. Breast-feeding after breast cancer in childbearing women. *Journal of Perinatal and Neonatal Nursing* 2007; 21(3):225-233.

Chang-Claude J, Eby N, Kiechle M, et al. Breastfeeding and breast cancer risk by age 50 among women in Germany. *Cancer Causes and Control* 2000; 11(8):687-695.

Cristofanilli M, Buzdar A, Hortobagyi G. Update on the management of inflammatory breast cancer. *The Oncologist* 2003; 8(2):141-148.

Collaborative Group on Hormonal Factors in Breast Cancer. Breast cancer and breastfeeding: collaborative re-analysis of individual data from 47 epidemiological studies in 30 countries, including 50302 women with breast cancer and 96973 women without the disease. *Lancet* 2002; 360(9328):187-195.

Coursey C, Frush DP, Yoshizumi T, et al. Pediatric chest MDCT using tube current modulation: effect on radiation dose with breast shielding. *American Journal of Roentgenology* 2008; 190:W54-W61.

Dahlbeck S, Donnelly J, Theriault R. Differentiating inflammatory breast cancer from acute mastitis. *American Family Physician* 1995; 52(3):929-934.

Danforth D. How subsequent pregnancy affects outcome in women with prior breast cancer. *Oncology* 1991; 5(11):23-35.

David F. Lactation following primary radiation therapy for carcinoma of the breast. *International Journal of Radiation Oncology, Biology, Physics* 1985; 11(7):1425.

Djuric Z, Visscher DW, Heilbrun LK, et al. Influence of lactation history on breast nipple aspirate fluid yield and fluid composition. *Breast Journal* 2005; 11(2):92-99.

Dow KH, Harris JR, Roy C. Pregnancy after breast-conserving surgery and radiation therapy for breast cancer. *Journal of the National Cancer Institute Monogram* 1994; (16):131-137.

Freudenheim J, Marshall J, Graham S, et al. Exposure to breastmilk in infancy and the risk of breast cancer. *Epidemiology* 1994; 5(3): 324-331.

Freund K. Rationale and technique of clinical breast examination. *Medscape Women's Health* 5(6), 2000.

Harper J, Franklin L, Jenrette J, et al. Skin toxicity during breast irradiation: pathophysiology and management. *Southern Medical Journal* 2004; 97(10):989-993.

Helewa M, Levesque P, Provencher D, et al. Breast cancer, pregnancy, and breastfeeding. *Journal of Obstetrics and Gynaecology Canada* 2002; 24(2):164-180.

Higgins S, Huffy B. Pregnancy and lactation after breast-conserving therapy for early stage breast cancer. *Cancer* 1994; 73(8):2175-2180.

Kasum M. Breast cancer treatment - later pregnancy and survival. *European Journal of Gynaecological Oncology* 2006; 27(3):225-229.

Kim Y, Choi JY, Lee KM, et al. Dose-dependent protective effect of breast-feeding against breast cancer among ever-lactated women in Korea. *European Journal of Cancer Prevention* 2007; 16(2):124-129.

Lind DS, Smith BL, Souba WW. 5 Breast Complaints. in Souba WW, Fink MP, Jurkovich GJ, et al. *ACS Surgery Online.* New York: WebMD Inc. 2004.

Love S. *Dr. Susan Love's Breast Book.* Cambridge, MA: Perseus Publishing, 2000; pp. 336-337.

Love S, Barsky S. Breast duct endoscopy to study stages of cancerous breast disease. *Lancet* 1996; 348(9033):997-999.

Martin RM, Middleton N, Gunnell D, et al. Breastfeeding and cancer: the Boyd Orr cohort and a systematic review with meta-analysis. *Journal of the National Cancer Institute* 2005; 97(19):1446-1457.

Moran MS, Colasanto JM, Haffty BG, et al. Effects of breast-conserving therapy on lactation after pregnancy. *Cancer Journal* 2005; 11(5):399-403.

Osuch J, Bonham V, Morris L. Primary care guide to managing a breast mass step by step workup. *Medscape/*womens.health/1998/v03.n05/wh3.

Patton S, Canfield L, Huston G, et al. Carotenoids of human colostrum. *Lipids* 1990; 25(3):159-65.

Petok E. Breast cancer and breastfeeding: five cases. *Journal of Human Lactation* 1995; 11(3):205-209.

Rohan T, McMichael A, Baghurst P. A population-based case-control study of diet and breast cancer in Australia. *American Journal of Epidemiology* 1988; 128(3):478-89.

Roy I, Fortin A, Larochelle M. The impact of skin washing with water and soap during breast irradiation: a randomized study. *Radiotherapy & Oncology* 2001; 58(3):333-339.

Shema L, Ore L, Ben-Shachar M, et al. The association between breast-feeding and breast cancer occurrence among Israeli Jewish women: a case control study. *Journal of Cancer Research and Clinical Oncology* 2007; 133(8):539-546.

Steyskal R. Minimizing the risk of delayed diagnosis of breast cancer. Medscape/womens.health/1996/v0.n07/w65.

Tan B, Sher M, Good R, et al. Severe food allergies by skin contact. *Annals of Allergy, Asthma, & Immunology* 2001; 86(5):583-86.

Willett W, Hunter D, Stampfer M, et al. Dietary fat and fiber in relation to risk of breast cancer. *Journal of the American Medical Association* 1992; 268(15):2037-2044.

World Cancer Research Fund (WCRF). Food, nutrition, physical activity, and the prevention of cancer: a global perspective. http://www.babyfriendly.org.uk/pdfs/World_Cancer_Research_Fund_2007-10.pdf. Accessed Feb. 2008.

Zheng R, Duan L, Liu Y, et al. Lactation reduces breast cancer risk in Shandong Province, China. *American Journal of Epidemiology* 2000; 152(12):1129-1135.

Twin, Triplet, and Tandem Breastfeeding

In the past decade, multiple births occurring in the United States and elsewhere have increased as the result of drugs used to treat infertility. Over 3 percent of infants born annually in the US result from a multiple gestation pregnancy (Geraghty 2004). Many of the women who deliver multiples want to breastfeed, and the benefits of breastfeeding can be extremely important to them. The lactation consultant may be called upon to assist with breastfeeding strategies when multiples arrive.

Increased Infant Risks Associated
with Multiple Birth

Mothers struggling with the challenges of integrating 2 or more babies into the family may worry about giving their babies less attention than a single child would receive. In fact, research suggests that this concern is valid, particularly in higher order multiples. Feldman (2005) reports that triplets scored lower than singletons and twins on developmental assessments at 6, 12, and 24 months. The smallest triplets showed decreased cognitive skills at 12 and 24 months compared with their siblings. See **Fig. 60** for an example of discordant twins.

Greater medical risk at birth, multiple-birth status, limited access to exclusive parenting, and reduced infant social involvement in the first 2 years were each predictive of lower cognitive outcomes at 2 years of age. Mothers of multiples may find it reassuring to know that the inter-action between mother and baby inherent in the activity of breastfeeding is a way to enhance infant stimulation and improve bonding and attachment. Human milk also provides nutrients vital for normal brain growth.

Prematurity is a frequent complication of multiple births. Additionally, multiples tend to be small for gestational age (SGA). Morley (2004) identified improved cognitive outcomes of SGA infants in breastfed versus formula fed babies. Given the higher risk of cognitive delay (especially in the smallest baby), breastfeeding is crucial for multiples and their mothers.

Depending on their size and condition, preterm babies often experience delays in going to the breast. Their behavioral cues are often indistinct, making it difficult for mothers to obtain positive feedback at feeding time, or to accurately identify infant stress cues.

Early interventions may be needed to support the milk supply and to encourage the mother to provide milk for her hospitalized babies. It is critical to ensure an abundant milk supply when the infants are too weak or small to stimulate the breasts. It is thus important for the LC to recommend double pumping with a hospital grade pump for at least 15 minutes at least 8 times a day as recommended by the AAP (2005). The transition to normal feeding will be easier if there is an ample milk supply.

Increased Maternal Risk Associated
with Multiple Birth

A large retrospective study comparing singleton with multiple-fetal pregnancies identified a higher incidence of maternal health complications in mothers of multiples (Walker 2004). These maternal risks included significant increases in cardiac morbidity, pre-eclampsia, gestational diabetes, postpartum hemorrhage, prolonged hospitalization, hysterectomy, and blood transfusion. Any of these conditions may delay the onset of lactogenesis II and thus negatively impact milk production. In addition, delivery at less than 28 weeks gestation may interrupt pregnancy-related breast development and may negatively impact lactation (Geddes 2007).

Research suggests that mothers of preterm multiples provide human milk less often than mothers of term singletons and term multiples. They are significantly at risk for providing milk for a shorter duration than other groups of mothers (Geraghty 2004).

Reasons for reduced incidence and duration of lactation in mothers of preterm multiples have not yet been well studied. Damato (2005) identified unique issues related to breastfeeding multiples that caused the early cessation of lactation. These included concerns about inadequate milk supply, the burden of extra pumping, and general maternal fatigue. Issues relating to infant behavior included sleepiness, poor suck, disinterest in feeding, illness, or poor infant weight gain.

McKenzie (2006) identified the need to understand and respect the fact that mothers pregnant with multiples require more resources during pregnancy than are now available to help them make informed infant feeding decisions. More breastfeeding education materials are required that are specifically adapted for mothers who are pregnant with multiples.

Mother of multiples require extra support to successfully breastfeed or to preserve lactation with pumping. Lack of support from her partner and increased maternal anxiety when informed of a multiple pregnancy were factors that were significantly associated with the decision to bottle feed in a large study of Japanese mothers of multiples, compared to a control of singleton mothers (Yokoyama 2004). Flidel-Rimon (2006) documented that mothers of multiples require the combined support of spouse, family and friends, and the medical team to make either full or partial breastfeeding possible. There is a case report of a woman who breastfed quadruplets (Berlin 2007). The LC may need to counsel families to help them realize the importance of their support and to identify concrete ways the family can assist.

Postpartum care of mothers of multiples must include instruction on how to protect the option to breastfeed if the mother is ill or requires extended recovery time before being able to provide a robust milk supply. In the event that ill health or lack of breast development precludes a full or even a partial supply of own mother's milk, the LC may wish to provide information about donor human milk from an approved milk bank.

While casual milk sharing is discouraged, owing to concern about the risk of transmission of incurable viruses from human milk, the risks of artificial formula, especially in preterm populations, have created a renewed interest in human milk banking as a method of providing safe milk for hospitalized infants whose mothers cannot produce a full milk supply.

In the US and Canada, milk banks are regulated by the Human Milk Banking Association of North America (HMBANA), an organization comprised of representatives from member banks. Founded in 1985, it developed guidelines to establish donor requirements, donor screening protocols, pasteurization policies, and bacteriological quality control standards for dispensed milk. HMBANA guidelines take into consideration guidelines developed by the US Centers for Disease Control, the US Food and Drug Administration, and the American Association of Blood Banks for other human donor tissues. The HMBANA guidelines can be viewed on-line at: www.hmbana.org.

Reducing Neonatal Necrotizing Enterocolitis in Preterm Populations

Research indicates that the use of human milk reduces the incidence of neonatal necrotizing enterocolitis (NEC) in populations of preterm infants (Lucas 1990). This issue is meaningful to mothers of multiples as many of these infants are preterm. NEC is a devastating inflammatory condition that destroys the lining of the intestinal wall (Luig 2005). The causes of this painful disease are

unclear, although 75 percent of cases occur in preterm infants. NEC accounts for a significant percentage of deaths in infants <1500 g. Many infants who develop NEC are treated surgically to remove affected sections of their bowels. The infants then develop short gut syndrome, which puts them at risk for life-time nutritional disability.

Lucas (1990) reported that NEC was rare in those preterm infants receiving at least some human milk feeds. He observed that the incidence of NEC was 20 times more common in formula-fed infants. Dvorak (2003) reported that maternal milk is the major source of trophic peptides with significant healing effects on injured gastrointestinal mucosa. Women who deliver preterm infants have higher concentrations of these peptides in their milk than are present in term milk or in formula. In the recent past, authorities were unclear whether donor human milk provided a protective effect similar to own mother's milk in the reduction of NEC. McGuire (2003) performed a meta-analysis of previous research and identified a significant association in reduction of relative risk of NEC in preterm infants fed *donor* human milk rather than formula. Evidence of improved neonatal outcomes in human milk-fed infants suggests an increased role of own mother's and donor human milk to reduce NEC and as a method to improve growth and development in preterm infants (Slusher 2003, Diehl-Jones 2004, Updegrove 2004). The LC has an obligation to share such information with the families who are pregnant with multiples. Such knowledge enables families to make informed decisions about how to advocate for their infants during hospitalization in the neonatal intensive care unit.

Resources for Families of Multiples

HCPs and mothers of multiples can find information, books, guidance about equipment, and support from organizations such as La Leche League International (LLLI) and the Australian Breastfeeding Association (ABA). See references for websites for LLLI and the ABA. Community organizations such as Mothers of Twins clubs and The Triplet Connection (which produces a newsletter) were founded to support the special needs of families with multiples. Both organizations have local chapters in many US cities. Internet searches can help parents locate resources in their communities.

The LC should review literature about breastfeeding multiples carefully before sharing it with parents. Inaccurate, unrealistic, or negative materials may undermine breastfeeding. Putting a mother in touch with a positive role model is helpful. Some LCs maintain a phone or email list of willing former clients who are available to talk to newly delivered mothers of multiples.

The LC may also be aware of other community resources that are available to help provide mothers of multiples with special types of assistance.

Simultaneous vs. Sequential Feeding

Time management is important to the family adjusting to more than one baby. It makes sense to breastfeed twins simultaneously, although newborns often require more postural support than a mother can manage with one hand. Small, immature, or weak infants require careful positioning at the breast in order to feed efficiently and to ensure adequate intake. Such increased positioning support may require both the mother's hands. In such cases, switching to sequential feeding (e.g., one baby at a time) may be an appropriate temporary strategy. Sequential feeding is often recommended if there is no helper available to assist the mother during latch on.

The LC assesses and, if necessary, assists the mother's positioning and latch technique. Special nursing pillows have been developed for simultaneous breastfeeding. A woman with multiples may find the pillow helpful to assist with postural support for the babies. As the babies grow stronger and require less physical support, breast-feeding positions become more casual and are often very creative!

One of the roles of the LC is to praise and encourage the mother's helpers in their support of the new mother and her babies. The LC can provide valuable, specific information to these helpers, showing them how to assist with positioning, pillows, and props to make things easier for the mother and babies. The LC emphasizes to the mother the wisdom of resting and utilizing the resources provided by these family helpers during the early weeks postpartum.

Breastfeeding Twins

The twins in **Fig. 293** were born at 36 weeks gestation, weighing 4 lb 15 oz (2245 g) and 5 lb 6 oz (2440 g) respectively. Their mother had previously breastfed 2 other children. She was confident about breastfeeding; however, she often found it difficult to get both babies well latched. The twin wearing the hat is sleeping at the breast. Observe the more alert affect of the twin who is better positioned. Because of their small size and stamina issues, these twins required short, frequent feedings. Because of difficulties getting them both well latched during the newborn phase, the mother often fed them sequentially. The LC and pediatrician coordinated weekly weight checks to reassure the family that the twins were growing well. Once the babies reached their due date and had

gained to approximately 7 lbs (3169 g), they became stronger feeders and needed less help from their mother to achieve positional stability. At this point, the mother increased the frequency of simultaneous breastfeeding.

Fig. 293 shows the mother positioning Baby A (wearing the hat) in a cradle position. Baby B, the larger twin, is beside her, placed in the football position. Note the use of the pillow that wedges Baby A in close and supports the mother's arm so that she does not have to strain to lift the baby. The mother places her hand at the back of Baby B's shoulders to stabilize the infant, keeping his body and chin pressed close to the breast. His nose is tilted away from the breast. This facilitates an open airway, and places the baby in an *en face* (face-to-face) gazing position with his mother. Whenever this mother breastfed simultaneously, she was encouraged by the LC to switch each baby to the opposite breast midway through the feeding. This permitted the larger, stronger twin to stimulate both breasts, facilitating overall milk production.

Fig. 294 also demonstrates the difficulty of positioning newborn, preterm twins for simultaneous breastfeeding. Neither twin is latched well enough to feed effectively. The twin in the background has fallen asleep. The nose of the twin in the foreground is buried in the breast. A few seconds after this photo was taken, she pulled away and began to cry. Repositioning, (seen in **Fig. 295**) improved their milk intake. The LC used test weighing to verify the improvement.

The 7 day-old twins (born near term) in **Figs. 296**, **297**, **298**, and **299** are being breastfed in various positions. The mother uses pillows under each elbow to support her arms (**Fig. 296**). The twin's legs come together in a "V" configuration, with support from the mother at their necks and hips to stabilize their bodies. It can be difficult to latch babies this way without help from a third person. Some mothers can accomplish simultaneous feeding by noticing which baby seems to need more assistance, and latching that baby first.

In **Fig. 297** the same mother uses a breastfeeding pillow to lift and support the babies so that her hands are free. This only works if both of the babies are fairly vigorous and stable. Weaker or smaller babies may require far more postural support to feed effectively without falling away from the breast.

In **Fig. 298**, both of the twins are in a clutch or football hold. This mother's breasts are ideally shaped for breast-feeding twins because they are widely spaced. While widely spaced breasts can be a marker for PCOS, this mother has no history of that condition. She has ample milk to feed 2 babies. The wide span between her breasts and the angle of her nipple placement permits her to position the babies for simultaneous breastfeeding while she rests in **Fig. 299**. Such a good "fit" between a mother and her twins is not always the case. A body pillow folded into a horseshoe shape and placed around this mother's shoulders provided arm support.

The 5 month-old twins in **Fig. 300** require far less physical support from their mother than they did as newborns. Here they are positioned on their knees, facing the breast. They use their hands to support the weight of the breast. Their mother leans slightly back, and stabilizes each baby with her arms. The twins have healing lesions on the backs of their heads. They are recovering from chicken pox.

In **Fig. 301**, 8 month-old twins are shown breastfeeding in a special sling. Older, stronger twins need little help from the mother in latching and staying on the breast, even if their mom is in motion.

Another view of the cradle-football combination hold is shown in **Fig. 302**. These 3 month-old twins have been exclusively breastfed and gaining well since birth. Their slender mother finds it challenging to obtain sufficient calories to maintain her own weight while breastfeeding.

The LC may discover that the mother of multiples needs dietary counseling. Caring for multiples is so time-consuming that meal preparation may be neglected. Breastfeeding mothers, especially mothers of multiples, may be protein deficient. This may manifest as an increased craving for sweets. Adding additional servings of protein to the daily diet provides a more stable source of energy, reducing the craving for sweets or carbohydrates. Strategies to help the mother obtain proper nutrition include:

- cooking and freezing meals during pregnancy
- organizing friends and family to bring meals during the first weeks postpartum
- using "rocking chair time" to mentally plan easy menus
- asking her partner to take over the responsibility of shopping and preparing meals
- having plenty of nutritious "finger foods" on hand such as fruit, carrots, yogurt, cheese, hard-boiled eggs, cold meats, etc.

Shopping lists may be drawn up with pre-planned menus in mind, and meals can be partially prepared during times when the infants are quiet or napping. The LC can remind mothers to keep a stash of non-perishable food in the house and in the car for nutritious snacking throughout the day.

Strategies to Increase Rest

The LC reminds the mother of multiples to take every opportunity to rest. Breastfeeding breaks can be relaxing for mother as well. A comfortable reclining chair, such as the one pictured in **Fig. 303**, became a useful tool for the mother of these 13 month-old twins. This mother put her feet up and relaxed at feeding times. Safe-sleeping practices caution against the mother falling asleep while breastfeeding on couches or recliners.

Older Babies

The 13 month-old twins, pictured breastfeeding while standing up in **Fig. 304**, are just learning to walk. The many bumps and bruises they sustain as toddlers create an ongoing need for reassurance from their mother. The easy and effective comfort provided from a brief breastfeeding session helps this woman appreciate the advantages of breast nurturing.

Breastfeeding Triplets

Two 8 month-old triplets are pictured breastfeeding in **Fig. 305**. Higher order multiple births may or may not result in the need for supplementation. Some women who deliver triplets are able to exclusively, or near exclusively breastfeed. Baby A and Baby B are put to the breast. After they finish, Baby C breastfeeds from both breasts. At the next feed, the babies are rotated, so that Babies B and C each breastfeed from a full breast, and Baby A breastfeeds afterwards. An alternative plan for triplets involves breastfeeding two at each feeding, and offering the third baby (on a rotation basis) a bottle of banked human milk or formula.

Higher Order Multiples

The value of human milk for all infants is well established. Mothers of higher order multiples should be encouraged to pump their breasts and to provide as much milk as possible for their infants, who often will require treatment for prematurity related issues in special care nurseries. If the mother requires medical care and is unable to pump, screened, pasteurized donor human milk may be prescribed for temporary use until the mother recovers. When the infants are able to directly breastfeed, mothers should be encouraged to attempt whatever level of breastfeeding is achievable.

Tandem Breastfeeding

While most twins are identified during the pregnancy, sometimes their arrival is a surprise. The woman in **Fig. 306** does not know she is pregnant with twins. She is pictured breastfeeding her 2 year-old son, who breastfeeds mostly at naptime and bedtime. An older daughter, 4 years of age, still breastfeeds occasionally as well. The mother in this photograph continued to breastfeed her 2 older children for comfort as well as fully breastfeeding her twins.

In **Fig. 307**, a mother is pictured tandem breastfeeding a 4 year-old and a 16 month-old toddler.

In **Fig. 308**, a 4 year-old and a 19 month-old child are shown breastfeeding together. Some women choose tandem breastfeeding as a way to permit child-led weaning when births are closely spaced and to promote feelings of closeness (Hills-Bonczyk 1994). The experience can be enjoyable for the mother, who then benefits from the quiet moments that breastfeeding provides. She may also feel that tandem breastfeeding reduces sibling rivalry, providing the children moments of peaceful intimacy with each other. However, some mothers report that tandem breastfeeding contributes to emotional strain and a sense of feeling "touched out." HCPs or family members, sensing this, often pressure these mothers to wean. At times, such advice and weaning assistance may be appropriate. At other times, the mother may merely need more support and encouragement.

The mother who is tandem breastfeeding generally has a robust milk supply, with ample milk for both children. The older child, responding to an increase in milk volume after the birth of the new baby, may temporarily increase breastfeeding, but typically returns to a pattern of less intense, less frequent breastfeeding over time. In some cases, however, it becomes important to ensure that the younger child gets sufficient nourishment for normal growth. Older children can obtain milk from the breast much faster than a newborn, and some mothers may need to ensure that the baby breastfeeds first. BWC has seen 2 cases where infants have failed to thrive owing to older siblings, in very short duration feeds, emptying the breast and jeopardizing the infant's intake. However, if the mother has oversupply or a forceful milk ejection, the older child can drain off some of the milk pressure so that feeding is more comfortable for the infant. Most mothers who are tandem breastfeeding soon work out the logistics of the activity.

Fig. 309 shows a 2 year-old and her almost 5 year-old brother relaxing with their mother. Images such as this can be startling in a culture where breastfeeding the older child often becomes a "closet" activity. However, older breastfeeding children such as the 3 year-old child shown in **Fig. 310** are not uncommon, even in the US. Health care providers benefit from seeing visual images of what

is a normal experience for many families (Dettwyler 1995, Sugarman 1995, AAP 1996, AAP 2005).

Legal Issues Related to Breastfeeding Past Infancy

Evidence associates the continuation of breastfeeding past the introduction of solids with reduced severity of infectious diseases, particularly in stressed environments (Prentice 1991). Many people in the US are unfamiliar with tandem and extended breastfeeding. Lactation consultants may receive requests for help from women accused of improper intimacy or sexual abuse of their children solely because they are breastfeeding older children. The LC can provide written documentation from medical and anthropological sources and may provide expert testimony that toddler nursing and breastfeeding older children is normal behavior (Wilson-Clay 1990, Corbett 2001).

Several books address breastfeeding past infancy: *How Weaning Happens* (Bengson 1999), *Mothering Your Nursing Toddler* (Bumgarner 2000), *Breastfeeding: Biocultural Perspectives* (Stuart-Macadam and Dettwyler 1995), and *The Nursing Mother's Guide to Weaning* (Huggins 1994). The AAP policy statement on breastfeeding states: "There is no upper limit to the duration of breastfeeding and no evidence of psychological or developmental harm from breastfeeding into the third year of life or longer" (AAP 2005).

AAP. Breastfeeding studies. *AAP News* 1996; 12(7):2.

American Academy of Pediatrics (AAP) Section on Breastfeeding. Breastfeeding and the use of human milk. *Pediatrics* 2005; 115(2):296-506.

Australian Breastfeeding Association: www.breastfeeding.asn.au

Bengson D. *How Weaning Happens*. Schaumburg, IL: La Leche League International, 1999.

Berlin CM. "Exclusive" breastfeeding of quadruplets. *Breastfeeding Medicine* 2007; 2(2):125-126.

Bumgarner NJ. *Mothering Your Nursing Toddler*. Schaumburg, IL: La Leche League International, 2000.

Corbett S. The Breast Offense. *New York Times Magazine* May 6, 2001; pp. 82-85.

Damato EG, Dowling DA, Standing TS, et al. Explanation for cessation of breastfeeding in mothers of twins. *Journal of Human Lactation* 2005; 21(3):296-304.

Dettwyler K. A Time to Wean: The hominid blueprint for the natural age of weaning in modern human populations, in P Stuart-Macadam, K Dettwyler (ed). *Breastfeeding: Biocultural Perspectives*. New York: De Gruyter, 1995; pp. 65-66.

Diehl-Jones W, Askin D. Nutritional modulation of neonatal outcomes. *AACN Clinical Issues* 2004; 15(1):83-96.

Dvorak B, Fituch C, Williams C, et al. Increased epidermal growth factor levels in human milk of mothers with extremely premature infants. *Pediatric Research* 2003; 54(1):15-19.

Feldman R, Eidelman A. Does a triplet birth pose a special risk for infant development? Assessing cognitive development in relation to intrauterine growth and mother-infant interaction across the first two years. *Pediatrics* 2005; 115(2):443-452.

Flidel-Rimon O, Shinwell ES. Breastfeeding twins and high multiples. *Archives of Diseases in Childhood Fetal and Neonatal Education* 2006; 91(5):F377-380.

Geddes D. Gross anatomy of the lactating breast, in *Hale and Hartmann's Textbook of Human Lactation,* Amarillo, TX: Hale Publishing, 2007; p. 23.

Geraghty SR, Pinney SM, Sethuraman G, et al. Breast milk feeding rates of mothers of multiples compared to mothers of singletons. *Ambulatory Pediatrics* 2004; 4(3):226-231.

Human Milk Banking Association of North America (HMBANA). www.hmbana.org. Accessed on April 30, 2006.

Hills-Bonczyk S, Tromiczsak K, Avery M, et al. Women's experiences with breastfeeding longer than 12 months. *Birth* 1994; 21(4):206-212.

Huggins K, Ziedrich L. *The Nursing Mother's Guide to Weaning*. Boston, MA: Harvard Common Press, 1994.

La Leche League International: www.lalecheleague.org

Lucas A, Cole T. Breast milk and neonatal necrotising enterolcolitis. *Lancet* 1990; 336(8730):1519-1523.

Luig M, Lui K; NSW & ACT NICUS Group. Epidemiology of necrotizing enterocolitis - Part I: changing regional trends in extremely preterm infants over 14 years. *Journal of Paediatric Child Health* 2005; 41(4):169-173.

McGuire W, Anthony M. Donor human milk versus formula for preventing necrotizing enterocolitis in preterm infants: systematic review. *Archives of Disease in Childhood Fetal Neonatal Education* 2003; 88(1):F11-F14.

McKenzie PJ. The seeking of baby-feeding information by Canadian women pregnant with twins. *Midwifery* 2006; 22(3):218-227.

Morley R, Fewtrell M, Abbott R, et al. Neurodevelopment in children born small for gestational age: a randomized trial of nutrient-enriched versus standard formula and comparison with a reference breastfed group. *Pediatrics* 2004; 113(3):515-521.

Prentice A. Breastfeeding and the older infant. *Acta Paediatrica Scandia/Supplement* 1991; 374:78-88.

Slusher T, Hampton R, Bode-Thomas F, et al. Promoting the exclusive feeding of own mother's milk through the use of hindmilk and increased maternal milk volume for hospitalized, low birth weight infants (<1800 grams) in Nigeria: a feasibility study. *Journal of Human Lactation* 2003; 19(2):191-198.

Sugarman M, Kendall-Tackett K. Weaning ages in a sample of American women who practice extended breastfeeding. *Clinical Pediatrics* 1995; 34(12):642-647.

The Triplet Connection, P.O. Box 99571, Stockton, CA, 95209.

Updegrove K. Necrotizing enterocolitis: the evidence for the use of human milk in prevention and treatment. *Journal of Human Lactation* 2004; 20(3):335-339.

Walker M, Murphy K, Pan S, et al. Adverse maternal outcomes in multifetal pregnancies. *BJOG: An International Journal of Obstetrics & Gynaecology* 2004; 111(11):1294.

Wilson-Clay B. Extended breastfeeding as a legal issue: an annotated bibliography. *Journal of Human Lactation* 1990; 6(2):68-71.

Yokoyama Y, Ooki S. Breast-feeding and bottle-feeding of twins, triplets and higher order multiple births. *Nippon Koshu Eisei Azsshi* 2004; 51(11):969-974.

Alternative Feeding Methods

Breastfeeding is the physiological way to feed human infants. However, some babies are unable to breastfeed immediately, or their mothers need assistance improving milk supply. While the health care team evaluates their situation, the baby must be fed so that growth and energy are protected. Ideally, the baby receives human milk supplementation when breastfeeding is delayed. Pumped, own mother's milk or donor human milk from a milk bank are the safest alternatives to formula. Whenever mothers cannot provide sufficient milk to meet all their infant's needs, or no donor milk is available, infant formula may be required.

Numerous infant feeding methods are available to deliver supplemental calories to infants. However, there is an absence of clear evidence demonstrating the superiority of one feeding method over another. All methods appear to have risks and benefits. Therefore, careful individual assessment helps determine the most suitable method for a specific baby. The primary consideration in selecting an alternative feeding method is the safety and enjoyment of the feeding experience for the baby. "The goal of any alternative feeding method is for restoration of full, direct breastfeeding wherever possible" (Wight 2001).

Legal and Ethical Concerns

It is important that practitioners understand that legal and ethical issues arise whenever equipment is involved in a care plan. Ethical principles require that equipment is selected because it serves a therapeutic purpose, is safe, and that profit motive is not placed before patient welfare. Legal principles (generally grouped under commercial code statutes) govern product liability. Consumers have the right to be informed about potentially negative outcomes with the use of products. The LC must make decisions about feeding equipment that are based on available research while being aware that research in this area is somewhat limited. Care should be taken to avoid unsupported claims that various methods of alternative feeding are "most like breastfeeding."

Because of the specific and limited nature of product liability protection, manufacturers stipulate that they are not liable for any harm to the consumer if their product is used in a way other than that described in the instructions. Consequently, the LC potentially assumes legal risk in counseling parents to use equipment in a way that it is not intended to be used (Bornmann 1993). Open dialogue between LCs and clients, signed consent forms that document informed parental decisions, carefully charted

documentation, and malpractice insurance are all vital aspects of an LC's practice (Hall 2002). These issues come into play especially when assisting in alternative feeding situations.

Criteria for Selecting an Alternate Method of Infant Feeding

- It does not harm the infant.
- It is a good match for the infant's size, stamina, physical condition, and level of maturity.
- It is easy for the parents to manage.
- It involves equipment that the parents can obtain, afford, and clean.
- It is a suitable intervention for the length of time needed to remediate the feeding problem. Long-term interventions are the most stressful to maintain.
- It may help the baby learn to breastfeed.

Spoon Feeding

Sometimes a baby needs only a brief period of supplementation, a "jump start" of caloric energy, to rouse sufficiently to latch on to the breast. Spoon feeding is an excellent way to capture and deliver colostrum or small volumes of milk to non-breastfeeding or sleepy infants (Hoover 1998). About half a ml at a time seems to be a comfortable volume for a newborn to swallow (Lawrence 2005). Because a spoon holds only a small amount of fluid, parents worry less about overwhelming the baby or causing the baby to choke. In **Fig. 311** a baby is shown receiving approximately half a ml of expressed milk.

In **Fig. 312** a sleepy 10 day-old infant who is losing weight and not latching is offered milk by spoon. In **Fig. 313** the same baby, already more alert, willingly takes milk from the spoon. Note the baby's engaged affect. Once aroused, her increased energy enabled her to latch on to the breast.

Cup Feeding

Infant cup feeding implements have been used throughout the ages to supplement nonbreastfeeding infants. Owing to cost issues and the increased risk of infant infection in settings where bottle teat hygiene cannot be assured, a resurgence of interest in cup feeding in the modern era has occurred (Fredeen 1948, Davis 1948). This interest is partly influenced in the present era by a philosophical reluctance to expose infants to artificial teats and what is commonly called "nipple confusion."

A review of the literature on cup feeding identifies some studies that suggest that cup fed infants are at lower risk for oxygen desaturation than are bottle-fed infants (Dowling 2002). Other studies (Freer 1999) describe physiological instability and oxygen desaturation of preterm infants during cup feeding. Dowling suggests that the better oxygenation noted in some studies in cup feeding infants may be secondary to the delivery of smaller intake volumes for the feeding. Small intake volumes may increase the risk of poor growth in cup fed populations.

Some, but not all, studies reviewed observed similar weight gain in cup and bottle-fed infants (Rocha 2002). However, Dowling (2002) observed that up to 48 percent of milk that was cup fed to a group of preterm infants was lost to spillage. This was not always apparent to their feeders, and was revealed only when careful test weights were performed on the infants and their bibs. Dowling recommends careful monitoring of intake and spillage in cup fed populations, especially preterm infants.

A Cochrane Review identified only 4 cup feeding studies rigorous enough for meta-analysis. These studies were examined to determine the effects of cup feeding versus other forms of supplemental feeding on infant weight gain and achievement of eventual successful breastfeeding. There was no statistical difference in incidence of not breastfeeding at hospital discharge in 3 of the 4 studies between cup and bottle-feeding groups. While there was no statistically significant difference in weight gain from the one study that reported this outcome, there was a significantly increased length of hospital stay in the cup fed infants. The cup fed infants remained hospitalized a mean of 10.1 additional days. The conclusion of the Cochrane review was that "Cup feeding cannot be recommended over bottle-feeding as a supplement to breastfeeding because it confers no significant benefit in maintaining breastfeeding beyond hospital discharge and carries the unacceptable consequence of a longer stay in hospital" (Flint 2007).

The Cochrane Review findings do not mean that infants cannot be or never should be cup fed. Cups provides a hygiene benefit whenever a family's ability to procure and clean bottles may be compromised. Short-term cup feeding may also be useful in situations when only a few supplemental feeds will be required. Reducing the focus on bottles in such situations may provide a psychological benefit for the mother and help keep the focus on transitioning quickly to breastfeeding.

There is wide consensus in the cup feeding literature that technique is important (Howard 1999, Marinelli 2001).

Thorley (1997) describes problems that can be created by incorrect use of cups. Malhotra (1999) cautions against "force feeding," citing concerns about the risk of aspiration with improper technique. Cup feeding can be a difficult skill to learn from a text. Some LCs practice the technique by taking turns cup feeding each other. Parents who want to cup feed should be taught the technique and then observed while feeding the infant to make sure they are doing it safely. Such *return demonstration* reduces risk to the infant and increases the confidence of the infant's feeders.

During cup feeding, the infant's head and body should be stabilized. Lang (1994) suggests placing the rim of the cup level with the infant's lips and allowing the infant to sip or lap the milk. Milk is not poured into the mouth. Dowling (2002) cautions the feeder to observe the infant's respiration, allowing the baby to control the intake, pausing when necessary to allow the infant to reorganize respiration.

Some LCs have theorized that cup feeding leads to the acquisition of skills that facilitate breastfeeding. While it is clear that infants may be fed by cup, it is less clear whether this is a developmentally desirable practice for human infants. Dowling (2002) observes that cup feeding is a "closed mouth" activity and questions whether lapping and sipping mimic or facilitate the development of the oral behaviors required for breastfeeding. It is the activity of sucking that provides state stabilizing benefits in addition to being the normal feeding method of infants. Therefore, depriving infants of the opportunity to suck during feeding may have unforeseen consequences.

Dowling differed from others who have described the technique of cup feeding as "easy," and noted that correct cup feeding technique required considerable skill on the part of the feeders. Dowling's observations of cup fed, preterm infants also noted that the infants appeared to require a great deal of stimulation from their feeders to keep them engaged in the cup feeding process. Without continuous arousal, the infants tended to fall asleep while cup feeding. Dowling attributed this to lack of intra-oral tactile stimulation.

It is possible to feed both full term and preterm infants. The full term infant shown in **Fig. 314** manifests stable state behavior while cup feeding. Note the open eyes, calm facial expression, and absence of stress cues. Certain protective reflexes (the cough) may be immature in some infants, placing them at heightened risk for silent aspiration (Wolf 1992). Thus, it is important to observe the infant's behavioral cues during cup feeding and to pause if the infant appears stressed.

The infant in **Fig. 315** is being fed with a traditional feeding implement called a *paladai*, which is widely used on the Indian subcontinent. The baby drank an ounce of expressed milk, but did not open his eyes or engage socially during the feeding. Malhotra (1999) documents less spillage with the paladai than with a cup, probably because the spout allows for greater directional control of the fluid. However, Malhotra also observed a tendency to pour milk from the paladai into the mouth of the baby, which increases the risk of aspiration. Note the infant's pursed lips. By slowing the delivery of fluids, the mother may help the baby experience a less stressful feeding.

Finger Feeding

Finger feeding is another method of supplementation for the non-breastfeeding baby; however, there is no evidence to support claims that finger feeding is "more like breast-feeding." Many LCs report that finger feeding provides them with valuable information about how the baby is moving the tongue, thus facilitating a more sensitive assessment. However, the belief that finger feeding facilitates breastfeeding mechanics has not been systematically evaluated.

Because the adult finger is narrow, it is more similar to the diameter of a bottle teat than it is to the rounded contour of the human breast. Even more rigid than a bottle teat, the finger is inserted into (rather than shaped and drawn into) the mouth of the baby. Thus, finger feeding differs markedly from breastfeeding. Ideally, the feeder uses sensitivity and respect when inserting the finger into the mouth of the baby. A benefit may derive from the narrow gape promoted by finger feeding, particularly if an infant has weak lip tone and cannot seal off on a wide base. Likewise, it may be advantageous to finger feed when firm pressure is needed to help an infant correctly pattern the tongue into a central groove. Finger feeding may benefit the baby who cannot create adequate suction to withdraw milk from the breast. The feeder can gently bolus small volumes to the baby. This may be useful, for example, when infants have clefts of the palate. However, until research systematically examines these issues, no claims can be made about the superiority of finger feeding over other feeding methods.

No safety data have been reported on the practice of finger feeding. While finger feeding is widely performed by LCs and frequently described in breastfeeding texts, only one research study on finger feeding has been published. Oddy (2003) examined breastfeeding rates in an Australian hospital before and after implementation of the Baby Friendly Hospital Initiative (BFHI). The study reports improved breastfeeding rates at discharge when staff discontinued use of artificial teats and began supplementing babies by finger feeding. However, the implementation of other aspects of BFHI rather than the specific intervention of finger feeding may explain the improved breastfeeding rates. Oddy did not investigate the respiratory stability of the infants during finger feeding or comment on safety issues.

Larger volumes of milk can be delivered via finger feeding than by spoon, facilitating efficiency of feeding. Unlike the cup, which encourages lapping but not sucking, the finger feeding infant receives superior proprioceptive stimulation along the tongue. This may help the infant organize the tongue into the central groove that is essential for safe swallowing (Wolf 1992).

Technique is also important during finger feeding. The caregiver's hands should be clean and nails clipped. HCPs should be gloved or wear finger cots. The finger is inserted pad side up. Take care to avoid inserting the finger too deeply into the baby's mouth. The tip of the finger extends to near the junction of the hard and soft palates. Inserting the finger beyond this point will trigger a gag reflex, a noxious stimulus. Repeated triggering of noxious stimuli may create feeding aversion.

Whether a curved-tip syringe or a feeding tube is inserted with the finger, feeders must be careful to avoid squirting liquids down the infant's throat. Anecdotal reports describe the practice of inserting a syringe filled with milk directly into the mouth of the infant. There is no advantage to inserting a narrow device such as a syringe into the mouth. The resulting pursed mouth configuration does not facilitate breastfeeding, and there is also increased risk of aspiration when milk is squirted into the mouth in this manner.

Fig. 316 shows the Monoject 412® curved-tip syringe resting along the side of the mother's finger at the corner of the baby's mouth. Prior to inserting her finger, the mother gently stimulates the baby's lips. Finger feeding may provide the sensation of skin rather than plastic inside the baby's mouth, one possible additional advantage of the method. As the baby draws in the finger and begins sucking, the mother inserts the curved tip of the syringe, stabilizing it against her finger. Finger feeding can be used to rouse a sleepy baby. If the mother can induce the infant to suck on her finger, she can gently give a few swallows of milk to help rouse the baby without the spillage that often occurs when using a spoon or cup for this purpose. The mother may allow the baby to suck for a few seconds before delivering the first bolus of milk. Briefly delaying the milk flow mimics the experience of sucking on the breast prior to milk ejection. Thus finger feeding becomes a behavior modification technique that may help the baby remain more patient when transferred to the breast.

The mother in **Fig. 316** delivers a small bolus (1/2 ml) of milk by gently pressing the syringe in response to the baby's sucking. Half a ml is about half the width of the black gasket. By pacing the delivery of milk in response to the baby's sucking, the mother rewards the baby for sucking effort. When teaching this technique to parents, the LC helps them carefully observe the baby's ability to coordinate sucking, swallowing, and breathing. Notice how the mother has positioned the baby against her breast, skin-to-skin. This helps the baby remain oriented to the breast and may assist in transitioning the baby from alternate feeding to breastfeeding.

In **Fig. 317** a feeding tube is placed on the thumb. If the aim of any alternative feeding method is to promote transition back to the breast, the LC has to consider that finger feeding will accustom the baby to holding the mouth in a rather narrow position compared to the wide jaw and flanged lip positions required to breastfeed. The wider diameter of the thumb may be useful to accustom the baby to a wider mouth position. Notice that this baby has a poor seal, as revealed by the milk around the baby's lips. The baby looks worried. Perhaps the narrower base provided by a finger would be a better option for this baby until lip tone improves.

Fig. 318 demonstrates a mother using a #5 French feeding tube attached to a Monoject 412® curved-tip syringe. A Band-Aid® has been taped to the mother's finger to help hold the tubing in place. Before attaching the Band-Aid®, the narrow sticky strip beside the pad was cut off on each side, so the tubing could easily be threaded through. When the baby naturally pauses, the mother stops the flow of milk. Once the baby begins sucking again, the mother delivers more milk. Swallowing too quickly may overwhelm some infants, causing vomiting. Parents should be encouraged to mimic the average feeding times of the breastfeeding infant, which range from 10 to 25 minutes (L'Esperance).

Fig. 319 demonstrates an LC providing emergency supplementation to an infant who is significantly under birth weight. The infant was delivered prematurely at 36 gestational weeks, and presented with poor skin tone and turgor. This infant weighed 5 lbs 2 oz (2320 g) at birth. She was discharged from the hospital within 36 hours, before adequate breastfeeding was established. On Day 6 postpartum, her mother became concerned that the baby was not stooling and brought her to the lactation clinic. The baby's weight on the LC's scale was 4 lb 8 oz (2037

g). The baby had lost slightly more than 8 percent of her birth weight, appeared lethargic, and was beginning to demonstrate signs of dehydration.

The LC contacted the pediatrician by phone. He directed the LC to provide immediate nutrition. The LC attempted to obtain expressed milk to feed the baby. Because the baby was sleepy and feeding poorly, the mother's breasts were understimulated and Lactogenesis II had not yet occurred. Hand expression and breast pumping yielded only drops of milk. With the mother's permission and the doctor's approval, the baby was finger fed formula. The mother made arrangements to take the baby to the pediatrician for evaluation the same day.

Note that the LC in **Fig. 319** is gloved. Gloves are not necessary when handling human milk, nor are they necessary for parents. Gloves are required when the LC places a finger into the baby's mouth. Fungi and bacteria under the fingernails have been implicated in nosocomial infections (Parry 2001). The LC has an ethical obligation to protect the infant from exposure to pathogens not part of the baby's normal environment.

Feeding Tube Devices

Feeding tube devices allow infants to be supplemented at the breast with pumped milk or formula. These devices work well if the infant is able to latch onto the breast. Feeding tube devices deliver a steady flow of milk to the infant who is capable of sucking normally. This provides an enticement to the baby to keep sucking when the milk supply is low. Thus, feeding tubes are useful in situations where a mother is relactating, attempting to induce lactation for an adopted infant (Gribble 2004), or when an infant (such as a baby with PKU) requires special supplementation. Whenever possible, an infant's sucking is helpful in stimulating increased milk production, and the skin-to-skin contact facilitates bonding.

Feeding tubes are less effective in stimulating the breast if the infant learns to suck the tube as if it were a straw and never actively latches onto the breast. Similarly, feeding tubes may not benefit a baby who cannot generate sufficient suction. Such infants may find feeding with a tube exhausting and may fail to obtain adequate calories, thus prolonging their problems. In this situation, it is more beneficial to recommend pumping to protect the milk supply and to find another way to feed the baby. The mother is advised to continue to offer the breast for comfort until the baby stabilizes. Non-nutritive sucking (NNS), while generally understood as sucking on a pacifier, can take place at the breast. NNS helps stabilize the baby, shortens hospital stays, and helps transition babies from tube feeding (Pinelli 2005). Another possible benefit of a feeding tube device might be to deliver the scent and taste of human milk to preterm babies as an impetus to suck. Raimbault (2007) reported that exposure to mother's milk prior to early breastfeeding trials had a positive effect on sucking behavior and milk ingestion of preterm infants. It also resulted in shortened hospital stays.

The use of a feeding tube device should be reconsidered if the infant takes an unacceptably long time (>30 minutes) to complete a feed, falls asleep while feeding, or fails to gain weight adequately while using the device.

The feeding tube device can be elevated to create a greater gravity drop. This will increase the milk flow rate. Some mothers learn to squeeze the feeding tube container to augment the milk flow rate. An augmented flow may help deliver more milk to a weakly sucking infant. However, an augmented flow may overwhelm a baby with respiratory or swallowing problems. These issues should be explored when mothers are learning to use the feeding tube device.

Fig. 320 demonstrates a Monoject 412® curved-tip syringe being used to supplement the baby at the breast in a way that closely mimics a feeding tube. This method may be appropriate for short-term use, and often assists in helping infants transfer to the breast after bottle, finger, or cup feeding. The mother latches the baby on to the breast and then stabilizes the curved tip of the periodontal syringe against her breast. She inserts the tip into the corner of the baby's mouth, and drips milk to entice the baby to suck.

Fig. 321 shows a #5 French feeding tube inserted in a bottle of infant formula for use as a homemade feeding supplementer.

Two commercially available feeding supplementers sold in the United States (and elsewhere) are the Medela® Supplemental Nursing System (SNS)™ and the Lact-Aid®. In Australia, the Supply Line® system (not pictured) is available through the Australian Breastfeeding Association. Supplementers may be reimbursable under some US insurance plans because they are classified as medical equipment. Mothers report a range of opinions when discussing their experiences using feeding tube devices (Borucki 2005). However, the consensus is that mothers sought an alternative when their infants were unable to breastfeed, and the feeding tube device provided choices.

Fig. 322 shows a mother finger feeding with an SNS™. Finger feeding in this manner allows greater volumes of milk to be available and is more efficient than repeatedly refilling a syringe. Additionally, finger feeding in this manner requires the baby to actively suck the fluid rather than merely responding to the mother's giving boluses of milk. This activity may help strengthen the infant's suck. Once the infant becomes accustomed to the sensation of the feeding tube attached to the finger, it may be easier to transition the baby to a feeding tube worn at the breast.

Fig. 323 shows a woman breastfeeding her healthy, term, adopted baby with an SNS™ taped to her breast. The woman had lactated 15 years prior, and was inducing lactation for the new baby. Her baby easily adapted to the feeding tube device. At the peak of production the woman made approximately 6-10 ounces (170-283 ml) of milk daily. She and her son enjoyed the bonding benefits of breastfeeding. She continued to supplement him at the breast with only occasional bottles until he was 2 months old. She then returned to full time employment and discontinued using the feeding tube. She offered her breasts for comfort and supplemented with a bottle.

In **Fig. 324**, the LC has suggested using 2 tubes of an SNS™ at the same breast. Opening up both tubes simultaneously increases the milk flow rate and may assist the infant who has difficulty creating sufficient suction to obtain milk (idea attributed to Kittie Frantz). The infant in the photo was born at 37 weeks gestational age to a G3 P3 L3 mother. The baby weighed 5 lb 10 oz (2551 g) at birth, and weighed only 5 lb 4 oz (2381 g) at 5 weeks. The LC observed a weak suck. The baby was unable to maintain continuous sucking bursts, took a long time to drain the SNS, and frequently lost suction. Using double tubes reduced the work of feeding and helped the baby complete feedings in a shorter period of time. Improved weight gain and increased energy strengthened the infant's feeding ability.

The infant pictured in **Fig. 325** is breastfeeding with a Lact-Aid®. Because this device features a soft plastic bag rather than a firm feeding bottle, some mothers feel that it is less obtrusive when worn under clothing and thus prefer it for discreet breastfeeding in more public situations. The bag does not have to be worn around the neck, and can be comfortably tucked between the mother and the baby. The feeding tube comes out of the top of the Lact-Aid®, requiring that the baby suck milk against the pull of gravity. This may assist in strengthening the suck more than the SNS™, which positions the tube at the bottom of the bottle, providing a gravity drop to augment milk flow. Some mothers may use both devices, or may progress from the SNS™ to the Lactaid®, depending upon the therapeutic plan.

In **Figs**. **321-325**, all of the feeding tubes are shown positioned in the traditional manner. That is, the tubing is inserted under the upper lip and enters the baby's mouth centered along the palate. For some babies, the feel of the tube against the palate is a distraction. In **Fig. 326** the feeding tube is taped in a reverse position, and when the infant is placed in a cradle position, the tube will lie on the lower lip. **Fig. 327** shows a baby breastfeeding from a homemade feeding tube device with the tube positioned along the tongue. The tube is now in contact with the tongue rather than the palate (idea credited to Peter Hartmann's team, Perth, Australia).

Nasogastric Tube Feeding

Research has demonstrated that breastfeeding is easier than bottle-feeding for preterm babies and that preterm babies can breastfeed before they can bottle-feed (Meier 1987, Meier 1988, Chen 2000). However, owing to the effect of maturation upon sucking, exclusive breastfeeding may not provide enough calories, and the baby may still need supplementation. Supplementation via nasogastric (NG) tube may be appropriate until the infant's sucking pattern matures.

Studies examining the use of NG feeding of preterm babies reveal that this type of feeding is an appropriate substitute for bottles when the mother is not present to breastfeed. The NG tube fed group was 4.5 times more likely to be breastfeeding and 9.4 times more likely to be fully breastfeeding at discharge. NG tube supplemented infants also were more likely to be breastfeeding at 3 months and at 6 months (Stein 1990, Kliethermes 1999).

Sometimes an infant is so premature, ill, or weak, that oral feedings are impossible. **Fig. 328** shows a 3 month-old baby who is recovering from infant botulism. A symptom of infant botulism is sudden onset of sucking dysfunction and lack of stooling. The baby is recovering from the illness and is being fed by a nasogastric tube.

Infants who have had lengthy periods of NG or oral gastric tube feeding may have erosions of the tissue surrounding the tube. Adults who experience these procedures often complain of sore throats and irritated nasal passages, and infants may be equally uncomfortable following gavage feeding. They may develop anxiety owing to this pain. Sometimes this contributes to sensory defensiveness and aversive behavior surrounding feeding as the child is transferred to oral feeds (Palmer 1998).

Some infants are unable to feed orally for extended periods of time Sucking in the absence of oral feeding stabilizes the rate of breathing and increases oxygenation (Dowling 2002).

Therefore, pacifiers are often provided to infants during NG or gastric tube feeding. Preterm infants who sucked on pacifiers during NG feeds discontinued NG feeds earlier, had better weight gain, and were discharged from the hospital earlier (Measel 1979, Pinelli 2005).

Bottle-Feeding

Supplementation of breastfeeding infants without medical reasons significantly reduced the duration of exclusive breastfeeding in both multiparas and primiparas in a Swedish study (Ekstrom 2003). The Ten Steps of the Baby-Friendly Hospital Initiative wisely suggest giving newborns time to learn to breastfeed without interference or unnecessary interventions, especially bottle-feeding (WHO/UNICEF 1991). Step 9 specifies that no artificial teats or pacifiers be given to breastfeeding infants. This step has been widely implemented in the absence of any definitive evidence of the superiority of one method of supplementation over another (Cloherty 2005). However, in the event that an infant requires medically necessary supplementation, Wight (2001) points out: "The main advantage of supplementing without a bottle is the non-verbal message to parents that the alternative method is temporary." It seems clear that more research must be conducted on the issue of how best to feed the non-breast-feeding infant.

Ekstrom (2003) observed that if parents were aware that supplementation was medically necessary, it did not undermine confidence in breastfeeding. For infants who are unable to breastfeed and will require long-term supple-mentation, a method of feeding must be selected that is manageable for both the infant and the parents. It is less clear in such instances whether the use of bottle teats constitutes a major risk to renewed breastfeeding.

Some parents object to feeding tube devices because of expense, unfamiliarity, or difficulty of use. Others object to frequent milk spilling and the time consuming nature of spoon or cup feeding. Finger feeding is not a well known technique and some parents may prefer a more "normal" feeding method. Physicians may object to some forms of alternative feeding on the grounds that there are few studies demonstrating the safety or developmental suitability of the various feeding methods (Dowling 2002). In such situations, bottles may constitute the most acceptable method of supplementation. In some situations, practitioners are beginning to reexamine the practice of bottle-feeding, adapting it to provide therapeutic advantages to the non-breastfeeding infant.

As with other feeding methods, the LC has an obligation to learn how to make bottle-feeding a safe and pleasant experience for the baby, and to advocate for the use of human milk in the bottle. Additionally, with the goal of eventual breastfeeding in mind, the LC assists in using the bottle as a therapeutic intervention to transition the baby to breastfeeding.

When a baby is not breastfeeding well, it is wise to avoid planting negative suggestions about "nipple confusion." Many parents believe that there is no point in trying to breastfeed after the baby has been exposed to bottles. It is important to reassure parents that the issue of nipple confusion is complex, and that it is not clear whether exposure to bottles or pacifiers prevents subsequent breastfeeding (Victoria 1997, Dowling 2001). It is important to remind parents that babies who initially are having difficulty *can* learn to breastfeed once their problems resolve (providing that the mother still has a robust milk supply).

It is vital to assess each infant as an individual and to identify those for whom some aspect of bottle-feeding is overwhelming. This includes infants with respiratory or swallowing problems. Many LCs find that observing infants during alternative feeding provides valuable clues into the nature of an infant's specific feeding problems. Stress cues (see Ch. 2 and 3) can be identified during bottle-feeding. In **Fig. 329** a 6 week-old infant with FTT struggles with a flow rate from a bottle that is too fast for him to control. Note his furrowed brow and closed eyes.

The infant shown in **Figs. 330** and **331** was born with abnormally small nasal passages. (See **Fig. 37**.) This infant was unable to breastfeed. When his mouth was filled by the breast, he was unable to draw in enough air through his nostrils to sustain normal respiration. He experienced similar problems while bottle-feeding. His typical bottle-feeding behavior is shown in **Fig. 330**. He gulped as much milk as he could while holding his breath. Then he fought to push the bottle away and panted in an attempt to reorganize his breathing. That is, the baby experienced apnea and became stressed during prolonged sucking and swallowing. His pulling away was an attempt to recover respiratory stability. Such stressful feeding causes physiological and psychological distress to the infant and the feeder.

External Pacing Techniques: Paced Feeding

Any cessation of breathing is termed *apnea*. Oxygen desaturation and *bradycardia* (slowing of the heart rate) may result from apnea. Infants who are at risk include those experiencing prematurity, illness, anatomic anomalies, or a history of respiratory problems. Infants who are experiencing respiratory distress while feeding can be identified

by behavioral cues. They will experience nasal flaring, stiffening of the extremities, or will begin spilling milk from the corners of their mouths. Their eyes may widen, they may grimace, or the skin around the baby's lips may turn blue. Some struggle to push away from the feeding device. Others appear to fall asleep in an attempt to end the feeding.

Special feeding techniques are recommended by Speech-Language Pathologists (SLPs) and Occupational Therapists (OTs) to help the infant who has difficulty maintaining respiratory stability during feeding (Wolf 1992, Alper 1996). Palmer (1998) described incoordination of sucking and arrhythmic breathing in immature or compromised infants. She proposed systematic pacing of feeds to promote better infant organization of feeding in populations of preterm infants. No matter the gestational age, when an infant is unable to appropriately self-regulate or "pace" breathing with sucking and swallowing, the feeder must assume responsibility for ensuring the stability of the baby's respiratory status. This is called "external pacing."

A perceived benefit of breastfeeding is that it allows the infant maximum control over his own food intake. A guiding principle of external pacing is that the feeder strives to partner with the infant, and attempts to return as much control as possible to the infant (Wilson-Clay 2005).

When employing pacing techniques, the feeder closely observes and counts the number of sucks and swallows (Law-Morstatt 2003). If the baby does not take a spontaneous breath by the third to fifth suck, the feeder interrupts the delivery of fluids to impose a three to five second pause for breathing. With normal infants who are bottle-feeding for non-medical reasons, feeders simply observe facial cues. Parents and other care providers can be taught that infant motor and behavioral cues reliably signal the need for a brief pause so that the baby can maintain respiratory stability. Pacing techniques are adaptable to a variety of feeding methods, including cup and finger feeding.

Bottles lend themselves well to paced feeding techniques because they do not spill and are relatively easy to control. The flow rate from bottle teats is dependent on the firmness of the teat material, the number and size of holes, and the shape of the teat (Mathew 1990). A feeding specialist or LC can select teats based on suitability of size, shape, and flow rate by observing carefully to see what works best for the baby.

Once the mother learned how to use pacing techniques **(Fig. 331)** the infant with the small nostrils relaxed. He was able to enjoy bottle-feeding because he no longer had to struggle to breathe.

A 37 week-old baby who was also small for gestational age, is shown in **Figs. 332**, **333**, and **334.** The baby had been exclusively breastfed from birth. Here he is learning how to bottle-feed with pacing techniques after being diagnosed with FTT on Day 19. His mother had a diminished milk supply, presumably owing to lack of adequate breast stimulation by her weak, small baby. The woman described breastfeeding "18 hours a day," but said that her baby mostly slept at the breast. The pediatrician recommended supplementation to stabilize the baby's energy and weight. The mother had been bottle-feeding for 2 days when the LC arrived. As part of her evaluation, the LC asked to observe the baby bottle-feeding. Because the baby manifested poor respiratory control, milk spilling, and stressed facial expression, part of the consultation involved teaching the mother to safely bottle-feed.

The LC explained that pacing with a bottle can be done 2 ways. Some feeders prefer to withdraw the bottle and rest it lightly on the upper lip of the baby, waiting for a cue that the baby is ready to suck again. This method is seen in **Figs. 331-334**.

Some practitioners note that as the bottle is removed, some infants will resist the withdrawal. They may suck harder to hold onto the bottle, and may then swallow excessive amounts of milk as a consequence. Instead of withdrawing the bottle, the feeder first drops the level of fluid out of the teat, leaving an empty teat in the baby's mouth. When the baby reorganizes and starts to suck again, the feeder lifts the bottle and offers more milk.

As with cup feeding, it is important during bottle-feeding to maintain fluid level with the infant's lips. Pouring milk into the baby's mouth is generally an unsafe practice. Undue concern over "air swallowing" has caused most parents and even some HCPs to elevate the bottle so that there is no air in the teat. This puts an excessive gravity drop on the fluids and increases the rate of flow so that it often overwhelms even normal, term infants. Milk spilling and choking result.

Simply holding the fluid horizontally in the bottle will slow the rate of milk transfer. This makes feeding more comfortable for the baby (**Fig. 335**). Parents can be reassured that air bubbles in the bottle are not reflective of dangerous amounts of air going into the baby's stomach. All infants swallow some air while feeding. Burping or "winding" will solve that problem. It is more dangerous for the baby to manage a too-rapid milk flow.

Since the goal of the lactation consultant is to transition infants to breastfeeding as soon as possible, it is useful to teach parents to bottle-feed in a breastfeeding position (**Fig. 336**).

Some feeding therapists contend that certain types of bottle teats can be useful to help transition poor feeders to the breast (Noble 1997, Kassing 2002). In their experience, BWC and KH find that an experimental approach is best. Some infants require a narrow based teat owing to poor lip tone and inability to seal to a wide base. Some infants will gag if the teat is too long. Other infants seem not to respond if the teat is too short and insufficient proprioreceptive stimulation is provided along the tongue.

The infant in **Fig. 337** is feeding from a special bottle that was formerly called a Haberman Feeder™. Renamed the Special Care Feeder™, it features a chambered teat with a valve that permits a controllable flow rate. Some feeding specialists prefer this bottle because infants with clefts of the palate can operate it with gum compression. That is, they do not have to create suction to get milk. The flow rate of this teat is rapid, however, and it may overwhelm some infants unless pacing techniques are also employed.

All alternative methods of feeding have benefits and drawbacks. Rationales for selecting one method over another will vary, even among experienced lactation consultants. No method is guaranteed to work well every time, and it is possible for any method to result in a preference in the infant for continuing to be fed that way. This is commonly termed "confusion," but may be more accurately described as the development of an altered expectation for a satisfying feeding (Wilson-Clay 1996).

Because selection of an alternate feeding method is affected by the debate over the issue of nipple confusion, further research into the phenomenon and into the safety of alternative feeding methods is required. Dowling (2001) points out: "The relationship between exposure to artificial nipples and pacifiers and the development of the aversive feeding behaviors associated with nipple confusion is neither refuted nor supported in the research literature."

What seems clear is that appropriate counseling can help parents move toward normalizing feedings for those infants previously unable to breastfeed. Buckley (2006) discussed reasons parents give for continuation of pumping and bottle-feeding. Such parents lack confidence, and may initially feel that bottles are both more convenient and easier to quantify. The time commitment of "triple feeding" serves to jeopardize lactation. The LC must help families see that the burden of pumping and bottle-feeding can be relieved as the infant is gradually transitioned to the breast.

The mother will need help learning to interpret the indistinct feeding cues of her baby, and counseled that things will improve as the infant matures and grows. Assistance in transitioning the baby to normal feeding (i.e., breastfeeding) is part of the intervention. It may require outpatient follow-up or referral to a community-based LC to complete, but no intervention should be prematurely abandoned just because the patient has been discharged. Adequate follow-up is routine in other areas of medicine, and should be regarded as such until the infant is successfully transitioned to breastfeeding.

Until definitive research establishes clear rationales for the selection of alternative feeding methods, feeding choices will be partly based on the parent's feeding preferences. Such choices must be tailored to the individual infant. It is important for lactation specialists to maintain follow-up with mothers in order to monitor outcomes. This permits the LC to hone her own craft and refine her techniques.

It has been the authors' experiences that infants who are merely mildly habituated to an alternate method of feeding can be transitioned to breastfeeding with patience and skill. The infant with a dysfunctional suck or other problem may not be able to transition if breastfeeding remains a skill beyond his or her abilities (Neifert 1995).

Alper B, Manno C. Dysphagia in infants and children with oral-motor deficits: assessment and management. *Seminars in Speech and Language* 1996; 17(4):283-309.

Bornmann PG. A legal primer for lactation consultants. in R Mannel, P Martens, M Walker, *Core Curriculum for Lactation Consultants* 2nd ed. Sudbury, MA: Jones and Bartlett. 2008; pp. 159-190.

Borucki LC. Breastfeeding mothers' experiences using a supplemental feeding tube device: finding an alternative. *Journal of Human Lactation* 2005; 21(4):429-428.

Buckley KM, Charles GE. Benefits and challenges of transitioning preterm infants to at-breast feedings. *International Breastfeeding Journal* 2006; 1:13.

Chen CH, Wang TM, Chang HM, et al. The effect of breast and bottle feeding on oxygen saturation and body temperature in preterm infants. *Journal of Human Lactation* 2000; 16(1):21-27.

Cloherty M, Alexander J, Holloway I, et al. The cup-versus-bottle debate: a theme from an ethnographic study of the supplementation of breastfed infants in hospital in the United Kingdom. *Journal of Human Lactation* 2005; 21(2):151-162.

Davis HV. Effects of cup, bottle and breastfeeding on oral activities of newborn infants. *Pediatrics* 1948; 2:549-558.

Dowling D, Meier P, DiDiore J, et al. Cup-feeding for preterm infants: mechanics and safety. *Journal of Human Lactation* 2002; 18(1):13-20.

Dowling D, Thanattherakul W. Nipple confusion, alternative feeding methods, and breast-feeding supplementation: state of the science. *Newborn and Infant Nursing Review* 2001; 1(4):217-223.

Ekstrom A, Widstrom AM, Nissen E: Duration of breastfeeding in Swedish primiparous and multiparous women. *Journal of Human Lactation* 2003; 19(2):172-178.

Flint A, New K, Davies M. Cup feeding versus other forms of supplemental enteral feeding for newborn infants unable to fully breastfeed. *Cochrane Database System Review* 2007; (2):CD005092.

Fredeen RC. Cup feeding of newborn infants. *Pediatrics* 1948; 2:544-548.

Freer Y. A comparison of breast and cup feeding in preterm infants: effect on physiological parameters. *Journal of Neonatal Nursing* 1999; 5:16-21.

Gribble K. Adoptive breastfeeding beyond infancy. *Leaven*, Oct-Nov. 2004; pp. 99-104.

Hall JK. *Law & Ethics for Clinicians*. Vega, TX: Jackhal Books. 2002; pp. 179, 275-279.

Hoover K. Supplementation of the newborn by spoon in the first 24 hours. *Journal of Human Lactation* 1998; 14(3):245.

Howard C, de Blieck EA, ten Hoopen CB, et al. Physiologic stability of newborns during cup and bottle-feeding. *Pediatrics* (Supplement) 1999; 104(5):1204-1207.

Kassing D. Bottle-feeding as a tool to reinforce breastfeeding. *Journal of Human Lactation* 2002; 18(1):56-60.

Kelly BN, Huckabee ML, Jones RD, et al. Nutritive and non-nutritive swallowing apnea duration in term infants: implications for neural control mechanisms. *Respiratory Physiology & Neurobiology* 2006; 154(3):372-378.

Kliethermes PA, Cross ML, Lanese MG, et al. Transitioning preterm infants with nasogastric tube supplementation: increased likelihood of breastfeeding. *Journal of Obstetric, Gynecologic, and Neonatal Nursing* 1999; 28(3):264-273.

Lang S, Lawrence CJ, L'e Orme R. Cup feeding: an alternative method of infant feeding. *Archives of Disease in Childhood* 1994; 71(4):365-369.

Law-Morstatt L, Judd D, Snyder P, et al. Pacing as a treatment technique for transitional sucking patterns. *Journal of Perinatology* 2003; 23(6):483-488.

Lawrence RA , Lawrence RM. *Breastfeeding: A Guide for the Medical Profession* (6th ed). Philadelphia, PA: Elsevier Mosby, 2005; p. 261.

L'Esperance C, Frantz K. Time limitation for early breastfeeding. *Journal of Obstetric, Gynecologic, and Neonatal Nursing* 1985; 14(2):114-118.

Malhotra N, Vishwimbaran L, Sundaram KR, et al. A controlled trial of alternative methods of oral feeding in neonates. *Early Human Development* 1999; 54(1):29-38.

Marinelli KA, Burke GS, Dodd VL. A comparison of the safety of cup feedings and bottlefeedings in premature infants whose mothers intend to breastfeed. *Journal of Perinatology* 2001; 21(6):350-355.

Mathew OP. Determinants of milk flow through nipple units: role of hole size and nipple thickness. *American Journal of Diseases of Children* 1990; 144(2):222-224.

Measel C, Anderson G. Non-nutritive sucking during tube feedings: effect on clinical course in premature infants. *Journal of Obstetrical, Gynecologic and Neonatal Nursing* 1979; 8(5):265-272.

Meier P. Bottle and breastfeeding: effects on transcutaneous oxygen pressure and temperature in preterm infants. *Nursing Research* 1988; 37(1):36-41.

Meier P, Anderson GC. Responses of small preterm infants to bottle and breastfeeding. *Maternal Child Nursing* 1987; 12(2):97-105.

Neifert M, Lawrence R, Seacat J. Nipple confusion: toward a formal definition. *Journal of Pediatrics* 1995; 126(6):125-129.

Noble R, Bovey A. Therapeutic teat use for babies who breastfeed poorly. *Breastfeeding Review* 1997; 5(2):37-42.

Oddy W, Glenn K. Implementing the Baby Friendly Hospital Initiative: the role of finger feeding. *Breastfeeding Review* 2003; 11(1):5-9.

Palmer MM. Sensory-Based Oral Feeding Disorders, presentation, Fourth Annual Breastfeeding and the High Risk Neonate Conference, Albuquerque, NM: University of New Mexico, March 6, 1998.

Parry M, Grant B, Ykna M, et al. Candida osteomyelitis and diskitis after spinal surgery: an outbreak that implicates artificial nail use. *Clinical Infectious Diseases* 2001; 32(3):352-57.

Pinelli J, Symington A. Non-nutritive sucking for promoting physiologic stability and nutrition in preterm infants. *Cochrane Database System Review* 2005; (4): CD001071.

Protecting, Promoting and Supporting Breast-feeding: The Special Role of Maternity Services, A joint WHO/UNICEF Statement. Geneva, Switzerland: WHO, 1989.

Raimbault C, Saliba E, Porter RH. The effect of the odour of mother's milk on breastfeeding behavior of premature neonates. *Acta Paediatrica* 2007; 96(3):368-371.

Ramsay DT, Mitoulas LR, Kent JC, et al. Milk flow rates can be used to identify and investigate milk ejection in women expressing breast milk using an electric breast pump. *Breastfeeding Medicine* 2006; 1(1):14-23.

Rocha N, Martinez F, Jorge S. Cup or bottle for preterm infants: effects on oxygen saturation, weight gain, and breastfeeding. *Journal of Human Lactation* 2002; 18(2):132-138.

Slusher T, Slusher IL, Biomdo M, et al. Electric breast pump use increases maternal milk volume in African nurseries. *Journal of Tropical Pediatrics* 2007; 53(2):125-130.

Stein MJ. Breastfeeding the premature newborn: a protocol without bottles. *Journal of Human Lactation* 1990; 6(4):167-170.

Thorley V. Cup-feeding: problems created by incorrect use. *Journal of Human Lactation* 1997; 13(1):54-55.

Victoria C, Behague D, Barros F, et al. Pacifier use and short breastfeeding duration: cause, consequence, or coincidence? *Pediatrics* 1997; 99(3):445-453.

UNICEF. Baby-Friendly Initiative 1991. http://www.unicef.org/programme/breastfeeding/baby.htm#10. Accessed July 17, 2008.

Wight N. Management of common breastfeeding issues, in RJ Schanler, (ed). *The Pediatric Clinics of North America,* Breastfeeding 2001, Part II, The Management of Breastfeeding 2001; 48(2):321-344.

Wilson-Clay B. Clinical use of nipple shields. *Journal of Human Lactation* 1996; 12(4):279-285.

Wilson-Clay B. External pacing techniques: protecting respiratory stability during feeding. Independent Study Module, Amarillo, TX: Hale Publishing, 2005.

Wolf L, Glass R. *Feeding and Swallowing Disorders in Infancy.* Tucson, AZ: Therapy Skill Builders, 1992; pp. 108, 115-116.

Donor Human Milk Banking

Wet nursing describes the practice of a woman breast-feeding a baby other than her own. Historically, wet nurses were employed either by choice or necessity as the only reliable method to ensure an infant's survival if the infant's own mother did not breastfeed. Wet nursing was a well-established custom in many cultures. Historical records include laws, codes of conduct, and contracts pertaining to the practice. Both wet nursing and hand feeding of infants persist into the modern era.

Obed (2007) assessed the mortality outcomes of infants born to mothers who died in childbirth in Nigeria. According to local customs, such infants are fed animal milk or breastfed by an aunt or grandmother. Only 31.3 percent of infants orphaned at birth survived to age 5. Factors favoring survival included surrogate breastfeeding.

Many cultures have set standards governing the selection of a suitable wet nurse (Fildes 1986). Likewise, infant feeding vessels, often found in graves, provide anthropological evidence that other infants were *dry nursed*; that is, fed by hand. These feeding implements were made out of various materials and some contain residue of substances including animal milks and what may be described as ritual beverages (Fildes 1995).

Artificial formulas have changed over time in an effort to more closely resemble human milk; however, formula cannot duplicate the composition of human milk. Defective, contaminated formula, and high levels of potentially toxic metals in formula pose additional risks to the preterm or otherwise fragile infant (Navarro-Blasco 2003, Iverson 2004, Fattal-Valevski 2005). These risks make the use of human milk more desirable. Today, most health authorities advise against the practice of casual human milk sharing, owing to the risk of virus transmission. The documented risks of formula and the theoretical risks of infection through casual milk sharing have created renewed interest in human milk banking as a method of providing safe milk for infants who cannot breastfeed directly.

The immunological benefits of human milk continue to be elucidated (Hamosh 2001, Hanson 2004). Evidence suggests that preterm and medically fragile infants especially benefit from human milk feedings (Oddy 2004, Shoji 2004, Ronnestad 2005). Yet, mothers of preterm infants may have difficulty initiating or maintaining milk supplies sufficient for their infant's needs. Infants with feeding intolerance, short gut syndrome,

burns, renal failure, and other medical illnesses, have been assisted with exclusive human milk feeds (Hanson 2004). Owing to the stress of caring for a sick child, many mothers of such children may struggle to maintain adequate milk supplies. Screened, pasteurized, donor human milk is being used in these populations as a safe nutritional and therapeutic alternative to formula, or to informal milk sharing.

Proponents of human milk banking have argued that receiving human milk is a human right of the infant (Arnold 2006). Lording (2006) observed that in spite of demonstrated cost-effectiveness, milk banking is "largely invisible from national breastfeeding policies." This observation prompted recommendations that human milk banking should become an integral component of national breastfeeding policies. Best practices for the operation of donor human milk banks are being developed on a country-by-country basis, and in association with milk banking organizations. These practices include screening and processing criteria, traceability, and maintenance of records of all processing and storage conditions (Hartmann 2007).

Neonatal Necrotizing Enterocolitis (NEC)

A Cochrane Review compared formula with donor human milk for feeding preterm or low birth weight infants (Quigley 2007). While formula produced a higher rate of short-term growth, it led to a higher rate of risk for the development of *necrotising enterocolitis*. NEC is a devastating inflammatory condition that destroys the lining of the intestinal wall (Luig 2005). The causes of this painful disease are unclear, although 75 percent of cases occur in preterm infants. NEC accounts for a significant percentage of deaths in infants <1500 g. Many infants who develop NEC are treated surgically to remove affected sections of their bowels. These infants then develop short gut syndrome, which puts them at risk for life-time nutritional disabilities.

Lucas (1990) reported that NEC was rare in those preterm infants receiving at least some human milk feeds. He observed that the incidence of NEC was 20 times more common in formula-fed infants. Dvorak (2003) reported that maternal milk is the major source of trophic peptides with significant healing effects on injured gastrointestinal mucosa. Women who deliver preterm infants have higher concentrations of these peptides in their milk than are present in term milk or in formula (Chuang 2005). In the past, it was unclear whether donor human milk provided a protective effect similar to own mother's milk in the reduction of NEC. McGuire (2003) performed a meta-analysis of previous reseach and identified a significant association in reduction of relative risk of NEC in preterm infants fed *donor* human milk rather than formula. Improved neonatal outcomes in human milk-fed infants suggest an increased role for own mother's (Stout 2008) and donor human milk to reduce NEC and to improve growth and development in preterm infants (Slusher 2003, Diehl-Jones 2004, Updegrove 2004).

History and Guidelines

Although some cultures impose prohibitions or restrictions on the use of both wet nursing and on the use of donor human milk, milk banking has been common in Western European countries, Scandinavia, South and Central America, and China since the early 1900's. However, the trend toward formula feeding, hospital budgetary crises, and the HIV/AIDs epidemic saw the closure of many North American milk banks (Jones 2003). Since the 1980s, there has been a resurgence of interest in donor human milk banking in the US using screened donors and pasteurized milk. This renewed interest led to the formation in 1985 of the Human Milk Banking Association of North America (HMBANA). This organization is comprised of representatives from member banks and has developed guidelines establishing donor requirements, screening protocols, pasteurization policies, and described bacteriological quality control requirements for dispensed donor milk. The HMBANA guidelines take into consideration similar guidelines developed for other human donor tissues by the US Centers for Disease Control, the US Food and Drug Administration, and the American Association of Blood Banks.

Ethical issues and policies regarding donors and recipients and the conduct of the milk banks are addressed by individual milk bank regulations and more broadly at the level of HMBANA. There currently is no regulation of donor milk banks by the US government; however, there is consensus among the existing milk banks to adhere to HMBANA standards. The HMBANA guidelines describe donor requirements and exclusions, processing, and storage policies. Policies can be viewed on the HMBANA website: www.hmbana.org.

As of July 2008, the HMBANA network includes one Canadian milk bank and 10 donor milk banks in the US. Other communities are in the process of investigating how to establish a local milk bank. Since 2000, the growth in milk banking in North America has resulted in a 185 percent increase in the distribution of donor milk; over one million ounces of milk dispensed (Flatau 2008).

Different communities have created different models for human milk banks. Some milk banks are associated with research institutions or universities. Some are hospital-based. Others are free-standing, not-for-profit corporations funded through grants, program fees, and donations. Some hospital-based programs collect and dispense *own mother's* milk to infants who are patients in the special care nursery. While often referred to as "milk banks," these do not meet the HMBANA definition of a milk bank. HMBANA guidelines refer to facilities that provide *donor* milk. Some milk banks also have a research component. These institutions may provide small milk samples to scientists studying topics relevant to human milk (Geraghty 2005). The studies might include investigating the best methods of processing, storing, labeling, and dispensing human milk. Some milk banks also provide milk for older children and even for adults who require nutritional support in special situations.

HMBANA milk banks do not sell milk; however, they do establish fees that are calculated to recover some of the costs of screening, processing, and distributing the milk. The costs of screening and processing (but not of distributing) donor milk is sometimes reimbursed by private US insurance companies or government programs such as Medicaid. The HMBANA member banks advocate for increased private and public funding resources for donor human milk. All HMBANA banks have agreed to supply physician-prescribed donor human milk regardless of ability to pay for patients who meet established criteria. HMBANA is committed to maintain a non-profit approach to human donor milk banking, and to avoid creating an "industry" whose investors profit from the free donation of a human tissue; in this case, milk.

Donor Recruitment, Screening, and Exclusions

As demand for donor human milk increases, recruitment of adequate numbers of donor mothers has become an issue in some countries. To facilitate donor recruitment, several studies have examined the characteristics of human milk donors. While altruism and concern for the health of fragile infants have been identified as qualities of milk donors (Osbaldiston 2007, Azema 2003) other research has identified encouragement of a health professional as the primary reason for donation (Pimenteira 2008).

The first step in establishing the safety of donor human milk involves the careful screening of donors. HMBANA milk banks follow this protocol. A preliminary questionnaire is administered during a telephone interview. The interview elicits general information about travel history, health history, and screens for life style risk factors. A more comprehensive written questionnaire is administered to prospective donors who progress beyond the phone interview stage.

Blood tests (paid for by the milk bank) screen for HIV, HTLV, Hepatitis B and C, and syphilis. Donors may not smoke, drink more than 2 alcoholic drinks daily, or use illegal drugs. A woman cannot donate if she or her partner is at risk for HIV, if she has obtained a tattoo in the past year, or received a blood transfusion or organ transplant in the past 6 months. Women from certain African countries are excluded as donors (see HMBANA website). Women who lived in the UK for more than 3 months prior to 1996, or who lived in specific areas of Europe for more than 5 years between 1980-1996 are also excluded owing to concerns about Creutzfeld Jacob disease (the human form of what is commonly called mad cow disease).

Donors may use either progestin-only birth control pills or low dose (a maximum of 20mcg estrogen) estrogen/prog-esterone pills (Hale 2003). Women who have received Depo Provera injections and IUDs are also acceptable as donors. Synthroid (thyroid replacement hormone), insulin, and prenatal vitamins are also permitted. Donors may not be regular users of other medications, herbal supplements or mega-vitamins. All mothers who wish to donate are asked to commit to donating a minimum amount of milk (generally 100 oz). The establishment of a minimum level of donation assures that the milk bank will not incur the expenses related to screening with no return benefit. Exceptions are made for bereaved mothers, from whom smaller amounts of milk may be accepted. Finally, the donor must be in good health. A pediatrician must certify that her own infant is growing at the expected rate for that infant. The donor screening process seeks to ensure that the milk is safe and that no monetary incentive (or other issue) will deprive an infant of his own mother's milk.

Of special interest to milk banks are donors who deliver prematurely and those who are on dairy-free diets. Milk from both special categories of donors is processed and stored separately. This milk is dispensed to preterm infants or to those who exhibit dairy protein intolerance. Preterm milk differs from term milk in a variety of ways (Ronayne de Ferrer 2000, Dvorak 2003, Bielicki 2004). Preterm milk has higher protein levels (for about 4 weeks after the birth) than term milk (Lemons 1982, Butte 1984). Milk may be mixed with fortifiers to obtain the ideal mix of protein, minerals, and calories to help very small babies grow.

For some mothers, donating to a milk bank becomes an important part of the grieving process if their own baby has died (Tully 1999). These women find comfort in being able to provide life giving assistance to another baby.

Processing Donor Milk

A screening program in a Chinese hospital tested the milk of mothers who were expressing breastmilk for their own hospitalized premature infants. Unusually high rates of pathogens were discovered in their milk, including *enterococci* and *Staphylococcus aureus* (*S. aureus*). Researchers suspected that bacteriological contamination may have resulted from cultural traditions that prohibit bathing for one month after childbirth (Ng 2004). This study suggests that anticipatory guidance on hygiene is an important part of the education provided to mothers who are expressing milk for their own or other babies.

According to HMBANA guidelines, once a woman has been accepted as a donor, she receives written instructions relating to the hygienic collection of her milk. The mother temporarily stores milk in her own freezer until she accumulates enough to take a quantity of it to a collection site or directly to the milk bank. The raw, frozen milk is labeled, carefully logged, and stored in large freezers (**Fig. 338**).

Pasteurization of human donor milk is undertaken to protect fragile infants from viral and bacterial illness. While the pasteurization of own mother's milk has been shown to reduce fat absorption and growth in some preterm infants compared to unpasteurized own mother's milk (Andersson 2007), most donor milk is pasteurized. Many benefits remain after pasteurization. Biologically active compounds such as oligosaccharides, for example, play an "emerging leading role" in protecting preterm infants (Bertino 2008). Holder pasteurization does not affect the concentration or pattern of oligosaccharides in human donor milk. New methods of high-temperature short-time pasteurization (HTST) are being studied. Research has concluded that HTST is effective in the elimination of "bacteria and certain important pathogenic viruses" (Terpstra 2007). As milk banks struggle to accommodate increasing demands, new technologies for processing donor milk are needed.

In some milk banks, for example the Mothers' Milk Bank at Austin (MMBA), raw milk is biologically sampled and tested *prior* to pasteurizing as well as afterwards. Pre-testing is performed owing to concerns of milk contamination from *S. aureus*. Some strains of *S. aureus* are capable of producing a highly heat-stable protein toxin that causes food poisoning-like symptoms in humans (USFDA 2005). Pasteurization kills most pathogens in human milk, but some concern remains that *S. aureus* enterotoxin may pose risks to fragile babies. Some neonatologists believe that raw milk that contains *S. aureus* (and a similar heat-loving organism called *bacillis)* should be discarded. All milk banks discard milk that grows bacteria following pasteurization.

Researchers continue to investigate the best method of milk storage. Length of storage time and storage temperature affect milk integrity (Ogundele 2002, Hanna 2004). Changes in milk antioxidant activity occur from chilling and freezing. This may be important in populations of preterm infants, whose poorly developed antioxidant systems put them at increased risk of tissue damage from oxygen free radicals. Human milk's antioxidant activity may be one of the mechanisms that protect preterm infants from NEC, chronic lung disease, and intraventricular hemorrhage (Shoji 2004). Freezing somewhat diminishes the antioxidant activity of human milk. The optimal methods for human milk storage constitute an important area for future research.

Cytomegalovirus

Newborn exposure to *cytomegalovirus* (CMV) may occur during delivery or afterward through virus shed in breast milk (Meier 2005). Very low birth weight infants may be more susceptible to the virus because they are born before the transfer of protective immunoglobulins and they have extremely immature immune systems. Some special care nurseries freeze own mother's milk for 3 days in order to minimize the risk of neonatal CMV infection. However, new research has demonstrated that while freezing can diminish the viral load, it does not kill CMV in human milk. Hamprecht (2004) reported that viral infectivity of CMV was preserved in milk that had been frozen. Heat treatment with pasteurization kills CMV; therefore, donor mothers are not specifically tested for the virus.

Informal milk sharers should be informed that women with reactivated CMV infection and even some women with primary cases may be asymptomatic or only mildly ill. Because CMV is often mistaken for a common cold, a casual milk donor may not think to withhold her milk from donation during such mild illness. However, virus is being shed into the milk (Vochem 1998). Unpasteurized milk may thus exposes a recipient infant to acute CMV infection (Meier 2005). CMV is sometimes fatal in extremely low birth weight premature infants.

In Norway, researchers have demonstrated the benefits of providing freshly frozen unpasteurized donor milk to hospitalized infants whose own mothers are temporarily unable to produce sufficient milk. However, the donors are carefully screened for CMV status before donating milk and are re-screened every 3 months (Lindemann 2004). When close screening is impossible, pasteurization is vital.

Milk Labeling

In donor milk banks, raw milk is thawed for processing on regularly scheduled pasteurization days. In some milk banks, milk from several mothers is *randomly* pooled in hopes of assuring homogeneous fat content and a wide variety of immune factors. In Texas, the Mothers Milk Bank at Austin (MMBA) sought more specific control of this process that led to the purchase of a Foss Milkoscan (**Fig. 339**). This machine, which is widely used in the dairy industry, conducts a full spectrum infrared nutritional analysis. MMBA neonatologists re-calibrated it for human milk values. Use of the Milkocscan permits *targeted* pooling of donor milk. In other words, the milk in each pool is specifically selected for optimal nutritional values. Each bottle of pooled milk is then labeled with the total caloric and protein content. This method also permits identification of milk that cannot meet optimal levels, and therefore is not adequate for use in populations of hospitalized infants with high growth requirements.

The MMBA dispenses milk to special care nurseries with caloric values of 20, 22, and 24 calories per ounce. Labeling assists in the feeding of hospitalized infants with differing nutritional requirements. Outpatients are generally able to receive milk that is 17 calories per ounce or higher. Controlling for the calorie content of human donor milk may prevent growth problems in compromised infants (Slusher 2003).

It is important to note that individual variations in the caloric value of own mother's milk are insignificant for the normal breastfeeding baby. Breastfeeding babies are able to regulate their milk intake to accommodate for variations in milk fat content that arises owing to time of day, relative breast fullness, or any other factor (Daly 1993). Consequently issues related to the calorie value of pumped milk are only relevant for the non-breastfeeding infant.

In **Fig. 340** pasteurization workers at the MMBA have performed targeted pooling of the milk of 3 mothers. The milk of these 3 donors was selected for pooled processing because the caloric and protein content of their milk will complement each other to satisfy minimum requirements. The workers shown in **Fig. 340** pour pooled milk from large, sterilized, glass beakers into sterilized 4-ounce glass bottles. The bottles are capped with sterilized metal caps and placed into pasteurizers (**Fig. 341**) for Holder pasteurization. That is, the milk will be held in a shaking water bath at a carefully monitored temperature of 62.5°C for 30 minutes (**Fig 342**). Following heat treatment, the bottles are plunged into an ice slurry to cool quickly.

Prior to re-freezing the milk, the worker shown in **Fig. 343** withdraws small samples of milk for post-pasteurization bacteriological testing. Bottles are labeled with the date of pasteurization, a coded number identifying the donors in the pool, and information about caloric and protein values. The processed bottles are frozen to await the results of bacterial testing (**Fig. 344**). Records are carefully maintained, and the milk is not available to be dispensed until bacteriological results are reviewed.

When bacteriological results are received, each bottle is labeled with an expiration date one year from the earliest pumping date of the milk in that batch. Freezers in the MMBA are equipped with sensors that alert staff during power outages. Emergency generators protect the integrity of the frozen milk (**Fig. 345**).

Processed milk is transported by car to various hospitals within the city or region served by specific milk banks. Other batches are packed to prevent thawing and tampering and are shipped by air for 24-hour delivery.

The Rewards

Developing a donor human milk bank is a rewarding undertaking with wide-reaching benefits to the community in terms of improved outcomes for preterm infants and shorter hospital stays. A case of NEC increases the length of a preterm baby's hospital stay and adds cost to the care provided to that infant. Each case of medical NEC is estimated to cost a hospital an additional $74,000 (US dollars). It costs an additional $186,000 to treat a case of surgical NEC (Bisquera 2000). Prevention of NEC with the use of donor human milk is clearly cost effective.

HMBANA milk banks share a commitment to provide information on how to start a milk bank. Individual milk banks provide additional resources to communities who wish to develop such a resource.

Fig. 346 shows members of the board of directors of the MMBA.* The Austin experience suggests that assembling a diverse board of directors is an important aspect of success. It is critical to have participation and support from medical care providers, especially neonatologists. However, by inviting diverse participation, a milk bank achieves "buy-in" from the community at large. Milk bank board members serve without pay, and each brings specific expertise to the project. The MMBA board includes La Leche League leaders, RNs, IBCLCs, researchers, representatives from the health department, and neonatologists. Other valuable members represent the arts, business, legal, insurance, computer technology, religious, and entertainment communities.

A creative mix of personalities and talents allows special board committees to address specific needs of the project. Some committees raise funds, others seek positive publicity. Legislative committees may lobby to seek state funding to serve indigent clients. Board committees help establish ethics policies, analyze business practices, and engage in strategic planning to meet future needs. Additionally, the board of directors works to develop educational outreach to familiarize the public with the benefits of donor milk and to recruit donors. Milk banks employ paid staff who manage the day-to-day operations. This staff should include an IBCLC to work with donor mothers and with recipient families. Milk banks also generally utilize a cadre of volunteers whose services are often critical to the success of the project.

Most communities depend upon local blood and tissue centers to meet the needs of their citizens. Similar widespread establishment of local donor human milk banks will allow more preterm and critically ill infants to receive the therapeutic benefits and superior nutritional support of human milk feeds.

Disclaimer: Barbara Wilson-Clay is a founding board member and serves as the Vice President of the board of directors of the Mothers Milk Bank of Austin. She receives no financial compensation and has no conflicts of interest to declare with regard to the information presented here.

Andersson Y, Savman K, Blackberg L, et al. Pasteurization of mother's own milk reduces fat absorption and growth in preterm infants. *Acta Paediatrica* 2007; 96(10):1445-1449.

Arnold LD. Global health policies that support the use of banked donor human milk: a human rights issue. *International Breastfeeding Journal* 2006; 1:26.

Azema E, Callahan S. Breast milk donors in France: a portrait of the typical donor and the utility of milk banking in the French breastfeeding context. *Journal of Human Lactation* 2003; 19(2):199-202.

Bertino E, Coppa GV, Guiliani F, et al. Effects of Holder pasteurization on human milk oligosaccharides. *International Journal of Immunopathological Pharmacology* 2008; 21(2):381-385.

Bielicki J, Huch R, von Mandach U. Time-course of leptin levels in term and preterm human milk. *European Journal of Endocrinology* 2004; 151(2):271-276.

Bisquera JA, Cooper TR, Berseth CL Impact of necrotizing enterocolitis on length of stay and hospital charges in very low birthweight infants. *Pediatrics* 2002; 109(3):423-428.

Butte N, Garza C, Johnson C, et al. Longitudinal changes in milk composition of mothers delivering preterm and term infants. *Early Human Development* 1984; 9(2):153-162.

Chuang C, Lin S, Lee H, et al. Free amino acids in full-term and pre-term human milk and infant formula. *Journal of Pediatric Gastroenterology and Nutrition* 2005; 40(4):496-500.

Daly SE, Owens RA, Hartmann PE. The short-term synthesis and infant-regulated removal of milk in lactating women. *Experimental Physiology* 1993; 78(2):209-220.

Diehl-Jones W, Askin D. Nutritional modulation of neonatal outcomes. *AACN Clinical Issues* 2004; 15(1):83-96.

Dvorak B, Fituch C, Williams C, et al. Increased epidermal growth factor levels in human milk of mothers with extremely premature infants. *Pediatric Research* 2003; 54(1):15-19.

Fattal-Valevski A, Kesler A, Sela B, et al. Outbreak of life-threatening thiamine deficiency in infants in Israel caused by defective soy-based formula. *Pediatrics* 2005; 115(2):e233-238.

Fildes V. *Breasts, Bottles and Babies: A History of Infant Feeding.* Edinburgh, Scotland: Edinburgh University Press, 1986.

Fildes V. The culture and biology of breastfeeding: an historical review of Western Europe, in P Stuart-Macadam, K Dettwyler (ed), *Breastfeeding: Biocultural Perspectives* New York, NY: Aldine de Gruyter, 1995; pp. 101-126.

Flatau G. Milk banks keep the milk flowing - HMBANA responds to increasing demand. *HMBANA Matters* 2008; 5:1.

Geraghty S, Davidson B, Warner B, et al. The development of a research human milk bank. *Journal of Human Lactation* 2005; 21(1):59-66.

Hale T. Medications in breastfeeding mothers of preterm infants. *Pediatric Annals* 2003; 32(5):337-347.

Hamosh M. Bioactive factors in human milk, in RJ Schanler, (ed). *The Pediatric Clinics of North America* 2001; 48(1):69-86.

Hamprecht K, Maschmann J, Muller D, et al. Cytomegalovirus (CMV) inactivation in breast milk: reassessment of pasteurization and freeze-thawing. *Pediatric Research* 2004; 56(4):529-535.

Hanna N, Ahmed K, Anwar M, et al. Effect of storage on breast milk antioxidant activity. *Archives of Disease in Childhood Fetal and Neonatal Edition* 2004; 89(6):F518-520.

Hanson L. *The Immunobiology of Human Milk.* Amarillo, TX: Pharmasoft Publishing, 2004.

Hartmann BT, Pang WW, Kell AD, et al. Best practice guidelines for the operation of a donor human milk bank in an Australian NICU. *Early Human Development* 2007; 83(10):667-673.

Iversen C, Lane M, Forsythe SJ. The growth profile, thermotolerance and biofilm formation of *Enterobacter sakazakii* grown in infant formula milk. *Letters in Applied Microbiology* 2004; 38(5):378-382.

Jones F. History of North American donor milk banking: one hundred years of progress. *Journal of Human Lactation* 2003; 19(3):313-318.

Lemons J, Moye L, Hall D, et al. Differences in the composition of preterm and term human milk during early lactation. *Pediatric Research* 1982; 16(2):113-117.

Lindemann P, Foshaugen I, Lindemann R. Characteristics of breast milk and serology of women donating breast milk to a milk bank. *Archives of Disease in Childhood Fetal and Neonatal Edition* 2004; 89(5):F440-441.

Lording RJ. A review of human milk banking and public health policy in Australia. *Breastfeeding Reveiw* 2006; 14(3):21-30.

Lucas A, Cole TJ. Breast milk and neonatal necrotising enterocolitis. *Lancet* 1990; 336(8730):1519-1523.

Luig M, Lui K; NSW & ACT NICUS Group. Epidemiology of necrotizing enterocolitis - Part I: changing regional trends in extremely preterm infants over 14 years. *Journal of Paediatric Child Health* 2005; 41(4):169-173.

McGuire W, Anthony M. Donor human milk versus formula for preventing necrotizing enterocolitis in preterm infants: systematic review. *Archives of Disease in Childhood Fetal and Neonatal Edition* 2003; 88(1):F11-F14.

Meier J, Lienicke U, Tschirach E, Kruger D, et al. Human cytomegalovirus reactivation during lactation and mother-to-child transmission in preterm infants. *Journal of Clinical Microbiology* 2005; 43(3):1318-1324.

Navarro-Blasco I, Alvarez-Galindo J. Aluminium content of Spanish infant formula. *Food Additives and Contaminants* 2003; 20(5):470-481.

Ng D, Lee S, Leung L, et al. Bacteriological screening of expressed breast milk revealed a high rate of contamination in Chinese women. *Journal of Hospital Infection* 2004; 58(2):146-150.

Obed JY, Agida ET, Mairiga AG. Survival of infants and children born to women who died from pregnancy and labour related complications. *Nigerian Journal of Clinical Practice* 2007; 10(1):35-40.

Oddy W, Sherriff J, de Klerk N, et al. The relation of breastfeeding and body mass index to asthma and atopy in children: a prospective cohort study to age 6 years. *American Journal of Public Health* 2004; 94(9):1531-1537.

Ogundele MO. Effects of storage on the physicochemical and antibacterial properties of human milk. *British Journal of Biomedical Science* 2002; 59(4):205-211.

Osbaldiston R, Mingle L. Characteristics of human milk donors. *Journal of Human Lactation* 2007; 23(4):350-357.

Pimenteira Thomaz AC, Maia Loureiro LV, da Silva Oliveira T, et al. The human milk donation experience: motives, influencing factors, and regular donation. *Journal of Human Lactation* 2008; 24(1):69-76.

Quigley MA, Henderson G, Anthony MY, et al. Formula milk versus donor breast milk for feeding preterm or low birth weight infants. *Cochrane Database System Review* 2007; 17(4):CD002971.

Ronnestad A, Abrahamsen T, Medbo S, et al. Late-onset septicemia in a Norwegian national cohort of extremely premature infants receiving very early full human milk feeding. *Pediatrics* 2005; 115(3):e269-276.

Ronayne de Ferrer P, Baroni A, Sambucetti M, et al. Lactoferrin levels in term and preterm milk. *Journal of the American College of Nutrition* 2000; 19(3):370-373.

Shoji H, Shimizu T, Shinohara K, et al. Suppressive effects of breast milk on oxidative DNA damage in very low birthweight infants. *Archives of Disease in Childhood Fetal and Neonatal Edition* 2004; 89(2):F136-F138.

Slusher T, Hampton R, Bode-Thomas F, et al. Promoting the exclusive feeding of own mother's milk through the use of hindmilk and increased maternal milk volume for hospitalized, low birth weight infants (<1800 grams) in Nigeria: a feasibility study. *Journal of Human Lactation* 2003; 19(2):191-198.

Stout G, Lambert DK, Baer VL, et al. Necrotizing enterocolitis during the first week of life: a multicentered case-control and cohort comparison study. *Journal of Perinatology* 2008; 28(8):556-560.

Terpstra FG, Rechtman DJ, Lee ML, et al. Antimicrobial and antiviral effect of high-temperature short-time (HTST) pasteurization applied to human milk. *Breastfeeding Medicine* 2007; 2(1):27-33.

Tully MR. Donating human milk as part of the grieving process. *Journal of Human Lactation* 1999; 15(2):149-150.

Updegrove K. Necrotizing enterocolitis: the evidence for the use of human milk in prevention and treatment. *Journal of Human Lactation* 2004; 20(3):335-339.

US Food & Drug Administration (USFDA/), Center for Food Safety & Applied Nutrition. *Foodborne Pathogenic Microorganisms and Natural Toxins Handbook* (The Bad Bug Book), 2005. www.cfsan.fda.gov/~mow/chap3.html. Accessed on July 31, 2008.

Vochem M, Hamprecht K, Jahn G, et al. Transmission of cytomegalovirus to preterm infants through breast milk. *Pediatric Infectious Disease Journal* 1998; 17(1):53-58.

Breastfeeding in Special Circumstances

Because breastfeeding is normal mammalian behavior, most newborns are capable of thriving at the breast. However, special circumstances and unusual problems can and do occur. Human milk provides superior nutrition while reducing infant energy expenditure (Lubetzky 2003), thus it is especially important for the compromised infant. The health care team must possess sufficient assessment skills to identify infants who need special breastfeeding assistance (Hill 2007). In the event that direct breastfeeding is delayed, HCPs will ideally work together to ensure human milk feeds for the infant (AAP 2005).

Sometimes breastfeeding support focuses on the infant; however, maternal issues must also receive evaluation. The mother who suffers from a chronic illness or physical impairment, for instance, may deeply desire to breastfeed. While it is commonly recognized that women grieve the loss of a pregnancy, grief over the loss of the breastfeeding experience is seldom acknowledged in those cultures where bottle-feeding is prevalent (Pryor 1973).

Whether it is the infant, the mother, or both who require assistance, research demonstrates that excellent breastfeeding support results in increased maternal self-esteem and strengthens the bond between mother and baby (Ekstrom 2006). It also appears to confer resilience against psychosocial stress (Montgomery 2006). Breastfeeding provides unique physical benefits for the mother as well. For example short- and long-term decrease in maternal blood pressure has been observed during lactation (Jonas 2008). Lactation appears to be a modifiable behavior that improves maternal metabolic profile in ways that may positively affect women's future risk of cardiovascular and metabolic diseases (Gunderson 2007). Thus, effective breastfeeding support protects women both physically and emotionally, important goals when mothers are already stressed or physically challenged.

Continuity of care is particularly essential for the at-risk dyad. Referrals to community-based lactation care and to mother support groups should be routinely provided at the time of hospital discharge. What follows is an overview of cases that require extra assistance to protect and preserve successful breastfeeding.

Down Syndrome

Down Syndrome (Trisomy 21) is a chromosomal abnormality that occurs approximately once in every 1000 births. Growth and development are affected to varying degrees. Most develop as do other children, though on a delayed timetable. Down Syndrome is marked by certain distinctive physical traits, low muscle tone, and retardation that ranges from mild to severe. It is common for infants with Down Syndrome to have cardiac defects, and to be more susceptible to respiratory infections and otitis media (Davenport 1990). For information and resources available for families in the US, contact the National Down Syndrome Society: www1.ndss.org.

Exclusive or near exclusive human milk feeding lowers the incidence of illness (Raisler 1999) and thus helps maintain health. Breastfeeding also positively affects neurological development. A group of Dutch infants was studied to examine the effect of breastfeeding on neurological development (Lanting 1994). Newborn neurological examinations classified the infants at birth as normal, slightly abnormal, or frankly abnormal. At 9 years of age, the children were reexamined, and their mothers described their infant feeding practices. Researchers identified a small but significant beneficial effect of breastfeeding on neurological status, even after the data were adjusted for confounding issues. The largest randomized trial ever conducted in the area of human lactation provided evidence that prolonged and exclusive breastfeeding significantly improves the cognitive development of children (Kramer 2008).

Gross motor skill attainment was also improved in infants who breastfed or who received human milk feeds (Sacker 2006). Sacker suggests that the protective effect is "attributable to some component(s) of breast milk or feature of breastfeeding and is not simply a product of [the mother's] advantaged social position, education or of parenting style..."

In a research study that matched 560 children with Down Syndrome with 2 groups of healthy control infants, Pisacane (2003) reported that infants with Down Syndrome were significantly less likely to be breastfed. The main reasons their mothers reported for choosing to bottle-feed were: infant illness, maternal frustration and depression, perceived milk insufficiency, and infant sucking problems. Specific breastfeeding support for such mothers should become a relevant point of health supervision for children with Down Syndrome. Information about potential improvements in the child's physical health and intellectual and motor development may motivate parents of children with Down Syndrome to persevere until early problems resolve.

Some infants with Down Syndrome breastfeed well from the start. Others may be slow, inefficient feeders who need extra time at the breast and careful postural support. Ultrasonographic images reveal that sucking deficiencies in infants with Down Syndrome result from hypotonicity of the perioral muscles, lips, and masticatory muscles, and from deficiencies in the smooth tongue movement (Mizuno 2001). These sucking problems appear to be related to developmental lag, and improve over time. Hopman (1998) observed normal breastfeeding behavior and normal milk intake in infants with Down Syndrome. He noted that they experienced a delay in the age at which solid food was introduced. Hopman advised pre-speech therapy for babies who appear to be experiencing oral motor deficits that interfere with acceptance of solids.

Severely affected infants with Down Syndrome, especially those with cardiac problems, require a comprehensive program of feeding interventions to protect normal growth and development.

These interventions include:

- careful evaluation of the infant's feeding capabilities
- decisions about how to supplement, if needed
- protection of the milk supply by pumping
- growth monitoring with growth charts specifically designed for the baby with Down Syndrome (Cronk 1988)
- periodic reassessment to normalize feeding as the baby matures

The infant in **Fig. 347** demonstrates some of the facial characteristics common in children with Down Syndrome. Note the flat face, the low or flat nasal bridge, and low-set ears positioned below the lateral canthal eyeline. The eyes have an almond shape with an epicanthal fold and slant upward. The tongue appears to protrude and may be flat and unable to adequately cup the breast. The baby has a "pear-shaped" trunk (**Fig. 348**). Other characteristics include: small nose, short neck, small oral cavity, and high palate. Due to muscular hypotonia, the face may appear expressionless.

Breastfeeding encourages appropriate use of the infant's facial muscles (Labbok 1987) and assists in improving facial tone and development. Therefore, even weakly feeding infants should be put to the breast and allowed to enjoy comfort sucking. Improved orofacial development impacts speech and may assist in minimizing the tongue protrusion seen in some children with Down Syndrome. Normalizing physical appearance may improve social interactions, and thus is an important issue for families of children with this condition.

Fig. 349 shows a *palmar* crease, formerly called a *simian crease*. A single crease on the palm is another characteristic trait of Trisomy 21. A single *plantar* crease is sometimes seen on the soles of the feet as well. Some individuals who do not have Down Syndrome may also have single creases on the hands and feet.

Both male babies in **Fig. 350** are 4 months old. The hypotonic infant with Down Syndrome pictured on the right cannot stabilize his head, while the neurologically healthy infant on the left can maintain head control when pulled to a sitting position. Hypotonia in the body extends to the muscles of the face, mouth, and throat, and may result in a weak suck. The baby's lips may lack the strength and tone to form a proper seal. The tongue may be unable to sustain the muscular effort needed to create suction. If the baby tires, discontinuing the feed too soon, intake will suffer. The mother can compensate for this by providing careful postural support, including supporting the breast in the baby's mouth using the *Dancer hand position* (Cerutti and Danner) seen in **Figs. 351** and **352**.

Gentle counter pressure applied to the cheeks is an element of the Dancer hand position (**Fig. 352**). Counter pressure on the cheeks decreases the intraoral space. Reducing the size of the oral cavity means the baby does not have to suck as hard to create a vacuum. Mothers can also use breast compression during breastfeeding (**Fig. 353**) to increase both the volume and caloric value of the feed (Stutte 1988).

Short, frequent feeds appear to be easier for a weak baby to manage. The baby may feed well at some feedings and poorly at others, depending upon fatigue level or state (see Ch. 3). Mothers should be instructed to express milk accordingly since effective milk removal is an essential factor in protecting milk production.

Low Tone and Feeding Problems

It is important to remember that feeding involves the coordination of sucking, swallowing, and breathing. Weakness and lack of coordination in low-tone babies increase the risk of aspiration. Low tone may prevent the epiglottis from sealing tightly, increasing the risk of milk spilling into the lungs (McBride 1987). The soft palate is a muscle. If the muscle tone of the soft palate is too poor to support tight closure at the base of the nasopharynx, nasal regurgitation may occur during feeding. Milk that enters the nasopharynx creates nasal congestion and impairs breathing. Aspiration into the nasopharynx or the lungs increases the risk of respiratory illness, including, in severe cases, aspiration pneumonia.

To facilitate safe swallowing and protect respiration in low-tone infants, use external pacing techniques when supplementing (see Ch. 14). Avoid hyperflexing or hyper-extending the baby's neck during bottle-feeding. Maintenance of a *patent* (open) throat protects swallowing and breathing. Allow the baby to come off the breast for a few moments during the let-down if the milk ejection is forceful or appears to overwhelm the baby. Positions that permit extension of the head during breastfeeding help stabilize low tone babies.

Reflux

Spitting up milk is common in infants. It is typically not considered to be a medical problem unless infant growth is affected or the infant frequently appears to be in pain. Low muscle tone can affect the lower esophageal sphincter and contribute to gastric reflux. To reduce spitting up, avoid bending the baby forward in a "V" position during burping (winding) as shown in **Fig. 354**. Bending the baby in this manner compresses the abdomen and increases intra-abdominal pressure causing reflux, especially if the baby's stomach is full.

Infants suffering from gastroesophageal reflux disease (GERD) grow poorly. They often cough between feeds and may fuss when placed in car seats or in positions that cause the baby to slump (Wolf and Glass 1992). Whenever a tight waistband pushes on the abdomen below the lower esophageal sphincter, compression can push the stomach contents into the esophagus. Babies with GERD are assisted when placed in open, elongated body positions or in baby seats that allow them to lean back. Some affected infants (**Fig. 355**) may benefit from being diapered while lying on their sides. Diapering on the side avoids abdominal compression that may occur when the baby's legs are lifted and pressed back toward the belly.

Sudden Loss of Tone as a Marker for Illness

Sometimes a baby who has previously breastfed well develops hypotonia and feeding-related problems. This is a marker for illness. Infants with Rett Syndrome, for example, may breastfeed normally for several months before progressive encephalopathy and loss of purposeful motor activity begin to interfere with feeding (Percy 2005).

The mother of the 9 month-old baby in **Fig. 356** became concerned about her baby, who previously breastfed well. His worsening body tone and weakening suck prompted the mother to seek medical evaluation. Her baby was subsequently diagnosed with a brain tumor.

Hydrocephalus

The 4 month-old baby in **Fig. 357** has *hydrocephalus*, a condition that results when an obstruction prevents the normal circulation and drainage of cerebrospinal fluid. Hydrocephalus is one of the most common birth defects, with an average occurrence similar to that of Down Syndrome (1 in 1000 births). The condition can be congenital or acquired, as the result of head trauma, brain tumor, or infection. Some individuals with the condition live normal lives, and function with normal intelligence. Hydrocephalus may occur as an aspect of a syndrome. Some individuals experience complications; the most common are motor and learning disabilities. A nonprofit organization called the Hydrocephalus Foundation, Inc. maintains a website that provides families with information, support, and resources: www.hydrocephalus.org.

Treatment of hydrocephalus involves draining excess cerebrospinal fluid from the brain through an artificial *shunt* to another part of the body, usually the abdominal cavity or the atrium of the heart, where it can then be eliminated. This prevents build-up of fluid, enlargement of the ventricles of the brain, and dangerously increased pressure inside the head (Eastwood 1986).

The baby pictured in **Fig. 357** was referred because he suddenly refused to breastfeed from his mother's left breast. The LC concluded that pressure from the mother's forearm on the shunt caused the baby discomfort. Because the baby previously had been willing to breastfeed on both sides, the mother had not considered that pressure on the shunt was the problem. The LC explained that around the age of 3 months, many babies begin to develop opinions about things. This baby appeared to have decided that feeding from the left breast felt uncomfortable. The LC demonstrated upright feeding positions that avoided putting pressure on this area of the baby's head. The baby then resumed feeding from both breasts.

Abnormal Posturing

Abnormal posturing of the limbs or body can reveal a temporary or enduring problem. Drug exposure, birth trauma, or neurological dysfunction can affect how a baby moves his body. Inability to move freely *in utero* (as in breech presentations) may result in atrophied muscles and torticollis (see Ch. 3 and **Figs. 53** and **54**). Similarly, restricted movement *in utero* may cause the newborn baby to move a limb abnormally.

Odd posturing is sometimes the result of injury caused by child abuse. Child abuse must be reported to the appropriate authorities; however, the LC carefully assesses the situation and rules out other causes first. The LC then should discuss such concerns with the family's HCP.

Excessive Tone and Feeding Problems

Hypertonicity (high muscle tone) caused the 6 week-old infant in **Fig. 358** to assume hyperextended body postures. His arching behavior made him difficult to position for feeding, and prompted his mother to seek help from an LC for painfully damaged nipples. The LC explained that arching contributes to jaw clenching. Hip flexion helps reduce arching and generally improves jaw stability. In the case of the infant pictured in **Fig. 358**, hip flexion also helped the mother bring the baby in closer to the breast, preventing jaw closure on the nipple shaft.

In the event of abnormal infant posturing, the LC should consider other conditions such as *laryngomalacia* and *tracheomalacia*. Both relate to collapse of the airway owing to structural malformation or muscular weakness. Affected infants typically manifest stridor and other types of respiratory stress (Genna 2008), and may assume hyperextended neck positions in order to hold the airway open. Unusual or noisy breathing should be reported to the infant's HCP.

Sensory Integration Issues

Some babies have difficulty integrating sensory stimulation. Light touch, sudden sounds, bright lights, and motion startle and overwhelm them. The arching baby in **Fig. 358** exhibited *sensory defensiveness* in addition to excessive muscle tone. Too much stimulation while feeding caused his arching to become more severe and worsened his tendency to clamp down on his mother's nipples (see Ch. 2).

The LC advised the mother to rest her nipples for a few days so they could heal. During this time, a hospital grade electric pump maintained her milk supply. The mother's doctor prescribed a topical antibiotic to treat a superficial skin infection on one of her nipples. As her nipples began to heal, the mother alternated breastfeeding with pumping. Eventually, the mother resumed exclusive breastfeeding. Although breastfeeding became tolerable, it was never completely comfortable. The mother noticed that her baby breastfed better in a quiet environment and when she paid careful attention to his postural stability.

Bonding Issues

During the months that they worked together, the mother of the arching baby in **Fig. 358** confided to the LC that she felt as if her baby did not love her because he was so difficult to cuddle. His stiff, rejecting body language jeopardized their bonding. When the LC pointed out that hypertonicity was the cause of the baby's behavior, the mother was able to deal with her own feelings more rationally. Over time, she became more sensitive about how best to assist him. Co-bathing in a warm tub and increased skin-to-skin contact helped relax the baby.

A different baby is pictured in **Fig. 359** being carried in the so-called "colic hold." Being held in a flexed position seems to soothe some infants. Carrying babies in slings can also promote physiological flexion.

Around the time of his fourth birthday, about 6 months after weaning, the child pictured in **Fig. 358** experienced a seizure that temporarily weakened his left arm. Was his abnormal posturing in infancy perhaps an early indication of an underlying neurological problem?

Failure to Thrive

Lawrence (2005) describes failure to thrive (FTT) as a medical diagnosis referring to the baby who: "continues to lose weight after 10 days of life, does not regain birth weight by 3 weeks of age, or gains at a rate below the 10th percentile for weight gain beyond one month of age." A weight gain of 20 g per day assigns an infant to the fifth percentile if observed between 2 and 6 weeks of age. Infants gain approximately 20 to 35 g a day (Hill 2007).

Failure to thrive presents complex issues that may be related to milk production problems, to illness in the mother or child, or to management and psychosocial problems. Typically, a *combination of factors* interact to cause FTT. Identifying them is vital in developing a plan to assist the infant with faltering growth.

The infant with FTT differs from the slow gaining baby, who will appear thin, but alert and healthy, and whose growth is slow but consistent. An infant who is FTT may be apathetic, with a weak cry, poor muscle tone, or poor skin turgor. Such infants produce few diapers, and their urine may be dark in color and have a strong smell. They stool infrequently and fail to produce adequate numbers of yellow milk stools by the end of the first week (see Ch. 4).

Because poor growth results in poor energy, the infant with FTT may have difficulty breastfeeding owing to lack of stamina. Weak feeding behavior generally persists until catch-up growth is achieved. Many infants who appear at first to have serious sucking problems feed normally once they recover lost weight and energy. Feeding the baby generously becomes the top priority; however, simultaneous attention must be directed to improving milk production.

Recovery from malnutrition ideally is achieved with human milk feeds (Graham 1996). Supplementation with donor milk or formula may be temporarily or permanently required if the mother has an insufficient milk supply. An infant with FTT who has never experienced a full feeding may not initially be able to consume all the supplement offered. It may take several days before the baby is able to take in appropriate volumes at each feeding. Small, frequent feedings will improve the baby's physiologic capacity (Powers 2001).

Increase in Breastfeeding Malnutrition and the Risks of Dehydration

Hypernatremic dehydration is a potentially devastating and life-threatening disorder that can damage the central nervous system. Breastfeeding infants who lose excessive weight after delivery are at risk. Unal (2008) retrospectively identified a 4.1 percent incidence of hypernatremic dehydration secondary to inadequate breastfeeding in a group of 169 hospitalized term infants.

Dehydration poses serious risks to the neonate including brain shrinkage, venous thrombosis, and subdural capillary hemorrhage. Unsupervised rehydration of the severely dehydrated infant without balancing electrolytes may cause cerebral edema, subsequent seizures, and death (Rand 2001). Riordan (2004) describes signs of severe dehydration:

- very sunken eyes
- pinched skin that returns very slowly (>2 seconds)
- dry mouth; absence of tears
- lack of wet diapers over many hours
- lethargic appearance
- cold limbs

Mothers are sometimes unable to recognize acute conditions such as dehydration, or chronic issues such as FTT. They may think that they have a very "good" baby, when, in fact, the baby is lethargic (Neifert 1996). Some parents mistake poor stooling for constipation and hunger cries for colic.

Because most breastfeeding mothers are released from the hospital on Day 2, before their milk supply has been established, it is important for all babies to receive appropriately timed post-discharge follow-up. Hospitals should provide clear instructions for parents describing the warning signs of poor intake (scant stooling, excessive crying, lethargy). At risk dyads should be promptly referred for breastfeeding support in the community (AAP 2005). Pediatricians must document the recovery of infants who lose excessive weight, utilizing weighing and referral to lactation support (Iyer 2008).

A reporting tool was designed to facilitate early follow-up of at-risk, breastfeeding dyads (Wilson-Clay 2002). The one page checklist may be faxed at the time of hospital discharge to alert the community based HCP that the dyad has risk factors for breastfeeding difficulty. A copy of the High Risk Report Form appears at the end of this chapter and may be reproduced.

Risk Factors for Failure to Thrive

- Prematurity
- Multiple births
- Physical anomalies of mother or baby
- Maternal or infant illness
- Breast surgery
- Retained placental fragment
- Transient or enduring infant neurological issues
- Difficulty latching and painful feedings
- Psychosocial or psychophysiologic issues
- Long labor
- History of sexual abuse
- Lack of social support
- Poor lactation management
- Scheduling and/or time limiting feedings

A careful history of both the mother and the baby must be taken to rule out organic reasons for poor growth. Failure to thrive beyond one month of age is associated with organic illness of the mother or the baby (Lukefahr 1990).

Telephone counselors must be alert to questions that may indicate that a baby is feeding poorly. Mothers who complain of sore nipples or severe engorgement may have infants who are not breastfeeding well. Some mothers express concerns that their diet does not agree with the baby, causing fussiness that they blame on "gas," rather than hunger. Other mothers call to ask how to help the baby sleep more or sleep less. Parents who request help to deal with excessive crying should be encouraged to seek a weight check, especially if inquiries about the infant's voiding and stooling pattern reveal low output (Neifert 1996). Test weights provide accurate milk intake information and do not increase maternal stress or undermine confidence (Hill 2007).

The use of galactagogues such as domperidone (where available) or metoclopramide may be considered to assist the woman's milk supply (da Silva 2001). However, blood tests may be prudent to first document low prolactin levels.

Ethical Issues Related to FTT

The LC who encounters an infant with apparent growth failure has an ethical obligation to refer the baby for medical evaluation. The LC assists the HCP by sharing information about the infant's feeding behavior and the mother's health history, which may be relevant and often is unknown to the baby's doctor. The LC shares information about the impact of difficult delivery on infant breastfeeding behavior (Chen 1998), and on conditions that affect milk production such as: maternal anemia (Henly 1995), postpartum hemorrhage (Willis 1995), previous breast surgery (Neifert 1990, Hughes 1993), breast and nipple anatomy (Neifert 1985), maternal illness (Neifert 1990), medications, and acute or chronic conditions (Neubauer 1993, Betzold 2004).

Consequences of FTT

A group of British researchers compared a group of 6 year olds who had failed to thrive in infancy. These children were below the third percentile for at least 3 months. At age 6, the children who had FTT were "considerably smaller than matched comparisons, in terms of body mass index, and height and weight." (Boddy 2000). Results correspond to past research indicating that non-organic failure to thrive is associated with persistent limitations in physical stature. Consequently, supplementation may be critical. Williams (2002) suggests that LCs should praise the mother's efforts while validating her grief over not being able to exclusively breastfeed. The LC should help the mother find additional methods of nurturing. For example, to promote intimacy, the mother may use a feeding tube worn at the breast, co-bathe, and wear the baby in a cloth carrier.

Management Strategies for the Infant with FTT

The infant in **Fig. 360** is 35 days old. He was examined by his pediatrician on the day the photo was taken. The baby had gained only 5 oz (142 g) above his birth weight (8 lb or 3629 g). The LC was called to assist with supplementation at the breast and to help the mother increase her milk supply. The LC showed the mother how to improve positioning and taught her how to use a feeding tube device. Her weak baby needed constant stimulation to continue sucking, but the feeding tube device improved his intake. After brief practice, the baby took

2.5 ounces (71 ml) of formula at the breast from the device. This supplementation plan was followed until the baby regained sufficient strength to breastfeed without the feeding tube. Pumping and more effective breastfeeding resulted in improved milk production.

A similar situation occurred with the 18 day-old baby in **Fig. 361,** who weighed one pound (454 g) below his birth weight of 6 lb 11 oz (3033 g). Someone had advised his mother to offer the baby a little water each day. She began feeding him 6 ounces of water daily. The LC speculated that excessive water intake decreased his appetite for milk. The mother was advised to discontinue water supplementation. She briefly used formula supplements to help stabilize the baby's growth. The LC helped the mother improve her breastfeeding technique and milk supply. Her baby then began to grow appropriately.

Fig. 362 pictures a 19 day-old infant with FTT. Born at 38 weeks, his birth weight was 7 lb 3 oz (3260 g). He weighed 6 lb 12 oz (3058 g) at a pediatric check-up on Day 10. When the LC weighed him on Day 19, he was still losing weight, and had lost another 3 oz (85 g). The baby was visibly jaundiced on his face, trunk, and extremities. The LC observed white lesions in the baby's mouth that were characteristic of infant thrush. However, the mother did not have sore nipples.

Note the baby's worried look, which is characteristic of infants who are failing to thrive. This first-time mother adhered to a rigid feeding schedule. She limited the baby to 10 minute feeds on each breast. The mother reported that her baby cried a lot with "colic" during his first week. Since then, he had appeared lethargic and was difficult to rouse for feedings. The picture shows marked lip retraction, a sign of poor lip tone. (See also **Fig. 29**). The baby typically closed his eyes early in the breastfeeding session, often a sign of weak or stressed feeding or lack of milk transfer. The infant's jaw excursions were short, choppy, and irregular. He was unable to sustain 10 to 30 sucks before pausing, and he paused more than he sucked. These are markers both of weakness and of an immature, disorganized suck (Palmer 1993).

A test weight revealed that the baby ingested less than one ounce (24 ml) of milk in a 15-minute feeding before becoming exhausted and falling asleep. The LC calculated that the baby needed a minimum of 19 oz (537 ml) of milk per 24 hours to regain his birth weight. If fed 8 times per 24 hours, milk intake volumes should average 2.3 ounces (66 ml) at each feeding. If a baby is below birth weight, calculate the volume of milk needed using the baby's *birth weight*, not the baby's present weight. This allows for catch-up growth. Powers (2004) provides guidelines for determining appropriate volumes of supplementation for the infant with low intake and poor growth. To determine the total volume of milk (or formula) required from one week to 3 months, take the baby's weight in pounds and multiply by 2.5. This gives the number of ounces of milk the baby needs during each 24 hours. Using grams, calculate 150-200 ml per kilogram (kg) per 24 hours.

The LC devised an intervention designed to simultaneously increase the infant's daily caloric intake and to improve maternal milk production. The mother of this FTT infant was a heavy smoker. The LC suggested she cut back to 10 daily cigarettes, and to smoke immediately after breastfeeding. Such timing allows metabolites of nicotine to decrease in breast milk prior to the next breastfeeding, theoretically reducing the exposure to the infant (Labrecque 1989).

In order to stimulate milk production, the mother began double pumping with a hospital grade electric pump for 15 minutes after breastfeeding. She offered 2 oz of pumped milk or formula by bottle at each feed. The baby had previously averaged 7 feeds per 24 hours. The LC recommended increasing his feeding frequency to 10 feeds per 24 hours. Half of the supplement was offered at the beginning of each feed to give the baby energy to attempt breastfeeding. The second ounce was offered when the baby appeared to tire at the breast, or if he acted unsatisfied after breastfeeding. Additionally, the mother was taught to use deep breast compression whenever the baby paused longer than 10 seconds while breastfeeding (see **Fig. 353**).

The LC addressed the issue of the infant's thrush, which was being treated with oral nystatin. The mother was encouraged to continue treating until all symptoms resolved. The LC additionally counseled the mother on the importance of self care, including rest and good diet.

A follow-up appointment was scheduled to take place in 36 hours to weigh the infant. The infant gained 6 ounces (170 g) by the next visit and was more alert. His color, tone, and skin turgor had improved, and he breastfed with greater stamina and more coordination. Serial test weights performed during the visit verified improved intake. The mother reported that post-feed pumping had successfully increased her milk supply; her breasts felt fuller. She had reduced her cigarette consumption, although not to the desired level, and was pleased at the over-all improvements in her situation. The pediatrician was satisfied with the infant's weight gain.

Follow-up and Outcome Monitoring

The LC maintained telephone contact with this mother for several weeks in order to monitor the effectiveness of the interventions. The baby's bilirubin level dropped quickly as milk intake increased and stooling became more frequent. Nystatin failed to resolve the oral thrush. The LC directed the mother to notify the pediatrician, who recommended gentian violet therapy. Within a week the thrush had cleared up. Supplements continued until the infant regained and surpassed his birth weight, and were *gradually* withdrawn. By 5 weeks of age the baby was breastfeeding without supplements and growing normally.

Follow-up is critical when an infant presents with FTT. As this case illustrates, care plans often require frequent adjustments. Close monitoring allows the LC to revise interventions as needed. The process of following a case over time provides opportunities for the LC to receive feedback that improves her own skills. The LC must maintain contact with the supervising HCP, alerting the HCP if problems do not resolve. If the infant does not start to gain weight appropriately with improved breastfeeding management and increased milk intake, further diagnostic evaluation is required to rule out underlying illness.

Case History of an Infant with Turner Syndrome

The baby whose unusually-shaped foot is pictured in **Fig. 363** has Turner Syndrome (TS), a rare chromosomal disorder of females. Girls with TS have growth stunting and typically do not achieve normal stature without growth hormones. They are infertile. Other problems may be associated with TS, such as heart, kidney, or thyroid disorders. Physical malformations associated with TS include puffy feet and toes without toenails, unusually shaped palates, and micrognathia. Weak muscle tone is common in infancy. Infants with TS typically experience feeding problems (Skuse 1994a), generally thought to result from palate abnormalities and low tone.

Fig. 364 shows a grooved (channel) palate. While some grooved palates are the result of erosion from intubation (see **Fig. 408**), many syndromes, such as TS, affect palatal formation. Abnormally formed hard palates may create feeding problems similar to those associated with cleft palate (see Ch. 18). Once babies become old enough for solids, parents should check the palatal grove to remove accumulated food. BWC worked with a baby with TS, whose mother called to report a nursing strike. BWC advised the mother to check the palatal groove. A wad of soggy paper was wedged in the groove. Once it was removed, the baby breastfed normally.

The same infant whose foot is pictured in **Fig. 363** is also pictured in **Fig. 21**. Note the tape covering her visible ear. Another characteristic of TS is rotated ears that fold over on themselves. The baby's pediatrician recalled hearing a lecture on the subject of auricular (ear) malformation. He contacted a plastic surgeon who splinted the baby's ears with a soft material (dental compound) held in place by tape. Ear cartilage is very malleable in the neonatal period due to increased estrogen activity. Auricular splinting for several weeks produces excellent cosmetic results in correcting malformed ears (Brown 1986). The parents of this infant wanted to normalize her appearance in every possible way, because girls with TS often suffer from low self-esteem owing to their short statures (Skuse 1994b).

The infant with TS pictured in **Figs. 21** and **363** was born vaginally at 38 weeks gestation, weighing 5 lb 14 oz (2665 g) to a G2 P2 L2 mother. The birth was difficult. The baby's weight suggests she was small for gestational age (SGA). Infants who are SGA have special nutritional and energy requirements. At 9 months, girls who were SGA (but not boys) fed enriched formula had a significant developmental disadvantage compared to a breastfed comparison group (Morley 2004). Breastfed infants of both sexes had scored significantly higher on mental and psychomotor assessment compared to formula fed infants at both 9 and 18 months of age, and at school age (Slykerman 2005). Breastfeeding may be especially beneficial for cognitive development of children who are born SGA.

The SGA baby with TS had additional challenges. She required aggressive suctioning at delivery owing to meconium aspiration. This temporarily damaged her vocal chords, producing hoarse vocalizations that persisted for several months. The infant's head was engaged in her mother's pelvis for some weeks prior to birth, contributing to the formation of large, bilateral cephalohematomas (seen in **Fig. 21**). Owing to cranial bruising, the baby had elevated bilirubin levels and jaundice-related lethargy. All of these issues increased the risk for poor early feeding. Luckily, this mother was extremely motivated to breastfeed.

The day before the LC visit, the baby was fitted for a hip harness to correct hip dysplasia, which the pediatrician attributed to low muscle tone caused by TS. The hip harness also complicated breastfeeding. It was difficult for the mother to find a comfortable feeding position that allowed her to draw the baby close. The baby is seen in **Fig. 365** breastfeeding in the cross-cradle position. This feeding position and a firm nursing pillow helped the mother hold the baby more comfortably.

Like many babies with TS, this baby had a heart defect, specifically, a coarctation (narrowing) of the aorta and a malformation of the aortic valve. The heart defect required surgery to correct. The doctor informed the parents that excellent early growth was necessary to stabilize the baby prior to surgery. Unfortunately, owing to the many risk factors in her case, the baby breastfed poorly. She fell asleep at breast after a few minutes, and her intake was low.

The mother of this infant had a history of milk oversupply. While this had been a problem for her first child, robust milk production and a strong milk ejection reflex compensated for the new baby's weak suck. A nipple shield was occasionally used to block forceful milk spray. The nipple shield increased the baby's oral responsiveness, and seemed to stimulate her to suck longer.

Careful attention to positioning and good postural support compensated for this baby's weak muscle tone and the interference caused by the hip harness. The mother used deep breast compression while she breastfed to help improve milk transfer. She pumped after some of the feedings to protect her milk supply. Hindmilk was used to supplement breastfeeding. A rental scale allowed the parents to carefully track the baby's growth, and helped them know how much supplemental milk to provide. The infant was diagnosed with reflux, not unusual in low tone babies. Frequent, small feeds appeared to be more comfortable for her than large, widely spaced feeds.

At the 2 month pediatric check-up the baby had grown at the rate of one ounce (28.35 g) per day on exclusive human milk feeds. This achievement surprised both the pediatrician and the endocrinologist who was working with the family. The baby nearly doubled her birth weight by 4 months. At 5 months the baby had surgery to repair the aortic arch. The baby weighed 13 lb 7 oz (6095 g) at 6 months, and was 26 inches long. After the surgery, her energy improved significantly and she was able to breastfeed with no further need for supplements.

Girls with TS demonstrate differences in mandibular growth (Simmons 1999). Because the activity of breastfeeding positively benefits orofacial development, extended breastfeeding may benefit the child with TS.

Additionally, because growth normally slows in the breastfed baby between 5 and 6 months, it is important for infants with conditions that impact physical stature to achieve excellent *early* growth. This may help such children realize their maximum growth potential. BWC has maintained contact with the mother of another girl with TS for many years. This child, while challenging to feed in infancy, achieved excellent early growth with exclusive human milk feeds. She was breastfed for 5 years. When the girl was 8 years old, her mother wrote: "Our daughter continues to surprise her endocrinologist by growing. She is in the 50th percentile. So far there is still no talk of growth hormones."

While TS is a rare syndrome, the LC will encounter other types of complicated cases. Such cases remind the LC that her assessment must address all relevant issues.

Infant Surgery

Human milk provides protection for the infant who is ill or who requires surgery in the neonatal period. Anti-inflammatory properties (Diehl-Jones 2004) and epidermal growth factor (Dvorak 2003) accelerate healing. Additionally, while many painful procedures are performed while caring for hospitalized infants, most are performed without analgesia (Carbajal 2008). A Cochrane Review concludes that "If available, breastfeeding or breast milk should be used to alleviate procedural pain in neonates..." (Shah 2006). Thus, human milk feeds are important for the 14 day-old infant pictured in **Fig. 366,** who is recovering from heart surgery. Post-operative pain is not the only issue to consider. Cardiac problems create risks for poor feeding before and after surgery. Babies with heart defects require careful monitoring to assure adequate intake.

Infant cardiac patients commonly display poor stamina for feeding. It is important to ensure that they are consuming sufficient calories; however, often their fluid intake is medically restricted. Their care thus requires careful medical supervision. Communication between the doctor and the LC is critical. It is important to protect the milk supply with post-feed pumping until the baby is stable.

Maternal stress may affect milk production (Chatterton 2000) or impair the milk ejection reflex. Such stress is common whenever an infant is hospitalized. Oxytocin spray or prolactin-stimulating drugs may assist the mother whose milk supply temporarily falters. Social support and relaxation techniques may also help. Temporary use of banked donor milk, if available, is an option until the situation stabilizes.

Prematurity and Breastfeeding

In 2004, 17.6 percent of black infants and 12.4 percent of all US infants were born prematurely (Martin 2006). Preterm birth in the US has been described as a "social disease," occurring at higher rates when the mother is poor, has a low educational level, is isolated, single, or too young (Snyder 2004). The percentage of incidence of preterm birth is also increasing in affluent women, owing to advanced maternal age at the time of delivery and multifetal pregnancies conceived with reproductive technology. These highly vulnerable infants and their mothers require specialized interventions to protect breastfeeding.

The benefits of human milk for preterm infants are reviewed in Ch. 15. In spite of increased awareness of these benefits, the percentage of preterm infants who are discharged breastfeeding is low. Siddell (2003) noted that 30 to 70 percent of mothers with babies in the NICU discontinue their efforts to breastfeed prior to the infant's hospital discharge. The period of time shortly after hospital discharge is especially difficult for families. Transitioning to full breastfeeding may be complicated. Women often report a lack of confidence in their own abilities to determine whether the baby is "getting enough."

The preterm infant has likely been separated from his mother and may experience stressful interventions that might create feeding aversion (Abadie 2001). Bonding opportunities are interrupted, creating the potential for attachment disorders. This may explain the higher reported rates of child abuse and abandonment in preterm infants. In one study, 30 mothers who delivered preterm infants all displayed at least one symptom of post-traumatic stress (Holditch-Davis 2003).

Fortunately, successful models exist that suggest how NICU staff may be better educated to provide optimal breastfeeding support for this vulnerable population of babies and mothers. Research demonstrates that education about the benefits and protective aspects of breastfeeding can change the knowledge and attitudes of NICU nurses. Siddell (2003) identified the most experienced nurses as being the ones who most benefited from such education. Ongoing education to update knowledge appears to prevent burnout and to promote positive attitudes among staff regarding breastfeeding.

Storing and Pumping Milk for Preterm Infants

Clear instructions on hygiene are important to prevent infection in the special care nursery environment. Mothers should be instructed to wash their hands and scrub under their fingernails prior to pumping. Pump exteriors should be disinfected between users. Pump kits should be washed carefully in soap and water after use. Bottles should be turned upside down to dry (D'Amico 2003). Mothers should rinse off their nipples with clear water prior to pumping (Hurst 2004a). These practices will prevent the spread of infection and prevent milk contamination.

Pumping to protect the milk supply is the key intervention in preserving the option to breastfeed for mothers with preterm infants. Even when preterm infants are given early access to the breast, which should be encouraged, they are seldom capable of initiating and maintaining a full milk supply. Nyqvist (2008) explored the breastfeeding behavior of very preterm infants and documented rooting and short sucking bursts in infants of 29 weeks. Full breastfeeding was attained between 32 and 38 weeks. Time to attainment of full breastfeeding may not occur until 40 weeks for some ill preterm infants. Palmer (1993) identified transitional sucking patterns in preterm infants that differ from those of term infants. Mothers should be counseled to maintain reasonable expectations of infant feeding behavior until the infant matures. Outcomes obviously depend on many factors. Careful growth monitoring is vital.

In general, mothers are advised to begin pumping as soon as their own condition permits. It appears to be optimal, especially in pump-dependent women, to pump for a reserve supply. Mothers are usually told to pump 8 to 10 times per day if the goal is to achieve a full milk supply at discharge. Mothers with large milk storage capacities may not require such frequent pumping. Some mothers may only feel able to commit to a short period of pumping for their hospitalized infants. These mothers may be advised to pump 6 times per 24 hours. Calculation of the individual mother's 24 hour milk production will help determine a reasonable pumping schedule (see Ch. 5, p. 30).

The preterm infant seen in **Fig. 367** is being held skin-to-skin, also called "kangaroo care." Hill (1999) identified time spent in kangaroo care and frequency of pumping as being significantly related to improved milk production.

Hill (1999) found that expressing milk a minimum of 6 times per day was associated with maintenance of 500 ml/day milk production. This volume is considered to be the minimum level of production to sustain a preterm infant at discharge. Mothers who pumped at lower frequencies were unlikely to produce adequate milk supplies. Hill observed that the level of milk production reached by week 3 is likely to be maintained in subsequent weeks. Double pumping in Hill's study did not produce more milk than sequential pumping; however, it was more efficient. Jones (2001) identified a significant increase in milk production with double pumping. Simultaneous breast massage during pumping increased pumped volumes in both modes of pumping.

Hill (2001) reported that average pumping time per session and time of initiation of pumping were less significant in influencing milk production than was frequency of pumping. However, Hill states that "...it behooves clinicians to get mothers of preterm infants off to the best start possible if they intend to provide mother's milk exclusively to their preterm infants, because this group is at risk for diminished milk production over time. This may mean not only encouraging early initiation of mechanical pumping, but also frequent breast pumping." Hill defines "early initiation" of pumping as starting before 48 hours, and "frequent" as 6 or more pumping sessions per 24 hours.

Evidence-based Interventions to Support Mothers of Preterm Infants

Programs such as the Rush Mothers' Milk Club (Rush-Presbyterian St. Luke's Medical Center, Chicago, Ilinois) have devised effective, evidence-based interventions to help mothers of preterm infants to provide sufficient milk (Meier 2003). Although the low income, predominantly African American mothers in this urban hospital have significant risk factors for weaning, they achieve the most positive breastfeeding outcomes for preterm infants reported in the literature. Lactation initation rates in this program are 73 percent, with a mean dose of own mother's milk over the first 15, 30, and 60 days postbirth of 81.7 percent, 80.1 percent, and 66.1 percent, respectively, of total volume fed.

The Rush Mothers' Milk Club interventions (Meier 2003) include:

- Education is provided at weekly luncheons for mothers that includes scientific explanations about how human milk protects the baby. Knowledge empowers mothers to make informed choices on behalf of their baby.
- Free transportation is arranged so that mothers may attend the weekly meeting.
- 24 hour access to an advanced practice nurse is provided.
- Trained peer counselors phone the mothers and make home visits if needed.
- Early initiation of breast stimulation with hospital grade pumps helps establish a milk supply of approximately 1000 ml/day. Robust milk production may provide a hedge against the gradual diminishment of milk supply seen over time in mothers who are pump-dependent.
- Mothers are taught to separate foremilk from hindmilk, perform creamatocrits, and perform test weights to determine infant intake during breastfeedings.

- Skin-to-skin care is encouraged (**Fig. 367**).
- Mothers breastfeed without regard to minimum weight or gestational age criteria.
- Nipple shields are used temporarily to help compensate for the preterm infant's weak suction and to increase milk intake. The shield is used until the infant demonstrates good weight gain patterns, and discontinued gradually when the infant demonstrates longer periods of wakefulness and longer sucking bursts.
- Discharge planning includes instructions on how to transition to cue-based feeding, with continued test weights on home-rental scales to permit careful monitoring of growth until the infant reaches term.
- Discharge instructions include pumping to protect milk supply until the infant is competent to maintain production. Mothers are taught to remove a portion of foremilk (usually one third of the estimated volume in the breast) and put the infant to the partially emptied breast. This practice increases the percentage of hind milk consumed, and assists growth until the infant is stronger and exhibits more organized feeding behavior.
- Interventions are discontinued on a time table that is based on the individual infant's progress.
- Peer counselors are selected from the mothers who "graduate" from the NICU. They are trained to assist other mothers of preterm infants entering the program.

Spatz (2004) reported similar success with the same protocol in Philadelphia. She devised a 10 Step model for staff that communicates the key elements of support. Her protocol also utilizes nipple shields, test weights, skin-to-skin care, and emphasizes close follow-up during the transition to home care. During 2003, 73 percent of the mothers in this hospital's special care nursery were either pumping milk or breastfeeding their preterm infants. Replication of the success of this protocol suggests that wide spread implementation of these evidence-based interventions promote improved breastfeeding outcomes in populations of preterm infants.

Because of infants' physiological immaturity and owing to maternal concerns about milk adequacy, the transition from special care nursery to the home can be stressful for the breastfeeding mother. Special support is required to overcome challenges and mothers may be motivated by information about specific benefits of at-breast feedings for these babies (Buckley 2006). If this support is deficient, the demands of pumping and supplementing often result in the abandonment of lactation.

Test Weighing

Because preterm infants lack predictable feeding behaviors and manifest indistinct behavioral cues, they require vigilance for weight gain. Concern about adequacy of feeding is a source of anxiety for their mothers. Families worry if the baby is "getting enough," especially during the vulnerable period of transition from hospital to home (Kavanaugh 1995). Clinical observation of breastfeeding (audible swallowing, changes in breast fullness, etc.) does not provide accurate or reliable information on the milk intake of preterm infants (Meier 1996). Weights taken on sensitive, reliable scales permit appropriate calculation of supplementation, and assist in the management of the preterm infant, especially after hospital discharge. Test weighing does not undermine maternal confidence (Hill 2007).

Hurst (2004b) examined maternal reactions and breastfeeding outcomes in a group of mothers performing in-home test weights compared to a matched group who did not use test weights in the 4 weeks following discharge. All of the women in the test weight group reported that in-home measurement of milk intake had been "very" or "extremely" helpful to them. Approximately 35 percent stated that the use of the scale made them "somewhat" nervous; however, they reported that weighing helped them transition to cue-based breastfeeding. In the group of mothers who did *not* weigh, 75 percent indicated that in-home measurement of milk intake would have been "somewhat" to "extremely" helpful to them. These women felt that weighing would have relieved the stress of trying to decide how much extra milk to provide. Thus, weighing appeared to improve maternal confidence in determining that the infants were getting enough.

Kavenaugh (1995) reported that in the absence of real information about intake, mothers gave extra bottles "just to be sure." The lack of evidence documenting increased maternal stress or anxiety as the result of test weighing indicates that the prejudice against it should be reexamined. Test weights appear to be a useful tool for HCPs and mothers, and can be used to evaluate intake when infants are immature, ill, or when they exhibit ambiguous feeding cues, as is often the case with preterm babies.

Abadie V, Andre A, Zaouche A, et al. Early feeding resistance: a possible consequence of neonatal oro-oesophageal dyskinesia. *Acta Paediatrica* 2001; 90(7):738-745.

American Academy of Pediatrics Section on Breastfeeding (AAP). Breastfeeding and the use of human milk. *Pediatrics* 2005; 115(2):496-506.

Betzold C, Hoover K, Snyder C. Delayed lactogenesis II: a comparison of four cases. *Journal of Midwifery and Women's Health* 2004; 49(2):132-137.

Boddy J, Skuse D, Andrews B. The developmental sequelae of nonorganic failure to thrive. *Journal of Child Psychology and Psychiatry* 2000; 41(8):1003-1004.

Brown F, Colen L, Addante R, et al. Correction of congenital auricular deformities by splinting in the neonatal period. *Pediatrics* 1986; 78(3):406-411.

Buckley KM, Charles GE. Benefits and challenges of transitioning preterm infants to at-breast feedings. *International Breastfeeding Journal* 2006; 1:13.

Carbajal R, Rousset A, Danan. et al. Epidemiology and treatment of painful procedures in neonates in intensive care units. *Journal of the American Medical Association* 2008; 300(1):60-70.

Cerutti E and Danner S. The Dancer Hand Position was devised by and named for Sarah Danner, CNM, IBCLC and Edward Cerutti, MD.

Chatterton R, Hill P, Aldag J, et al. Relation of plasma oxytocin and pro-lactin concentrations to milk production in mothers of preterm infants: influence of stress. *Journal of Clinical Endocrinology & Metabolism* 2000; 85(10):3661-3668.

Chen D, Nommsen-Rivers L, Dewey K, et al. Stress during labor and delivery and early lactation performance. *American Journal of Clinical Nutrition* 1998; 68(2):335-345.

Cronk C, Crocker AC, Pueschel SM, et al. Growth charts for children with Down Syndrome: 1 month to 18 years of age. *Pediatrics* 1988; 81(1):102-110. For information about Down Syndrome, contact the National Down Syndrome Society, 666 Broadway, New York, NY 10012 800-221-4602 fax 212-979-2873. www1.ndss.org

da Silva O, Knoppert D, Angelini M, et al. Effect of domperidone on milk production in mothers of premature newborns: a randomized, double-blind, placebo-controlled trial. *Canadian Medical Association Journal* 2001; 164(1):17-21.

D'Amico C, DiNardo C, Krystofiak S. Preventing contamination of breast pump kit attachments in the NICU. *Journal of Perinatal and Neonatal Nursing* 2003; 17(2):150-157.

Davenport S. The child with multiple congenital anomalies. *Pediatric Annals* 1990; 19(1):23-33.

Diehl-Jones W, Askin D. Nutritional modulation of neonatal outcomes. *AACN Clinical Issues* 2004; 15(1):83-96.

Dvorak B, Fituch CC, Williams CS, et al. Increased epidermal growth factor levels in human milk of mothers with extremely premature infants. *Pediatric Research* 2003; 54(1):15-19.

Eastwood S (editor). *About Hydrocephalus: A Book for Parents.* San Francisco: University of California Press, 1986.

Ekstrom A, Nissen E. A mother's feelings for her infant are strengthened by excellent breastfeeding counseling and continuity of care. *Pediatrics* 2006; 118(2):e309-314.

Genna CW. *Supporting Sucking Skills in Breastfeeding Infants.* Sudbury, MA: Jones and Bartlett, 2008; p, 218.

Graham G, MacLean W, Brown K, et al. Protein requirements of infants and children: growth during recovery from malnutrition. *Pediatrics* 1996; 97(4):499-505.

Gunderson EP, Lewis CE, Wei GS. Lactation and changes in maternal metabolic risk factors. *Obstetrics and Gynecology* 2007; 109(3):729-738.

Hall R, Mercer A, Teasley S, et al. A breast-feeding assessment score to evaluate the risk for cessation of breast-feeding by 7 to 10 days of age. *Journal of Pediatrics* 2002; 141(5):659-64.

Henly S, Anderson C, Avery M, et al. Anemia and insufficient milk in first-time mothers. *Birth* 1995; 22(2):87-92.

Hill P, Aldag J, Chatterton R. Effects of pumping style on milk production in mothers of non-nursing preterm infants. *Journal of Human Lactation* 1999; 15(3):209-216.

Hill P, Aldag J, Chatterton R. Initiation and frequency of pumping and milk production in mothers of non-nursing preterm infants. *Journal of Human Lactation* 2001; 17(1):9-13.

Hill PD, Johnson TS. Assessment of breastfeeding and infant growth. *Journal of Midwifery and Womens Health* 2007; 52(6):571-578.

Holditch-Davis D, Bartlett T, Blickman A, et al. Posttraumatic stress symptoms in mothers of premature infants. *Journal of Obstetric, Gynecologic, and Neonatal Nursing* 2003; 32(2):161-171.

Hopman E, Csizmadia C, Bastiani W, et al. Eating habits of young children with Down Syndrome in The Netherlands: adequate nutrient intakes but delayed introduction of solid food. *Journal of the American Dietetic Association* 1998; 98(7):790-794.

Hughes V, Owen J. Is breast-feeding possible after breast surgery? *Maternal Child Nursing* 1993; 18(4):213-217.

Hurst N, Meier P. Breastfeeding the preterm infant, in J Riordan, *Breastfeeding and Human Lactation* (3rd edition), Sudbury, MA: Jones and Bartlett, 2004a; pp. 367-406, (see p. 380, Table 13-3).

Hurst N, Meier P, Engstrom J, et al. Mothers performing in-home measurement of milk intake during breastfeeding of their preterm infants: maternal reactions and feeding outcomes. *Journal of Human Lactation* 2004b; 20(2):178-187.

Iyer NP, Srinivasan R, Evans K. Impact of an early weighing policy on neonatal hypernatraemic dehydration and breast feeding. *Archives of Disease in Childhood* 2008; 93(4):297-299.

Jones E, Dimmock P, Spencer S. A randomized controlled trial to compare methods of milk expression after preterm delivery. *Archives of Diseases in Children* 2001; 85(2):F91-F95.

Jonas W, Nissen E, Ransjo-Arvidson AB. Short- and long-term decrease of blood pressure in women during breastfeeding. *Breastfeeding Medicine* 2008; 3(2):103-109.

Kavanaugh K, Mead L, Meier P, et al. Getting enough: mothers' concerns about breastfeeding a preterm infant after discharge. *Journal of Obstetric, Gynecologic, and Neonatal Nursing* 1995; 24(1):23-32.

Kramer M, Aboud F, Mironova E, et al. Breastfeeding and child cognitive development. *Archives of General Psychiatry* 2008; 65(5):578-584.

Labbok M, Hendershot G. Does breastfeeding protect against malocclusion? An analysis of the 1981 child health supplement to the national health interview survey. *American Journal of Preventative Medicine* 1987; 3(4):227-232.

Labrecque M, Marcoux S, Weber J, et al. Feeding and urine cotinine values in babies whose mothers smoke. *Pediatrics* 1989; 83(1):93-97.

Lanting C, Fidler V, Huisman M, et al. Neurological differences between 9-year-old children fed breast-milk or formula-milk as babies. *Lancet* 1994; 344(8933):1319-22.

Lawrence RA, Lawrence RM. *Breastfeeding: A Guide for the Medical Profession* (6th edition), Philadelphia, PA: Elsevier Mosby, 2005; pp. 435-449.

Lubetzky R, Vaisman N, Mimouni F, et al. Energy expenditure in human milk -versus formula-fed preterm infants. *Journal of Pediatrics* 2003; 143(6):750-753.

Lukefahr J. Underlying illness associated with failure to thrive in breast-fed infants. *Clinical Pediatrics* 1990; 29(8):468-470.

Martin JA, Hamilton BE, Sutton PD, et al. Births: final data for 2004. *National Vital Statistics Reports* 2006; 55(1):21-23.

McBride M, Danner S. Sucking disorders in neurologically impaired infants: assessment and facilitation of breastfeeding. *Clinics in Perinatology* 1987; 14(1):109-130.

Meier P. Supporting lactation in mothers with very low birth weight infants. *Pediatric Annals* 2003; 32(5):317-325.

Meier P, Engstrom J, Fleming B, et al. Estimating milk intake of hospitalized preterm infants who breastfeed. *Journal of Human Lactation* 1996; 12(1):21-26.

Mizuno K, Ueda A. Development of sucking behavior in infants with Down's Syndrome. *Acta Paediatrica* 2001; 90(12):1384-1388.

Montgomery S, Ehlin A, Sacker A. Breast feeding and resilience against pyschosocial stress. *Archives of Disease in Childhood* 2006; 91(12):990-994.

Morley R, Fewtrell M, Abbott R, et al. Neurodevelopment in children born small for gestational age: a randomized trial of nutrient-enriched standard formula and comparison with a reference breast-fed group. *Pediatrics* 2004; 113(3):515-521.

Neifert M. Early assessment of the breastfeeding infant. *Contemporary Pediatrics* 1996; 13(10):142-166.

Neifert M, DeMarzo S, Seacat J. The influence of breast surgery, breast appearance, and pregnancy-induced breast changes on lactation sufficiency as measured by infant weight gain. *Birth* 1990; 17(1):31-38.

Neifert M, Seacat J, Jobe W. Lactation failure due to insufficient glandular development of the breast. *Pediatrics* 1985; 76(5):823-828.

Neubauer S, Ferris S, Chase C, et al. Delayed lactogenesis in women with insulin-dependent diabetes mellitus. *American Journal of Clinical Nutrition* 1993; 58(1):54-60.

Nyqvist KH. Early attainment of breastfeeding in very preterm infants. *Acta Paediatrica* 2008; 97(6):776-781.

Palmer M. Identification and management of the transitional suck pattern in premature infants. *Journal of Perinatal and Neonatal Nursing* 1993; 7(1):66-75.

Percy AK, Lane JB. Rett Syndrome: model of neurodevelopmental disorder. *Journal of Child Neurology* 2005; 20(9):718-721.

Pisacane A, Toscano E, Pirri I, et al. Down Syndrome and breastfeeding. *Acta Paediatrica* 2003; 92(12):1479-1481.

Powers N. How to assess slow growth in the breastfed infant, in RJ Schanler (ed.). *The Pediatric Clinics of North America Breastfeeding 2001.* Part II The Management of Breastfeeding 2001; 48(2):345-363.

Powers N. Low intake in the breastfed infant: maternal and infant considerations, in J Riordan. *Breastfeeding and Human Lactation* (3rd edition), Sudbury, MA: Jones and Bartlett, 2004; p 297-307.

Pryor K. *Nursing Your Baby.* New York: Simon and Schuster, 1973; p. 7.

Raisler J, Alexander C, O'Campo P. Breast-feeding and infant illness: a dose-response relationship? *American Journal of Public Health* 1999; 89(1):25-30.

Rand S, Kolberg A. Neonatal hypernatremic dehydration secondary to lactation failure. *Journal of the American Board of Family Practice* 2001; 14(2):155-158.

Riordan J. *Breastfeeding and Human Lactation* (3rd edition). Sudbury, MA: Jones and Bartlett, 2004; pp. 553-554.

Sacker A, Quigley MA, Kelly YJ. Breastfeeding and developmental delay: findings from the Millennium Cohort study. *Pediatrics* 2006; 118(3):e682-689.

Shah PS, Aliwalas LI, Shah V. Breastfeeding or breast milk for procedural pain in neonates. *Cochrane Database System Review* 2006; July 19; 3.

Siddell E, Marinelli K, Froman R, et al. Evaluation of an educational intervention on breastfeeding for NICU nurses. J*ournal of Human Lactation* 2003; 19(3):293-302.

Simmons K. Growth hormone and craniofacial changes: preliminary data from studies in Turner's Syndrome. *Pediatrics* 1999; 104(4):1021-1024.

Skuse D. Feeding difficulties among infants and older children with Turner Syndrome, in J Rovet (ed.) *Turner Syndrome Across the Lifespan: Proceedings from the 3rd International Turner Syndrome Contact Group Meetings*, Toronto, Canada, 1994a; pp. 17-26, 151-164.

Skuse D, Percy E, Stevenson J. Psychosocial functioning in the Turner Syndrome: a national survey, in B Stabler, L Underwood (eds). *Growth, Stature, and Adaptation: Behavioral, Social, and Cognitive Aspects of Growth Delay.* Chapel Hill: University of North Carolina Press, 1994b; pp. 151-164.

Slykerman RF, Thompson AM, Becroft DM. Breastfeeding and intelligence of preschool children. *Acta Paediatrica* 2005; 94(7):832-837.

Snyder U. Preterm birth as a social disease. Medscape Ob/Gyn & Women's Health 2004; 9(2):1-6.

Spatz D. Ten steps for promoting and protecting breastfeeding for vulnerable infants. *Journal of Perinatal and Neonatal Nursing* 2004; 18(4):385-396.

Stutte P, Bowles B, Morman G. The effects of breast massage on volume and fat content of human milk. *Genesis* 1988; 10(2):22-25.

Unal S, Arhan E, Kara N. Breast-feeding-associated hypernatremia: retrospective analysis of 169 term infants. *Pediatrics International* 2008; 50(1):29-34.

Willis C, Livingstone V. Infant insufficient milk syndrome associated with maternal postpartum hemorrhage. *Journal of Human Lactation* 1995; 11(2):123-126.

Williams N. Supporting the mother coming to terms with persistent insufficient milk supply: the role of the lactation consultant. *Journal of Human Lactation* 2002; 18(3):262-263.

Wilson-Clay B, Maloney B. A reporting tool to facilitate community-based follow-up for at-risk breastfeeding dyads at hospital discharge, in K Auerbach ed. *Current Issues in Clinical Lactation* 2002; pp. 59-67.

Wolf L, Glass R. *Feeding and Swallowing Disorders in Infancy.* Tucson, AZ: Therapy Skill Builders, 1992; pp. 340-343.

Notes:

High Risk Reporting Form

Date: _____

From: Hospital Lactation Dept: _____

RE: Baby's name and DOB: _____

Mother's name/current Phone No: _____

Dear Doctor _____:

Some lactation problems do not present until after discharge.
Risk factors have been identified that predict early weaning. (Hall, *J Peds*, 2002.)
The hospital lactation consultants have identified the following red-flags for breastfeeding problems in the mother and baby being discharged. This dyad may need community-based support to insure that breastfeeding is well-established.

Maternal Risk Factors Noted:

___ History of previous breast surgery_____

___ Anatomic breast variations (hypoplasia, marked asymmetry)

___ Minimal breast changes during pregnancy/hormonal disorders (PCOS)

___ Medical illness (hypertension, anemia, blood loss, infection)

_____

___ Flat/inverted nipples, long or large nipples

___ Long/difficult labor – primiparous mother (associated in the medical lit. with delays in onset of copious milk production (Chen, *Am J Clin Nutr* 1998.)

___ Latch on difficulties

___ Young maternal age or history of previous breastfeeding failure

Infant Risk Factors Noted:

___ Prematurity or IUGR

___ Twins or other multiples

___ Jaundice

___ Vacuum assisted delivery (Hall, *J Peds* 2002)

___ Oral cleft/other oral anatomic variations including tongue-tie_____

___ Medical illness/neuromotor problems _____

___ Loss of >7% of birthweight at discharge

___ Suppl. feed by bottle/cup/SNS/other due to hypoglycemia/non-alert/separation/jaundice

Notes:_____
_____
_____.

Community Resources for Breastfeeding:

Free phone counseling: La Leche League (accredited volunteers) Hotline # _____

Income eligible LC services (WIC) _____

Out-patient LC services at this hospital _____

Private Practice Lactation Consultants:_____

Developed by: B. Maloney, RNC, IBCLC, B. Wilson-Clay, IBCLC, Revised by B. Wilson-Clay, 2005
May be copied freely if kept in its original form
Originally published in *Current Issues in Clinical Lactation 2002,* Jones and Bartlett, Boston.

Ankyloglossia

The tongue plays an important role in infant feeding, and later, in speech and dental health (Fernando 1998). Anatomical variations, especially if they affect how the tongue moves, may interfere with normal breastfeeding owing to changed sucking mechanics (Ardran 1958, Ramsay 2004a, Geddes 2008a). *Ankyloglossia* is a congenital oral abnormality, commonly called tongue-tie. The condition refers to a thin webbing of tissue (the *lingual frenulum*) that attaches the tongue tip to the floor of the mouth. A short, tight, or anterior lingual frenulum may prevent normal tongue lift, extension, lateralization, and grooving.

The incidence of ankyloglossia in neonatal populations is unknown. Reported ranges vary from less than 1 percent to to 4.8 percent of infants (Flinck 1994, Messner 2000, Ballard 2002, Lalakea 2003, Ricke 2005, Wallace 2006). Tongue-tie affects individuals to varying degrees (Amir 2005), and the problems it causes are often underestimated (Wright 1995). While some tongue-tied infants breastfeed without difficulty, a subset of infants appear to experience significant feeding difficulties (Ballard 2002). The restricted tongue may cause a variety of problems including reduced milk transfer, maternal nipple pain, prolonged feeding, and latch on problems (Hogan 2005, Geddes 2008b).

Some tongue-tied infants slide off the breast frequently. Mothers may report a sensation like a "snap-back" of the tongue as the baby releases the breast (Hazelbaker 1993). These abrupt releases may be painful to the mother and can be observed when the baby breastfeeds. Instead of wide, regular jaw excursions, the chin seems to jerk. Flicking of the tongue as it snaps back can be abrasive to the underside of the nipple shaft. When the baby loses suction, clicking sounds may be heard.

Ultrasound visualization of tongue-tied infants during breastfeeding sessions has identified differences in the sucking mechanics of tongue-tied infants compared to infants with unrestricted tongue mobility (Geddes 2008b).

Functional Assessment of Tongue-tie

Tongue-tie requires a *functional assessment* as well as visual identification. To rule out other problems, the examiner must take a careful history and observe a feeding. Since most LCs do not have access to ultrasound equipment, visual assessment includes evaluation of the ability of the infant to lift, extend, cup, and lateralize the tongue. Lift should be assessed with the mouth open wide. If the tongue cannot lift past the mid-line plane,

and the tongue tip notches as the tongue lifts, impairment of mobility is presumed to be occurring.

Because the forward position of the tongue pads the teat from the full force of lower jaw compression, the degree of tongue extension may impact sore nipples. The tongue normally extends beyond the infant's lower gum ridge, and ideally extends beyond the lower lip line. The infant should be able to maintain tongue extension without a "snap-back."

Inability to form a central groove with the tongue may impair the infant's capacity to organize fluids for safe swallowing. Breastfeeding and (if applicable) bottle-feeding should be directly observed. This permits the LC to identify milk spilling and to assess swallowing. Wet breathing may be an indication of aspiration.

Inability to latch onto the breast, frequent loss of the breast, maternal complaint of nipple pain, infant respiratory problems, prolonged feeding, and low milk intake are signs that a tongue-tied baby requires further evaluation and referral for possible release of the tongue.

The Mechanics of Breastfeeding

Milk can be removed from the breast using only positive pressure (hand expression). Pumping utilizes negative pressure to remove milk. During breastfeeding, the baby uses the lips and the cupped tongue to seal the oral cavity. Using suction, the baby shapes the breast tissue into an elongated teat that extends nearly to the junction of the hard and soft palates. During milk ejection, the downward movement of the baby's posterior tongue and lower jaw creates negative pressure that facilitates milk flow from the breast. When the tongue rises, it compresses the teat. When the teat is maximally compressed against the hard palate by the elevated tongue, milk flow slows or is interrupted (Ramsay 2004b). It is during this phase of the cycle that the infant pauses to take a breath (Meier 2003). When the tongue drops again, the level of negative pressure increases and the mouth refills with milk.

For an infant to breastfeed, the mobility of the tongue must be adequate to seal the oral cavity and to rise and drop to create and stop the milk flow. Owing to the size of the holes in most bottle teats, bottle-feeding requires less effort in terms of eliciting milk flow. The bigger challenge for the bottle-feeding infant involves controlling rapid milk flow and the protection of respiratory stability (Meier 2003).

Geddes (2008a) has demonstrated that minimal distortion of the nipple occurs during successful, established breastfeeding. Infants with ankyloglossia display differences in sucking when assessed by ultrasound (Ramsay 2004a). Two "distinct patterns of sucking" were observed in tongue-tied infants prior to frenotomy (Geddes 2008b). One group of tongue-tied infants positioned the tip of the nipple farther from the hard and soft palate junction (HSPJ). They humped the posterior tongue, pinching the nipple to a point. This group appeared to have difficulty sustaining enough suction to form an adequate seal. A second group of infants appeared to hold the nipple tip closer to the HSPJ, but compressed or bit the base of the nipple. Both patterns appear to be compensations employed by infants who are unable to attach well to the breast or perform the normal sucking mechanics for successful, pain-free breastfeeding. Both variant sucking patterns were associated with higher maternal pain scores and ineffective infant milk transfer.

After frenotomy, ultrasound revealed that these issues resolved or lessened. The infants in the study displayed significantly increased rates of milk transfer in shorter feeds and their mothers reported improved comfort during breastfeeding (Geddes 2008b). While only ultrasound provides direct visualization of these sucking mechanics, published case series have also reported improved maternal comfort and improved infant feeding following frenotomy (Srinivasan 2006, Wallace 2006).

Normal and Abnormal Range of Motion of the Tongue

Clinicians lack a tool with established reliability that objectively measures the degree to which anklyglossia will cause impaired feeding in an individual infant. Lalakea (2003) describes a novel method of determining lingual mobility in children who are old enough to cooperate with assessment. Measurements of tongue protrusion were calculated in millimeters of tip extension past the lower teeth. Tongue elevation was measured by recording the distance between the incisors with the tongue tip lifted as high as the child could manage, ideally touching the upper teeth. The researchers used a series of such measurements to help define degrees of tongue restriction. They found that protrusion and elevation values are typically in the range of 15 mm or less in children with ankyloglossia, and 20 to 25 mm or greater in normal children.

Fig. 368 shows the normal range of motion of the tongue. Note how this adolescent girl can lift her tongue tip to touch her upper teeth with her mouth open wide. Compare this to the woman in **Fig. 369** whose frenulum attaches near the tip of her tongue. Because the tongue tip is tethered

to the floor of the mouth, her tongue cannot fully lift to touch her upper teeth. Note that the tongue tip assumes a distorted heart shape as she attempts to elevate it. (Tongue lift is assessed with the mouth open because the baby has to open wide to accommodate the shape of the breast.)

The man in **Fig. 370** is the father of a tongue-tied infant. Note how his tongue tip curls under as he attempts to lift it. Distortions such as this have a cosmetic effect on the appearance of the tongue, and may create social problems, especially in adolescents. The LC photographed the father after assessing his infant. This man is unable to touch the tip of his tongue to his upper teeth. Inability to move the tongue and place it behind the upper teeth inhibits, in some individuals, the formation of certain sounds, and is implicated in certain speech disorders.

Ankyloglossia occurs most frequently as an isolated anatomic variation, but it often runs in families. It may occur with increased frequency in association with various congenital syndromes (Gorski 1994, Lalakea 2003). Often a family member will reveal to an LC that they (or other family members) are or were tongue-tied. BWC and KH have both had conversations with parents who had their tongues clipped as children to remediate speech or dental problems. Many parents of tongue-tied babies report that *their* mothers weaned to formula owing to breastfeeding difficulties. Since tongue-tied infants often drink more easily from bottles, pediatricians have commonly recommended that mothers abandon breastfeeding.

In spite of the fact that studies have identified ankyloglossia in adults (Lalakea 2003), physicians may delay interventions to remediate tongue-tie in infants because they believe that the condition will resolve spontaneously. The infant skull rapidly elongates during the first year after birth, causing the lower jaw to grow forward. Clinicians often hope that the forward growth of the jaw will stretch the lingual frenulum. Parents may be told that a tongue-tie will "disappear." What commonly occurs is accidental cutting of the frenulum. Toddlers may tear the frenulum in a fall, often biting through it with their sharp, new teeth, or a toy. BWC has had several families describe toddlers tearing a frenulum. Photos of adults with tongue-ties, as pictured in **Figs. 369** and **370,** document that the condition can endure beyond infancy.

The belief that time or fate will resolve tongue-tie often causes delays in correcting ankyloglossia that is severe enough to impair breastfeeding. Sadly, later concerns about the social implications of speech disorders, dental problems, or appearance supercede concerns regarding dysfunctional breastfeeding. Tongue-ties often are clipped when children start school to correct speech defects.

Fletcher (1968) found a significant increase in the number of articulation errors in the "limited lingual freedom" group compared with controls, and attributed these differences to ankyloglossia.

Lalakea (2003) reported that current opinion among speech therapists is evenly divided: 49 percent believe that ankyloglossia is *not* associated with speech problems, while 51 percent believe it is. Delaying remediation past early infancy, when frenotomy is generally performed as an office procedure, increases health risks owing to the loss of the protection of breastfeeding. Because toddlers and some pre-school age children cannot be depended upon to remain still, they may require general anesthesia for frenotomy. Anesthesia increases the risk of the procedure. Frenotomy is not reported to be particularly painful and does not cause excessive bleeding (Amir 2005).

Fig. 371 pictures a tongue-tied infant. Note how the baby's tongue tip forms a distorted, notched "V" shape. The heart-shaped tongue tip is characteristic of tongue-tie. Often the restriction at the tip of the tongue prevents the individual from adequately forming a central groove. This has implications for respiratory health, because the central groove channels and organizes fluids for safe swallowing. Severely tongue-tied infants may have difficulty swallowing during breast and bottle-feeding. Fernando (1998) documents tongue-tied older children with excessive salivation and difficulties managing solids as the result of poor organization of swallowing.

Fig. 372 illustrates the variability of tongue lengths. The photo shows a married couple. The woman (on the left) has normal tongue extension. The man has a short tongue which limits his range of motion. For instance, he could not lick an ice cream cone.

The 12 year-old boy in **Fig. 373** is tongue-tied. While his breastfeeding experience was uneventful, he could not extend his tongue. The boy's tongue tip was attached just behind his lower gum ridge. The forward placement of the lingual frenulum caused his tongue tip to roll under. At age 17, the boy's orthodontist performed a frenotomy to preserve the beneficial effect of braces used to correct his malformed teeth. While frenotomy was not painful, the boy complained that his recovery was more uncomfortable than he had been led to expect. For a week after his frenotomy, his tongue hurt at the site of the incision. Frenotomy is a relatively common procedure in orthodontia patients, where the influence of the tongue on teeth spacing is widely appreciated (Palmer 1998).

The baby in **Fig. 374** has an unusually long tongue. Her siblings nicknamed her "Giraffe Tongue!" The length of the baby's tongue may have contributed to sore nipples in the mother, which persisted in spite of interventions to adjust positioning and latch. The mother described breastfeeding this infant as very different from what she had experienced with her other 2 children. This case suggests that differences in tongue length may impact breastfeeding comfort.

When tongue mobility is restricted by a tongue-tie, the tongue distorts as the individual attempts to perform normal oral mechanics such as removing food particles from side or back teeth.

Note the bunching and distortion as the tongue-tied infant in **Fig. 375** attempts to extend her tongue.

Fig. 376 illustrates normal lateralization in an adolescent girl. Her younger sister, seen in **Fig. 377**, has a tight lingual frenulum that attaches at the mid-section of the tongue. Note how the tongue-tied girl demonstrates a limited ability to lateralize. Her tongue distorts as she attempts to move it toward her lateral incisors. This may negatively effect dental health, because the ability of the tongue to perform dental hygiene is impaired. Such impairment may also restrict the ability to efficiently clear food from the tongue during swallowing.

The infant pictured in **Fig. 378** demonstrates normal tongue mobility. She is able to easily move her tongue from side to side. If the LC wishes to assess lateralization, touching the side of the tongue should produce a lateral tongue-seeking response.

Fig. 379 shows a baby girl with a tongue-tie. Note the mother's nipple damage. The LC assisted with improving the latch, but the baby was unable to draw in enough breast tissue for her mother to experience pain-free breastfeeding. Once the baby's frenulum was clipped, breastfeeding became comfortable.

Contrast the limited lift of the tongue in the baby shown in **Fig. 379** with that of the baby pictured in **Fig. 380**. Note how this infant can position her tongue tip behind her upper gum ridge.

Positioning Interventions

A breastfeeding position that pulls the chin very close to the breast shortens the distance the tongue must reach to cup and hold the breast. Thus, an extended head position that brings the chin close helps compensate for the somewhat receding chin of the average newborn. It may be even more important to chose feeding positions that help the tongue-tied infant extend the tongue. For example, prone positions that helps drop the tongue forward may be useful.

Ranly (1998) describes the rapid forward growth of the mandible during the first 4 months after birth. Changes in the orientation of the lower jaw may indeed explain some of the cases where breastfeeding a tongue-tied baby becomes, over time, less painful. The forward jaw growth may stretch the frenulum or pull the tongue slightly forward, assisting the infant's ability to latch. Mothers may find it helpful to support the breast with a hand to help the baby stabilize and hold onto the breast. Breast support may be especially useful for infants who bite the base of the nipple (Geddes 2008b). When the baby's nose is tipped away from the breast (as in **Fig. 116**), it indicates that the chin is sufficiently close.

Fig. 381 shows a normal infant breastfeeding. The mother pulls back on the breast to reveal the wide gape of a well-latched infant. The tongue is seen cupping the underside of the breast. Note how the curled lateral edges of the tongue assist the lips in forming a seal around the breast. The sides of the tongue fill the gaps at the corners of the lips when the mouth is open wide. Tongue-tied infants are challenged to create the lateral curl because of limited mobility and the tendency of the tongue to distort. When the tongue cannot seal the gap at the corners of the mouth, suction is impaired. Any impairment in the infant's ability to create negative pressure compromises breastfeeding.

Messner's (2000) prospective study described ankyloglossia as a relatively common finding in the newborn population, which "adversely affects breastfeeding in selected infants." She found that breastfeeding difficulties were experienced by 25 percent of the mothers of tongue-tied babies as compared with only 3 percent of the mothers in the control group. There is a greater prevalence of males with the condition (Messner 2000, Lalakea 2003). Messner suggests that frenotomy should be considered when breastfeeding difficulties occur. Lalakea remarks that "...complications of frenotomy and frenuloplasty are rare." (p. 395) Ballard (2002) describes frenuloplasty, when indicated, as a "successful approach to the facilitation of breastfeeding in the presence of significant ankyloglossia."

Powers (2001), in an overview on the management of the slowly gaining infant, states that slow growth in the presence of a "short frenulum" requires "careful evaluation of tongue function by a lactation specialist or infant feeding specialist...Consider frenotomy."

Neifert (2001) identifies ankyloglossia as an "early breast-feeding risk factor." Lawrence (2005) suggests it as a pos-

sible cause of nipple pain, and recommends that the physician should consider cutting the frenulum if the diagnosis is confirmed by oral examination.

Wight (2001) states that while the "clinical significance of ankyloglossia is controversial and much broader than just breastfeeding, most lactation consultants and some physicians have found that tongue-tie can make breastfeeding difficult, causing sore nipples, poor infant weight gain, low milk supply with early weaning, and maternal fatigue and frustration." Wight describes frenotomy as a "simple procedure...and complications are extremely rare."Amir (2005) states that "Frenotomy is a safe and easy procedure."

Jain (1996) produced a video to instruct pediatricians in the procedure of frenotomy. In the video she discusses how tongue-tie impacts breastfeeding.

Articles in peer reviewed journals may be useful to share with HCPs who wish to learn more about the impact of ankyloglossia on breastfeeding.

Frenotomy and Frenuloplasty

Frenotomy and *frenuloplasty* are terms that describe procedures to free the tongue from the restriction of ankyloglossia, permitting it to move normally.

Lalakea (2003) describes frenotomy as a simple release of the tongue, generally performed in newborn infants and older individuals without anesthesia or topical analgesia. The procedure is performed by pediatricians, ear, nose and throat specialists (ENTs), dentists, oral surgeons. and other physicians. Two gloved fingers or a forked tool are placed below the tongue on either side of the mid-line to lift the tongue and expose the frenulum. Small, sterile scissors make a cut directly adjacent to the tongue to avoid injuring the submandibular ducts in the floor of the mouth. Occasionally, more than one cut is needed to fully release the tongue. Bleeding is slight, although because blood mixes with saliva, it may sometimes seem as if there is more bleeding than really occurs. Slight pressure for a minute or so generally causes bleeding to subside.

Frenuloplasty involves more invasive resectioning of the underside of the tongue and requires general anesthesia. It typically is performed on children over 1 to 2 years of age (Lalakea 2003). In frenuloplasty, the frenulum is released as it is in frenotomy. Sometimes the genioglossus muscle requires resectioning to obtain an adequate release of the tongue. The wound is closed with sutures. While more involved, frenuloplasty takes only minutes to perform and bleeding is generally minimal. Following the surgery, older patients are asked to perform tongue exercises to strengthen the tongue.

Masaitis (1996) comments that because of increased awareness of the importance of breastfeeding and the low risk of frenotomy, physicians are beginning to reconsider the practice of delaying frenotomy. Griffiths (2004) identified 215 tongue-tied infants in the UK who were younger than 3 months and were experiencing breastfeeding difficulties. Following release by frenotomy, there were no significant complications. Within 24 hours, 80 percent were feeding better. Overall, 64 percent of this group breastfed for at least 3 months. The UK national average is 30 percent breastfeeding at 3 months.

The Genetics of Ankyloglossia

Research into the nature of orofacial abnormalities has uncovered an association between the location of the gene for ankyloglossia, cleft palate, and other mid-line defects seen as part of a cluster of symptoms in syndromic conditions (Forbes 1996). Japanese researchers (Mukai 1991) have noted an association of tongue-tie with abnormalities of the epiglottis and larynx. Infants whose mid-line defects extend to the throat may experience breathing problems (apnea) as well as feeding difficulties.

Because of the role that the tongue plays in shaping the palate during the prenatal period, there is speculation that disorders of the tongue may contribute to unusually shaped palates. Certainly it is often the case that infants with severely restricted tongues present with high, narrow, or arched palates.

BWC helped a 2 month-old infant who was experiencing breastfeeding problems. A digital assessment identified a high, bubble-shaped palate, causing BWC to comment that she seldom felt such a palate unless the baby was tongue-tied. When the infant subsequently began to cry, a tongue-tie was identified.

Because mid-line defects may be linked with other genetic syndromes that have the potential to affect an infant's general health, it is crucial to look at the whole baby, not just the tongue-tie. Sucking impairment can have more than one cause, and some tongue-tied babies continue to have feeding problems even after the tongue is released.

Hypospadias is another mid-line defect that sometimes appears in families with a history of tongue-tie or as part of a cluster of defects in an individual. Hypospadias refers to an atypical location of the urethral opening on the shaft or base of the penis, scrotum, or perineum (Stokowski

2004). Hypospadias is a common developmental disorder of the urogenital tract occurring in approximately 1 in 125 male births.

The urethral opening of the boy shown in **Fig. 382** was located at the base of the penis. His father and a male cousin were tongue-tied. The child underwent successful surgical repair at one year of age. Because the infant faced surgery and there were general concerns about his urogenital health, the low renal solute load of breast milk was considered to be beneficial for him. He breastfed well after an LC consult corrected positioning and latch problems.

Case Study of a Tongue-tied Infant With FTT

Fig. 383 shows a 10 day-old infant one pound (452 g) below birth weight as she attempts to latch onto her mother's breast. Note her expression of distress. Her lips are retracted. Even though her chin is placed close to the breast, she seems unable to draw in enough breast tissue to latch on. Her mother told the LC that each breastfeeding session was marked by frustration. If the baby managed to latch, the mother heard a few minutes of noisy sucking during milk ejection. As soon as the milk ejection subsided, the baby's eyes closed, and she fell asleep. When the mother tried to lay her down, the baby would awaken, cry frantically, and the cycle would begin again. The infant appeared robust owing to her large birth weight, when in fact her energy and growth were seriously impacted by excessive early weight loss and poor feeding.

Fig. 384 reveals a tight, rather fleshy lingual frenulum attached to the infant's tongue tip. Such a thick membrane is unlikely to stretch. Note how flat the tongue appears. During the initial evaluation, the LC observed that the baby had difficulty forming a central groove with her tongue. This affected her ability to feed from a cup and bottle, as well as to breastfeed. When offered a bottle, the baby struggled, spilling milk. She appeared to have difficulty swallowing and occasionally coughed while feeding. The baby became very agitated when cup fed, spilling more milk than she swallowed.

The LC recommended referral to a pediatric ENT. Three days later, after numerous attempts at supplementation, the baby had gained only 2 ounces (57 g). The pediatrician referred the infant for evaluation by a pediatric ENT.

Fig. 385 shows a pediatric ENT manipulating the baby's tongue. He agreed that the frenulum was unlikely to stretch on its own, and observed that the baby had poor ability to lift, cup, or extend her tongue. The baby was 18

days old, still feeding poorly, and was not back to birth weight. The ENT recommended frenotomy to release the tongue. The infant was seated on her mother's lap, and held still by the mother and a nurse. The doctor, wearing a visor with a spot-light on it, carefully visualized the frenulum to locate any blood vessels. He lifted the tongue with his fingers and snipped the frenulum twice (**Fig. 386**).

In **Fig. 387** the doctor applies pressure on the underside of the tongue with a gauze pad. Within a few minutes of the procedure, the infant began rooting for the breast. Within 10 minutes she latched onto the breast more deeply than ever before (**Fig. 388**), and breastfed until she fell asleep.

Fig. 389 shows the underside of the tongue almost a week after the frenotomy. Note the small white lesion, which has not yet healed. Unlike many babies who have their tongue-ties clipped and immediately feed well, this baby continued to have problems gaining weight. Perhaps the thickness of her frenulum or the delay of almost 3 weeks created tongue patterning problems that took time to resolve. Within 2 weeks of the frenotomy (**Fig. 390**) the tongue completely healed. Note the cupped shape of the tongue. **Fig. 391** shows the baby breastfeeding 3 weeks after the procedure. She now was able to coordinate swallowing fluids from both breast and bottle. Her stamina improved, allowing her to sustain longer, more effective feedings. Her growth rate improved.

A Tongue-tied Baby Who Breastfed Normally

Fig. 392 shows a tight frenulum that distorts the baby's tongue into the characteristic heart shape so often seen in tongue-tied individuals. However, this baby was able to breastfeed without causing his mother discomfort. His weight gain was appropriate. This case emphasizes how difficult it is to predict the breastfeeding ability of a tongue-tied infant.

Case Study of Severe Nipple Damage Caused by a Tongue-tied Infant

A 33 year-old primiparous mother of a 9 day-old infant was advised by her obstetrician's office staff to phone BWC to discuss remedies for a "yeast infection." Neither the doctor nor a nurse had seen the mother since her last office visit. The mother's description of persistent, severe deep breast pain, a "burning" sensation, and white material on the surface of the nipples led both the mother and the phone nurse to conclude that she had a fungal infection.

BWC insisted on seeing the mother and the infant. She immediately observed that the infant was tongue-tied. The infant was unable to lift her tongue past the mid-line plane of the mouth when she opened her mouth wide. When the tongue lifted, a thick lingual frenulum pulled against it, notching the tongue tip (**Fig. 393**). The infant had regained birth weight by Day 9, but the mother was offering bottles of formula owing to reduced milk supply and pain while breastfeeding.

Both nipples were badly abraded, the left nipple (**Fig. 394**) more severely than the right. The left nipple was inflamed and red. The red area spread past the areolar margin onto the breast itself. The Montgomery glands around the left areola were swollen, with white heads. Yellow, crystallized material appeared as crusts on the nipple wounds on both breasts. Blood and pus oozed from open lesions on the left nipple.

BWC and the mother decided that it would be too painful to practice latching. The mother agreed to express her milk with a hospital grade electric pump to allow the nipples to rest. Milk volumes were low; the mother pumped only 15 ml total during a double pumping session of approximately 12 minutes. The pumped milk was stained with blood and contained clumps of pus. The appearance of the milk so upset the mother that she understandably did not wish to feed it to the baby.

BWC phoned the mother's OB to report these symptoms. Even though the mother was afebrile, there were more signs and symptoms of bacterial infection than there were of a fungal infection. Interestingly, this mother had shared that she almost never developed an elevated temperature when ill. The OB prescribed an oral and a topical antibiotic. Within several days of beginning antibiotic therapy, the woman's nipples began to heal, and the appearance and volume of her pumped milk returned to normal.

BWC also faxed a written report to the baby's pediatrician, describing the mother's extreme nipple damage. She recommended assessment of the infant by a pediatric ENT. The ENT evaluated the baby on Day 21 and noted moderate ankyloglossia with poor tongue elevation. In his report to the LC, the ENT stated, "It seemed as if the 2 sides of the tongue were moving in opposition." The ENT performed a frenotomy in his office, and noted immediate improvement in the way the baby moved her tongue.

Fig. 395 shows the baby 15 days after the initial assessment, 2 days after frenotomy. The baby's tongue was able to lift and extend normally.

At this point, the mother had been exclusively pumping for the past 15 days. Her right nipple was healed, and her more damaged left nipple was almost healed (**Fig. 396**).

The mother confided during a phone call that she was afraid to latch the baby onto the breast. She asked for a follow-up visit to practice latching. BWC assisted the mother in finding a comfortable position, and the baby self-attached. The relieved mother exclaimed that it was no longer painful to breastfeed. The baby was still breastfeeding at 19 months, when this mother called BWC to refer a cousin whose new baby was also tongue-tied.

Frenotomy at Age Forty

The adult woman whose tongue-tie is seen in **Fig. 369** had considered a frenotomy for some years. She had a slight speech impediment that she disguised well, and she disliked the appearance of her tongue. A speech pathologist gave her a mirror and asked the woman to chew a red pill used by dentists to help patients identify dental plaque. The speech pathologist asked the woman to observe how many swallows it took to clear the chewed up red pill from her tongue. In this way, the speech pathologist demonstrated how dysfunctionally her tongue performed. The woman's dentist agreed to perform the frenotomy. She described the procedure as essentially painless. "It felt strange; like dull scissors cutting through wet wool." Because her frenulum was thick and fibrous, it took the dentist 3 snips before the tongue was freed. She felt a slight "burning sensation" on the last clip.

In the weeks following the frenotomy, the woman performed simple exercises suggested by the speech pathologist. She was initially unable to lateralize her tongue. It quivered and became extremely tired when she tried to hold it in an elevated position. One of her exercises involved balancing a small, round plastic ring on the front of her elevated tongue. After several months of exercising, she was able to move her tongue in any direction, and it functioned normally. Her tongue after frenotomy is pictured in **Fig. 397**. Note that while she can now lift it freely, the heart-shaped tongue tip remains.

It may be that some infants experience similar weakness of the tongue muscle following frenotomy. They may also require a period of rehabilitation. A parent might imitate the simple exercises used by the woman in **Fig. 397,** by placing a clean finger at the corners of the lips to trigger lateral tongue seeking behavior. Sucking on a finger or on a soft air- or gel-filled pacifier might encourage the infant to do "push-ups" with the tongue. A hollow, collapsible pacifier is not as useful as it offers too little resistance. Tapping lightly on the tongue tip will elicit tongue protrusion, thus encouraging the baby to extend the tongue. Breastfeeding, itself, is physical therapy for the muscles of the mouth. The activity of breastfeeding will help strengthen the tongue. Parents should be reminded that while some babies will breastfeed immediately following frenotomy; others will need time for healing and strengthening. A baby has spent many months practicing sucking *in utero*. It may take a while for some babies to repattern the tongue. In general, it appears that the longer the baby waits to have the frenotomy, the longer the period of rehabilitation.

Amir LH, James JP, Beatty J. Review of tongue-tie release at a tertiary maternity hospital. *Journal of Paediatric and Child Health* 2005; 41(5-6):243-245.

Ardran G, Kemp F, Lind J. A cineradiographic study of breast-feeding. *British Journal of Radiology* 1958; 31(363):156-162.

Ballard J, Auer C, Khoury J, et al. Ankyloglossia: assessment, incidence and effect of frenuloplasty on the breastfeeding dyad. *Pediatrics* 2002; 110(5): e63.

Coryllos E, Genna CW, Salloum D. Congenital Tongue-tie and its impact on Breastfeeding. American Academy of Pediatrics, Section on Breastfeeding newsletter, Breastfeeding: Best for Baby and Mother Summer 2004; 1-7.

Fernando C. *Tongue Tie: from Confusion to Clarity*. Sydney, Australia: Tandem Publications, 1998.

Fletcher S, Meldrum J. Lingual function and relative length of the lingual frenulum. *Journal of Speech, Language, Hearing Research* 1968; 11(2):382-390.

Flinck A, Paludan A, Matsson L, et al. Oral findings in a group of newborn Swedish children. *International Journal of Paediatric Dentistry* 1994; 4(2):67-73.

Forbes A, Brennan L, Richardson M, et al. Refined mapping and YAC contig construction of the X-linked cleft palate and ankyloglossia locus (CPX) including the proximal X-Y homology breakpoint within Xq21.3. *Genomics* 1996; 31(1):36-43.

Geddes DT, Kent JC, Mitoulas LR, et al. Tongue movement and intraoral vacuum in breastfeeding infants. *Early Human Development* 2008a; 84(7):471-477.

Geddes DT, Langton DB, Gollow I, et al. Frenotomy for breastfeeding infants with ankyloglossia: effect on milk removal and sucking mechanism as imaged by ultrasound. *Pediatrics* 2008b; 2(1):e188-194.

Gorski S, Adams K, Birch P, et al. Linkage analysis of X-linked cleft palate and ankyloglossia in Manitoba Mennonite and British Columbia native kindreds. *Human Genetics* 1994; 94(2):141-148.

Griffiths D. Do tongue ties affect breastfeeding? *Journal of Human Lactation* 2004; 20(4):409-411.

Hazelbaker A. *The Assessment Tool for Lingual Frenulum Function*. Master's Thesis, Pasadena, CA: Pacific Oaks College, 1993.

Hogan M, Westcott C, Griffiths M. Randomized, controlled trial of division of tongue-tie in infants with feeding problems. *Journal of Paediatric and Child Health* 2005; 41(5-6):246-250.

Jain E. Tongue-tie: Impact on breastfeeding (video). Calgary, Alberta, Canada T3E 5R8: 6628 Crowchild Trail, 1996.

Lalakea M, Messner A. Ankyloglossia: does it matter? *Pediatric Clinics of North America* 2003; 50(2):381-387.

Lawrence RA, Lawrence RM. *Breastfeeding: A Guide for the Medical Profession (6th edition)*. Philadelphia, PA: Elsevier Mosby 2005; p. 303.

Masaitis N, Kaempf J. Developing a frenotomy policy at one medical center: a case study approach. *Journal of Human Lactation* 1996; 12(3):229-232.

Meier P. Supporting lactation in mothers with very low birth weight infants. *Pediatric Annals* 2003; 32(5):317-325.

Messner AH, Lalakea ML, Aby J, et al. Ankyloglossia: incidence and associated feeding difficulties. *Archives of Otolaryngology - Head & Neck Surgery* 2000; 126(1):36-39.

Mukai C, Mukai S, Asaoka K. Ankyloglossia with deviation of the epiglottis and larynx. *Annals of Otology, Rhinology, and Laryngology Suppl.* 1991; 153:3-20.

Neifert M. Prevention of breastfeeding tragedies. in RJ Schanler (ed.) *Pediatric Clinics of North America* 2001; 48(2):273-297.

Palmer B. The influence of breastfeeding on the development of the oral cavity: a commentary. *Journal of Human Lactation* 1998; 14(2):93-98.

Powers N. How to assess slow growth in the breastfed infant. in R Schanler, (ed). *Pediatric Clinics of North America* 2001; 48(2):345-363.

Ramsay D, Langton D, Gollow I, et al. Ultrasound imaging of the effect of frenulotomy on breastfeeding infants with ankyloglossia, Abstract of the 12th International Conference of the International Society for Research in Human Milk and Lactation, Sept. 10-14, 2004; Queen's College, Cambridge, UK, 2004a; p. 52.

Ramsay D, Mitoulas L, Kent J, et al. Ultrasound imaging of the sucking mechanics of the breastfeeding infant. Abstract of the 12th International Conference of the International Society for Research in Human Milk and Lactation, Sept. 10-14, 2004, Queen's College, Cambridge, UK, 2004b; p. 53.

Ranly D. Early orofacial development. *Journal of Clinical Pediatric Dentistry* 1998; 22(4):267-275.

Ricke L, Baker N, Madlon-Kay D, et al. Newborn tongue-tie: prevalence and effect on breastfeeding. *Journal of the American Board of Family Practice* 2005; 18(1):1-7.

Srinivasan A, Dobrich C, Mitnick H, et al. Ankyloglossia in breastfeeding infants: the effect of frenotomy on maternal nipple pain and latch. *Breastfeeding Medicine* 2006; 1(4):216-224.

Stokowski L. Hypospadias in the neonate. *Advances in Neonatal Care* 2004; 4(4):206-215.

Wallace H, Clarke S. Tongue tie division in infants with breast feeding difficulties. *International Journal of Pediatric Otorhinolaryngology* 2006; 70(7):1257-1261.

Wight N. Management of common breastfeeding issues, in RJ Schanler (ed.) *Pediatric Clinics of North America* 2001; 48(2):321-344.

Wolf L, Glass R. *Feeding and Swallowing Disorders in Infancy.* Tucson, AZ: Therapy Skill Builders, 1992; pp. 16-18.

Wright J. Tongue-tie. *Journal of Paediatric Child Health* 1995; 31(4):276-278.

Orofacial Variations

The relationship between appearance and social stereotyping has been established as one of the most consistent research findings in social science. In earlier times, a bodily difference was referred to as a *stigma*. Cleft disorders have been considered in many cultures to be stigmatizing. Even in more sophisticated eras and locales, the appearance of an infant with an orofacial abnormality may initially be shocking. While intellectually aware that the condition is repairable, on an emotional level, a new mother may feel distress at her child's appearance. For a time, until she adjusts, she may painfully re-experience the impact of this distress each time a new person looks at her child.

Emotional Attachment

Because feeding involves both nutrition and nurture, it is crucial to consider the bonding implications connected with the activity of feeding. Success in feeding often determines how women judge their competency as mothers (Ramsay 1996).

Experts in the field of attachment and bonding observe that the mother provides a "mirror" for her baby (Klaus 1996). Her responsiveness to the baby's appearance, her sensitivity and success in handling, holding, and feeding, and how much she smiles at her baby, all influence the baby's responses to her. These mutual responses create an ongoing feedback loop. Parents of children with orofacial abnormalities realize that surgery will most likely correct the facial defect. However, care providers must be aware that parents of "sick" infants process information anxiously, and respond to their children differently. For example, parents of infants who are hospitalized in special care nurseries smile less at their infants. Their infants, in turn, smile less at 3 months (Minde 1982).

The birth of a child with special needs contributes greatly to increased family stress. Financial issues, transportation logistics, and even marital stress are compounded. Comprehensive social services may be required to assist the family. HCPs must seek ways to reduce additional sources of stress. Human milk protects the health of infants, and is especially important to prevent compromised infants from becoming ill (Wright 1998). Therefore systematic support for human milk feeds for infants with cleft defects can provide a meaningful method of lessening the burden of additional illness for struggling families.

Parents of children with orofacial abnormalities deal with what has been described as "chronic" grief. They worry about how to provide the baby and themselves with a normal experience. Over time, most families find a way to integrate the image of the ideal baby dreamed of during pregnancy with the real baby who has been born. During this adjustment phase, social support for the mother may help her provide a more positive "mirror" for her newborn. She may need counseling, and she will certainly need nurturing of her own needs. The quality of her responsiveness may have important long-term effects on the baby's cognitive and behavioral outcomes (Ainsworth 1982).

Human Milk for Infants with Cleft Defects

Early failure-to-thrive (FTT) is common in infants with cleft defects (Glenny 2004), and it has generally been attributed to feeding difficulties. However, FTT appears to be linked to cleft type and to the presence of other anomalies (Beaumont 2008). Infants with cleft lip had similar birth weights when compared to the general population. Infants with cleft lip and palate, or those with isolated cleft palate were significantly lighter at birth and had significantly more early growth delay. Therefore, infants with cleft palate require specialized feeding support to protect growth. Their growth often influences the timing of surgical repair. Consequently, more systematic support for these infants could improve nutritional intake and move the schedule for surgical repair forward (Amstalden-Mendes 2007).

The infant with cleft palate is at high risk for poor ventilation of the eustachian tube, a contributing factor for development of *otitis media* (middle ear infection). The eustachian tube is opened and closed by muscles that cross the palate, the tensor muscle, supported by the levator veli palatini muscle. Because the palatal plates have failed to form normally, these muscles are also abnormally formed. The impaired ventilation of the eustachian tube is not fully corrected either by surgery or tubes in the ears (Aniansson 2002). Thus, the infant with a cleft palate is at risk for chronic ear infection.

No difference in hearing sensitivity per se was found in a study that compared children with cleft lip and palate to children in a control group. However, perhaps because of a greater *frequency* of middle-ear disease, the children with cleft lip and palate had lower language comprehension scores, and lower scores on tests of cognition and expressive language (Jocelyn 1996). Consequently, it is crucial to identify other preventive methods of reducing episodes of ear infections in this population. Paradise (1994) and Aniansson (2002) identified that longer duration of human milk feeding is significantly correlated with a reduction in acute and secretory otitis media in children with cleft palate.

BWC has worked with 2 infants with clefts of the palate who were exclusively fed human milk for 5 and 6 months respectively. Neither infant was capable of obtaining sufficient milk while directly breastfeeding. Their mothers put them to breast for comfort and to help stimulate milk supply, but these babies were primarily fed pumped breast milk by bottle. Neither baby experienced any ear infections until formula or solid food was introduced into their diets. Ethically, parents should be informed of the risk of formula in the development of otitis media in infants with cleft defects. If a mother's milk supply is not adequate, donor milk from an accredited human milk bank is an option to ensure exclusive human milk feeds.

HCPs may wonder if promoting breastfeeding or the use of human milk will increase maternal stress. HCPs may conclude that giving "permission to wean" spares women the extra work of extended pumping. Research studies indicate, however, that lactation reduces physiologic stress, improves maternal mood, and increases immune strength in women. Thus, lactation protects maternal as well as infant health (Groer 2004).

The Role of the Lactation Consultant on the Orofacial Team

In order to advocate for the important protections conferred by lactation (for the mother) and human milk (for the infant), an LC should be a member of the cleft palate care team. The LC advises the mother on how to provide breast milk, whether or not the baby is able to breastfeed. She instructs the mother on how to pump her milk, and encourages skin-to-skin holding as a way to assist milk production and enhance bonding.

Infants with cleft palate defects are challenging to feed no matter what feeding method is used. They may choke, experience nasal regurgitation, and spill milk. These challenges may put the infant at risk for reduced positive social contact during feeding (Morris 1977).

There are few documented cases of effective breastfeeding in infants with cleft palate. Because of the cleft, these babies cannot create suction, and hence are unable to transfer sufficient amounts of milk. It is doubtful that they have the ability to empty the breast adequately enough to sustain a full milk supply. "Practical information related to breastfeeding the infant with a cleft defect is lacking," (Crossman (1998).

While being realistic about the need for supplementation, the LC should encourage the mother to experiment with breastfeeding. If a palatal cleft is small and located on the hard palate only, a mother with soft, elastic breasts may find that her breast tissue plugs the cleft. If she has an ample milk supply, a responsive milk ejection reflex, and erect nipples, her infant may be able to breastfeed better than expected. Older infants may become more adept over time, as has been reported in the anthropological literature.

Because the breast may obscure the facial defect, breastfeeding gives the mother a chance to look at the baby without the visual intrusion of the facial abnormality. Even though breastfeeding attempts may not produce much intake of milk, more than one mother has shared that the only time her infant looked "normal" was when placed at breast. Because of the beneficial effect on bonding, such experiences should be encouraged. The LC also models acceptance by commenting upon the beautiful features and strengths of the baby.

While many claims are made for various feeding devices and methods, a Cochrane Review of research related to feeding infants with cleft defects (Glenny 2004) found no statistical difference between feeding outcomes in infants who were fitted with maxillary plates compared to no plate. Nor did they discover any statistical difference in growth outcomes when comparing the available bottle types used to feed infants with clefts. The Cochrane Review found no evidence to support any type of current maternal advice and/or support for these babies. Since evidence-based protocols do not yet exist to provide guidance for feeding children with clefts, common sense approaches aim to maximize growth while reducing the risk of aspiration.

The LC, along with other feeding specialists such as occupational therapists (OTs) assist in teaching mothers alternative feeding methods. Given the lack of evidence to demonstrate the superiority of one method over another, the team must experiment to discover which method of feeding works best for the individual infant. Mothers who learn about the protective benefits of human milk are often relieved to discover that there is something crucial they can contribute to the baby's well being. Maternal self-esteem is enhanced when the care team takes into account the mother's perceptions of how her infant reacts to various feeding interventions.

Counseling skills such as active listening and validation of feelings help establish trust and rapport between the mother and the LC. Being aware of her own emotional reactions helps the LC avoid adopting a crisis mentality when helping families of infants with birth defects. Just as tension can be "catching," so can calm. Tone of voice is important, and the skillful LC deliberately pitches her voice to help soothe anxious parents. Some parents worry that they will not be able to master special feeding instructions or learn to use the equipment involved in caring for the baby. The LC seeks to reduce parental stress by calmly repeating details, giving written instructions, and providing follow-up until the feeding plan is established.

What Causes Cleft Lip and Palate?

Clefts of the lip and palate are among the most common birth defects. They occur roughly once in every 700 births, affecting both boys and girls. Clefts occur most often among Asian and American Indian races, and whites are almost twice as likely to be affected as blacks. Information and resources are available from the American Cleft Palate-Craniofacial Association: http://www.acpa-cpf.org (accessed August 2008).

Clefts form early in pregnancy, often before women are aware they are pregnant. Clefts of the lip appear between the 5th and 8th gestational weeks when the masses of the median maxillary and premaxillary process fail to fuse. Clefts of the palate form during the 6th to 12th weeks when the mesenchymal masses of the palatine fail to fuse.

No single factor has been identified that causes cleft defects; however, a positive association has been identified between maternal smoking during the first trimester of pregnancy and cleft lip and palate (Little 2004, Bille 2007). Treatment with excessive amounts of Vitamin A during pregnancy induces fetal malformations in mice, most notably, cleft palate (Inomata 2005). Folic acid supplements and a diet high in folate (fruits and vegetables) seem to reduce the risk of isolated cleft lip (Wilcox 2007). Genetic studies have mapped the chromosomal locus for some forms of cleft palate and ankyloglossia, and have identified these two mid-line defects in certain families as a recurrent genetic trait (Gorski 1994).

There are isolated clefts, and clefts associated with other birth defects and syndromes. Clefts have been identified as a feature of over 300 syndromic conditions. When clefts occur as part of a broader problem, other effects of the specific disease or syndrome must also be considered in the feeding plan.

For instance, a certain syndrome may be associated with muscle weakness. Cardiac abnormalities may affect infant feeding stamina or require restriction of fluid intake. Feeding a child with a combination of medical issues requires careful planning to ensure that adequate nutritional support is provided in a way that addresses all the child's special needs. A team approach ensures that the LC is guided by others and tailors her suggestions appropriately.

Genetic Counseling

When a couple gives birth to a child with a cleft defect, the risk of delivering another child with similar problems is increased 2 to 4 percent. Genetic counseling can help parents identify whether their child has an isolated cleft, or if the cleft defect has occurred as part of a syndrome. Counseling also helps determine the odds of bearing another at-risk child (Cleft Palate Foundation 1987).

Cleft Lip

The lips stabilize the breast in the mouth, and work with the tongue to form a seal (see Ch. 3). Maintenance of a tight seal creates negative pressure and allows the baby to generate suction (Geddes 2008). Since suction is the main mechanism of milk removal, gaps or breaks in seal are problematical. A small, *incomplete* cleft of the lip (**Figs. 398** and **399**) generally does not impede breastfeeding if it can be sealed in some manner. Cleft lip is classified as *complete* if the cleft extends from the lip into the nasal cavity (as in **Fig. 407**). Complete clefts of the lip are more disfiguring and harder to seal.

To plug or seal a cleft lip, the mother holds the infant close to her breast. She draws up breast tissue between 2 fingers (similar to grasping a cup handle) and presses it into the gap in the lip. The so-called "teacup hold" is demonstrated in **Fig. 400**). Or, the mother may place her finger over the cleft to create a seal. Once a seal is achieved, the baby can create suction. If the cleft lip extends into the nasal cavity, it is more difficult for the mother to help the infant achieve a seal. Surgical repair of a cleft lip usually takes place within a few days, weeks, or months of the birth, depending on the preferences of the surgical team and the family, and on the size and health of the baby.

Types of Cleft Palate

Clefts of the palate vary greatly. Some involve small, isolated perforations of the hard or soft palate; other cleft formations are more extensive and create severe facial disfigurement. The size and location of the cleft influence feeding in different ways. Clefts of the palate can be *bilateral*, that is, affecting both sides of the mouth on each side of the midline. **Figs. 401-403** show clefts of the soft palate. Note the absence of the uvula.

Clefts can be *unilateral*, on one side only. Clefts can be *complete*, from uvula to nostrils. They can be *incomplete*, that is, the cleft does not extend to the gum ridge.

Sub-mucosal clefts are relatively uncommon clefts of the palate that occur in 1 in 1,200 children (McMillan 1999). Skin covers the cleft, thus, they are not easily detected by casual visualization. They can be detected with a gentle digital exam, by shining a light on the palate, or by a light probe placed within the nose. About 30 percent of individuals with a sub-mucosal cleft will have a *bifid* (cleft) uvula. "A cleft uvula should raise suspicion of a palatal defect" (Rudolph 2003). The severing of the muscles of the soft palate creates dysfunctional swallowing. Some infants with sub-mucosal clefts present with nasal regurgitation and most have feeding problems of some degree.

It is tempting to assume that small clefts will not affect feeding, but a small cleft of the hard or soft palate poses considerable problems for feeding, especially in early infancy. The 3 week-old girl in **Fig. 403** has a centrally located cleft of the soft palate. She cannot seal the oral cavity and is thus unable to create suction. Her breathing sounds wet after feeding, and feeding appears stressful.

Weighing 9 lbs (4075 g) at birth, this baby appeared robust; however, she had severe feeding problems. No matter what oral feeding method was tried, the baby demonstrated distress after consuming approximately one ounce (28 g) of milk. In **Fig. 404**, the baby has been flexed at the hips for feeding. She is feeding from a Mead cleft palate feeder, a soft bottle that allows the feeder to squeeze milk to the baby. The baby flared her lips often during feeding, allowing milk to spill out. The baby consumed about an ounce of milk, and then she demonstrated feeding refusal behavior. She arched her back, and when that failed to signal her mother to remove the bottle, the baby appeared to fall asleep (**Fig. 405**).

At the time the photos were taken, this infant was 30 days old and not back to her birth weight. The LC had been working with this dyad and reporting to the pediatrician since Day 4. The mother had tried various types of feeding implements, including spoons, cups, Special Needs Feeder™, and the Pigeon™ feeder. A feeding tube at the breast was also tried. The baby demonstrated the same tendency to limit her intake no matter how she was fed. The LC informed the pediatrician that feeding was not successful for the infant. The pediatrician, concerned about the lack of weight gain, ordered a nasogastric tube (NG) to be placed. The infant is shown in **Fig. 406** sucking on a pacifier (to protect oral feeding skills and to calm her) while being fed fortified human milk via the NG tube.

Because of this infant's inability to feed normally and her poor growth, her pediatrician referred her to a surgical team in another city for evaluation for early repair of the cleft defect.

Early Surgical Repair

Traditional repair of cleft defects are scheduled for the lip at 3 months; soft palate repairs are usually done around 6 to 8 months. Hard palate repairs have occurred between 12-18 months. *Early* repair of both lip and palate can occur in some infants within the first 2 weeks after birth, with larger, wider clefts repaired at 2 to 3 months of age (Denk, personal communication 2002).

Early repair is based on the idea that during the first 28 days after birth, neonates retain fetal wound healing capabilities. Rapid healing is desirable in itself, and enhances cosmetic effect, helping to improve appearance. Additionally, younger babies have enhanced immunologic status as the result of breast milk feeds and transplacentally acquired immune factors, enabling them to better withstand the stress of surgery.

Because surgeries such as hernia repair and bowel resectioning of infants with NEC are now widely performed on newborns, anesthesiologists are experienced in providing sedation for neonates. Greater skill in managing neonatal anesthesia is thought to reduce the level of risk of early repair surgery. Some surgical teams have been performing early repair of cleft lips in neonates for close to a decade. To date, their results have been favorable. (Denk 2001).

Breastfeeding is sometimes interrupted after lip surgery for fear the sutures will tear, although there is little clinical evidence to support this. Weatherly-White found evidence of better weight gain, shorter hospital stays, fewer complications, and no apparent difference in the operative results when he compared breastfed infants with cup- or syringe-fed term infants following lip repair (Weatherly-White 1987). In a prospective, randomized trial, Darzi (1996) showed that early postoperative breastfeeding after cleft lip repair is safe, results in more weight gain at 6 weeks after surgery, and is less labor intensive than spoon feeding.

Not all babies are willing to breastfeed immediately following surgery. Some parents report that their infants refused to breastfeed for several days, apparently owing to discomfort. Some infants will put their mouths close to the breast but will not suck. Other babies breastfeed immediately.

Interestingly, the infant pictured in **Figs. 403-406**, experienced a successful and uneventful surgical repair of her cleft of the soft palate. However, while she was recovering in the special care nursery, she suffered a complete bowel rotation. The neonatologists caring for her speculated that her early self-limitation of intake had more to do with the undetected partial bowel rotation than to her cleft defect. When the bowel rotation fully manifested, it required emergency surgery. The infant slowly recovered and began feeding at breast with a feeding tube device by the time she was 3 months old. Her stressed mother had difficulty maintaining a full milk supply, and the baby was supplemented with human donor milk whenever necessary.

Defects of the Hard Palate: Clefts and Grooved Palates

Fig. 407 shows an infant with a complete cleft of the lip and hard palate. Note the involvement of the nose. Complete clefts of the hard palate create problems with dental formation. These infants not only require surgery to repair the cleft, they will also need extensive dental correction with surgery and orthodontia (Redford-Badwal 2003).

Fig. 408 shows the palate of an infant who was intubated for many weeks, causing re-shaping of the palate and the formation of a groove or channel. This palatal formation can mimic many of the feeding problems created by a cleft of the hard palate. The infant may have difficulty positioning the nipple against the palate (Snyder 1997). Some instances of unusual palate formation occur as part of syndromic conditions (Rovet 1995). **Fig. 409** shows the abnormally-shaped palate of a 12 year-old with Down Syndrome. This boy was unable to breastfeed exclusively as an infant. (See also **Fig. 364** and the discussion of Turner's Syndrome in Ch. 16.)

Case Study of an Infant With a Cleft of the Lip and Palate

The infant in **Figs. 410-414** was referred by the mother's midwife. The infant had a complete (nose to soft palate) unilateral cleft (**Fig. 410**). His mother had previously breastfed another child and had normal, well-everted nipples. Her breasts were firmly engorged at the time of the LC visit. The hospital nurses helped the mother initiate breastfeeding, and the baby received no supplementation during the first 4 days after birth. The baby's birth weight was 7 lb. 6 oz. (3345 g). He had lost approximately 8 percent of his body weight at the time of the lactation consultation on Day 4. He appeared jaundiced and had produced only one small, dark stool in the past 36 hours (**Fig. 411**).

The hospital staff had taught the mother to use up right feeding positions to protect the baby from choking. They correctly encouraged her to carefully support the weight of her breast in her hand, and to use breast compression to help transfer milk to the baby (**Fig. 412**). The hospital LCs

assumed that the baby was breastfeeding well because he made many "swallowing sounds." However, this impression was not validated by test weights on an accurate scale, and the baby was discharged without documentation that he was transferring milk.

When BWC visited the mother at home, she also shared an initial impression that the baby was breastfeeding well. The mother demonstrated good positioning and excellent breastfeeding technique. The baby sounded as if he were swallowing milk. However, test weights revealed no evidence of intake. The first weight indicated that the baby actually lost 1 g during the feeding. Three subsequent test weights were performed after positioning changes. All the test weights indicated zero intake.

Based on the lack of measurable intake, reduced stooling, dark, scant urine, rising bilirubin levels, and continued weight loss, the LC advised the mother to begin pumping her breasts and to use this milk to supplement the baby. The mother had a small quantity of hand-expressed colostrum in the refrigerator. The colostrum was warmed and offered to the baby by spoon and then by cup. He seemed unable to organize swallowing from these utensils. In **Fig. 413** the baby is shown drinking this colostrum from a Medela Special Needs Feeder™ (formerly called the Haberman Feeder™). The baby's feeding affect was depressed at this feeding, but improved over the next 24 hours. The baby was soon feeding reasonably well from the special bottle.

The LC discussed the options available to the family, including early repair. The parents visited the website of a plastic surgeon who specializes in early repair. On Day 18, the family traveled out of state for the surgery. The surgery was uneventful, and the baby is pictured in **Fig. 414** several days after the surgery (photo courtesy of K. Bird). The initial surgery closed the lip and partially repaired the palate.

One of the factors that motivated the parents to seek early repair was their goal of preserving breastfeeding. However, even this highly motivated mother experienced great difficulty maintaining her milk supply. She took domperidone, used herbs believed to increase milk supply, pumped at recommended levels, and used a feeding tube device at breast. The baby had great difficulty obtaining milk from any method that required creation of suction, and soon refused to breastfeed.

The mother told the LC, "He gets so angry when I try to nurse him, and I feel really sad and rejected." The mother had problems achieving a milk ejection when she pumped. Shortly after returning home from the hospital where the surgery was performed, both the baby and his older sibling developed respiratory syncytial virus (RSV). "Between caring for the baby and the 2 year-old, pumping, doing the nebulizer and oxygen treatments, I felt just a little bit insane." The mother decided to wean. She described feelings of depression as she dealt with the loss of the lactation. Successful surgery to finish the repair of the cleft palate was performed when the baby was 2 months old. At this time, the mother considered, but did not undertake, relactation.

This case serves to remind HCPs of the enormous stress involved in caring for such infants. Stress may impact the decision to continue to maintain lactation (Lau 2001). In spite of help from an LC, and good social support, breastfeeding was not successful. However, the infant had the benefit of colostrum and of several weeks of exclusive human milk feeds. In such situations, the LC helps the mother process her feelings, praises her for her efforts, and answers questions accurately, including details about relactation or assistance with weaning.

Nasal Regurgitation

Inability to create suction is only one problem caused by cleft defects. The breach of the barrier between the oral and nasal cavities exposes the nasal tissues to contact with food when the infant swallows. An infant with a cleft palate may experience frequent nasal regurgitation, spilling milk out of the nose with each swallow. The experience worries parents and is uncomfortable and unpleasant for the baby. An upright feeding position may help. The LC reassures parents that feeding ability improves with practice. The baby will eventually learn to swallow more effectively. Human milk is a physiological and non-irritating substance. It contains anti-inflammatory agents (Goldman 1986) and will not irritate sensitive nasal tissue as much as formula will. This issue may be especially important during the time the infant is recovering from surgery, when extensive suturing increases inflammation of the tissues.

Palatal Obturators

If the baby cannot breastfeed, how should the milk be delivered? The chapter on alternate feeding methods describes various options available. Babies with cleft palates may try to obtain milk by compressing with their jaws and tongue because they cannot milk the breast in the normal manner (using suction). While the infant may obtain some milk using compression, many devices have been evaluated to see if breastfeeding might be improved. Some cleft palate teams use a soft silicone prosthesis called an *obturator* to simulate an intact hard

palate (Markowitz 1979, Curtin 1990). Some infants appear to be able to breastfeed more effectively using such devices, although the evidence for this is unclear. Obturators are created from a mold taken of the infant's palate, generally by the pedodontist member of a cleft palate team. New obturators are made as the infant grows.

Another device used in the treatment of infants with clefts is a palatal prosthesis created by an orthodontist to align the palatal segments and nasal cartilage to aid surgical correction. These plates are sized and changed weekly. The baby wears the plate all the time until the repair takes place. The mother removes it once a day to clean it. Glenny (2004) found no statistically significant difference in outcomes for infants fitted with a maxillary plate compared to those with no plate.

Special Bottles

The Medela® Special Needs Feeder (formerly the Haberman Feeder™) is a bottle with a chambered teat that is controlled by compression rather than suction. Thus it can be manipulated by an infant who cannot successfully create suction. It is designed to have a controllable flow rate. The soft teat chamber can be squeezed to assist the infant. However, some infants find the flow rate too fast, especially if the teat is squeezed too fast. Three lines of varying length on the teat indicate flow rate. At the start of the feeding, insert the teat so that the shortest line is under the baby's nose. The tip of the teat is positioned under the intact part of the palate. The teat can then be rotated to position the middle or the longest line under the baby's nose. If the infant seems overwhelmed by the milkflow rate, rotate the teat until the shortest line is under the nose.

The Pigeon Cleft Palate Nurser™, is a specially designed bottle with a chambered teat that controls the milk flow rate. The Pigeon teat has a Y cut in the tip of the nipple, and a V notched at the base of the nipple. The V indicates an air vent, which must be rotated so that it is positioned under the infant's nose in order to work properly. One side of the Pigeon teat is softer than the other. The harder side is held against the palate. The soft side is placed in contact with the tongue. Simply touching the teat with the tongue initiates milk flow. If the teat frequently collapses, it may help to slightly enlarge the Y cut, or use a vented bottle system. The mother in **Fig. 415** holds her baby close to her naked breast while he drinks from a Pigeon Feeder™.

Feeding Tube Devices

Feeding tube devices may be useful in feeding some infants with cleft palate. However, in order to work, the infant must be able to create some suction. Some infants with cleft defects become easily exhausted during feedings and will be unable to obtain adequate milk volumes using feeding tube devices. Therefore, intake must be carefully monitored. A gravity feed may increase flow rate and help the infant who is unable to create sufficient suction to draw milk into a feeding tube. If using a Supplemental Nursing System™, for example, the bottle can be elevated (strung on a pole lamp or a hook on the wall) to take advantage of a greater gravity drop. The tube is taped as usual to the mother's breast or to a parent's finger. A parent can also squeeze the device to increase the milk flow rate.

Nipple Shields

Soft silicone nipple shields, which enlarge the diameter of the mother's nipple, may simulate the effect of a palatal obturator. The excess tissue of the shield may help plug a small cleft of the hard palate. The infant will probably not be able to breastfeed normally, but this intervention may help the baby stay on the breast longer, thus assisting the process of bonding.

One Mother's Experience

The mother of an infant born with a simple cleft of the lip wrote the following letter to BWC some months after the surgical repair was performed. The infant's surgical team was firm in instructing this mother that damage to the sutured lip would occur if she breastfed her son within 2 weeks of his lip repair.

"It's been nearly a year since I first asked you for help in planning the surgery for my son's cleft lip repair. I guess I didn't realize it would take this long for me to talk about it.

"His surgery was done at 5 months and was very smooth, but certainly emotionally draining. He looked like a little refugee from a war-torn country when he came to, and stayed like that for about 24 hours. He didn't make any indication for the first 3 days of wanting to nurse, although once on each of those days I did nurse him because I couldn't stand it. He refused the syringe feedings with extreme vigor and never did accept them except at night when he was so sleepy he didn't realize it. I'm sure the little nursing I offered him made it harder for him, but I found I couldn't make a stand either way.

"At 36 hours after surgery, he began to grab food off my plate (although he still didn't try to nurse). At 48 hours, I finally began to mix a little pureed sweet potato with lots of breast milk and spoon-fed him. He wouldn't accept a syringe from the nurses either. Dr. — witnessed one of the feeding attempts at length at about 48 hours after surgery. And then at last he very quietly said, "You know, I guess I've never seen a breastfed baby." I could tell it had sunk in that there was something very different going on here. After 72 hours I couldn't pump enough to keep up with feeding, so I began to nurse to build up the supply again. The baby nursed well with no physical complications, although I was nervous for a few days. And it was not until the first long nursing at home that he made eye contact with me — the first time since the surgery.

"So it was hard, mostly because of my emotional quandary over being instructed not to nurse the baby. I still haven't told Dr. — that we nursed so early on. He wanted me to wait 2 weeks, which would have been impossible for both of us."

Other Orofacial Issues

Because of the shape of the infant's skull, babies have slightly recessed chins. As normal growth occurs, the skull elongates and the chin pulls forward. However, some infants, for various reasons, have abnormally receding chins. **Fig. 416** shows a baby with a normal chin beside an infant with *retrognathia* (abnormal development) of the lower jaw. A familial tendency toward a receding chin or retrognathia caused by a syndromic condition such as *Pierre Robin Sequence*, can pose significant, often unrecognized, feeding challenges. The mother of such an infant often experiences sore nipples. While it appears as if the baby is well-positioned at breast, the bottom jaw, being recessed, is not close enough to the breast. Jaw closure occurs on the shaft of the nipple and causes pain for the mother. Poorly positioned jaw closure may also obstruct milk flow to the infant, compromising intake.

Parents of infants with receding chins should be informed that the activity of breastfeeding, itself, promotes optimal development of the jaw. One large study found that a significant percentage of malocclusions could be prevented by an extended duration of breastfeeding (Labbok 1987).

Pierre Robin Syndrome

Pierre Robin Syndrome (or Sequence) is an autosomal, recessive, genetic condition marked by significant retrognathia (receding chin) and downward displacement of the tongue. It can result in serious swallowing disorders, respiratory compromise, and poor feeding. Pierre Robin Syndrome is often associated with cleft defects, and may further compromise feeding.

The Labial Frenum

A *frenum* is a membrane that connects two body parts and controls or limits movement. There are several *frena* in the human mouth: under the tongue (called the lingual frenulum), between the cheeks and gums, and between the lips and gums. **Fig. 417** shows an infant whose upper labial frenum attaches to the gum ridge. If the frenum is tight, short, and non-elastic, the infant may have difficulty flanging the lips. Rolled-in lips may reduce the stability of the latch and create frictional abrasion of the nipple. The mother generally can correct this by manually flanging the lips once her baby has latched.

Generally, tight labial frena do not significantly interfere with breastfeeding; however, there is one case report of an infant whose tight upper labial frenum did impair breast-feeding until it was released (Wiessinger 1995). As in tongue-tie, the upper labial frenum may be surgically incised, or ablated with a technique called laser frenecto-my. Correction of this mild mid-line defect can be per-formed by a dentist, involves little bleeding, and requires no anesthesia. Muscle activity influences bone placement. Dentists are aware that this frenal anomaly results in the creation of a gap between the top 2 teeth, requiring ortho-dontia to close. **Fig. 418** pictures an adult with such a gap. Like tongue-tie and cleft palate, this trait may run in families. This man's daughter had a similar gap caused by a tight labial frenum. She cut her labial frenum in an accident at age 12. The gap between her upper teeth closed over the next 6 months, and she did not require previously planned orthodontia.

Ainsworth M. Early caregiving and later patterns of attachment, in M Klaus, M Robertson, (eds), *Birth, Interaction and Attachment: Exploring The Foundations for Modern Perinatal Care,* 1982; Johnson & Johnson, Pediatric Round Table:6, pp. 35-43.

American Cleft Palate-Craniofacial Association: www.acpa-cpf.org Accessed August 2008.

Amstalden-Mendes LG, Magna LA, Gil-da-Silva-Lopes VL. Neonatal care of infants with cleft lip and/or palated: feeding orientation and evolution of weight gain in a nonspecialized Brazilian hos-pital. *Cleft Palate and Craniofacial Journal* 2007; 44(3):329-334.

Aniansson G, Svensson H, Becher M, et al. Otitis media and feeding with breast milk of children with cleft palate. *Scandinavian Journal of Plastic and Reconstructive Surgery and Hand Surgery* 2002; 36(1):9-15.

Beaumont D. A study into weight gain in infants with cleft lip/palate. *Paediatric Nursing* 2008; 20(6):20-23.

Bille C, Olsen J, Vach W, et al. Oral clefts and life style factors - a case-cohort study based on prospective Danish data. *European Journal of Epidemiology* 2007; 22(3):173-181.

Curtin G. The infant with cleft lip or palate: more than a surgical problem. *Journal of Perinatal & Neonatal Nursing* 1990; 3(3):80-89.

Crossman K. Breastfeeding a baby with a cleft palate: a case report. *Journal of Human Lactation* 1998; 14(1):47-50.

Darzi M, Chowdri N, Bhat A. Breastfeeding or spoon feeding after cleft lip repair: a prospective, randomized study. *British Journal of Plastic Surgery* 1996; 49(1):24-26.

Denk M. Bridging the gap: working with a baby with a cleft. Conference presentation, ILCA Conference, Acapulco, Mexico. July 18, 2001.

Denk M. Personal communication, Feb. 2002.

Geddes DT, Kent JC, Mitoulas LR, et al. Tongue movement and intra-oral vacuum in breastfeeding infants. *Early Human Development* 2008; 84(7):471-477.

Glenny A, Hooper L, Shaw W. et al. Cochrane Oral Health Group, Cochrane Database System Review, 2004; (3): CD003315.

Goldman A, Thorpe L, Goldblum R. Anti-inflammatory properties of human milk. *Acta Paediatrica Scandia* 1986; 75(5):689-695.

Gorski S, Adams K, Birch P, et al. Linkage analysis of X-linked cleft palate and ankyloglossia in Manitoba Mennonite and British Columbia Native Kindreds. *Human Genetics* 1994; 94(2):141-148.

Groer M, Davis M. Health, mood, stress, and immune benefits of lac-tation. Poster, Proceedings of the12th International Conference of the International Society for Research in Human Milk and Lactation. Sept 10-14, 2004; Queen's College, Cambridge, UK, p.. 79.

Inomata T, Kiuchi A, Yoshida T, et al. Hypervitaminosis A resulting in DNA aberration in fetal transgenic mice. *Mutation Research* 2005; 586(1):58-67.

Jocelyn L, Penko M, Rode H. Cognition, communication, and hearing in young children with cleft lip and palate and in control children: a longitudinal study. *Pediatrics* 1996; 97(4):529-534.

Klaus M, Kennell J, Klaus P. *Bonding.* Reading, MA: Addison-Wesley Publishing, 1996; pp. 122-127.

Lau C. Effects of stress on lactation. in R Schanler, (ed). *Pediatric Clinics of North America* 2001; 48(1):221-234.

Labbok M, Hendershot G. Does breast-feeding protect against malocclu-sion? An analysis of the 1981 child health supplement to the national health interview survey. *American Journal of Preventative Medicine* 1987; 3(4):227-232.

Little J, Cardy A, Arslan M, et al. Smoking and orofacial clefts: a United Kingdom-based case-control study. *The Cleft Palate-Craniofacial Journal* 2004; 41(4):381-386.

Markowitz J, Gerry R, Fleishner R. Immediate obturation of neonatal cleft palates. *The Mount Sinai Journal of Medicine* 1979; 46(2):123-129.

McMillan J, DeAngelis C, Feigin R, et al. *Oski's Pediatrics: Principles and Practice* (3rd edition). New York: Lippincott Williams & Wilkins, 1999; p. 391.

Minde K. The impact of medical complications on parental behavior in the premature nursery, in M Klaus, M Robertson (eds), *Birth, Interaction and Attachment: Exploring The Foundations for Modern Perinatal Care,* 1982; Johnson & Johnson, Pediatric Round Table:6; pp. 98-104.

Morris S. Interpersonal Aspects of Feeding Problems, in J Wilson (ed), *Oral Motor Function & Dysfunction in Children,* University of North Carolina at Chapel Hill, Division of Physical Therapy, Conference proceedings May 25-28, 1977; pp. 106-113.

Paradise J, Elster B, Tan L. Evidence in infants with cleft palate that breast milk protects against otitis media. *Pediatrics* 1994; 94(6):853-859.

Ramsay M, Gisel E. Neonatal Sucking and Maternal Feeding Practices. *Developmental Medicine and Child Neurology* 1996; 38(1):34-47.

Redford-Badwal D, Mabry K, Frassinelli J. Impact of cleft lip and/or palate on nutritional health and oral-motor development. *Dental Clinics of North America* 2003; 47(2):305-17.

Rovet J (editor). *Turner Syndrome Across the Lifespan.* Markham, Ontario: Kelin Graphics, 1995; p. iv.

Rudolph C, Rudolph A. *Rudolph's Pediatrics (21st edition).* New York: McGraw Hill, 2003; p. 88.

Snyder J. Bubble palate and failure to thrive: a case report. *Journal of Human Lactation* 1997; 13(2):139-143.

The Genetics of Cleft Lip and Palate: Information for Families. Cleft Palate Foundation, 1218 Grandview Ave, Pittsburgh, PA 15211, 1987.

Weatherly-White R, Kuehn D, Mirrett P, et al. Early repair and breast-feeding for infants with cleft lip. *Plastic and Reconstructive Surgery* 1987; 79(6):879-885.

Wiessinger D, Miller M. Breastfeeding difficulties as a result of tight lingual and labial frena: a case report. *Journal of Human Lactation* 1995; 11(4):313-316.

Wilcox AJ, Lie RT, Solvoll K, et al. Folic acid supplements and risk of facial clefts: national population based case-control study. *British Medical Journal* 2007; 334(7591):433-434.

Wright A, Bauer M, Naylor A, et al. Increasing breastfeeding rates to reduce infant illness at the community level. *Pediatrics* 1998; 101(5):837-844.

Notes:

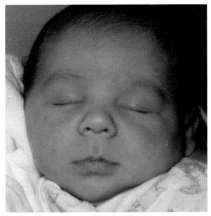

Fig. 1 Deep sleep -- good facial tone

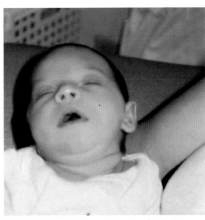

Fig. 2 Deep sleep -- poor facial tone

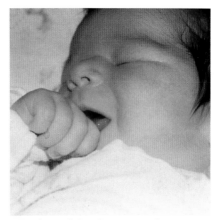

Fig. 3   Light sleep -- early feeding cue

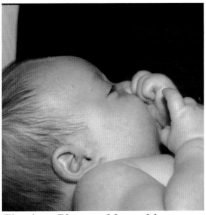

Fig. 4   Pleasurable sucking -- drowsy state

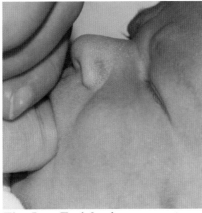

Fig. 5   Facial grimace -- a stress cue

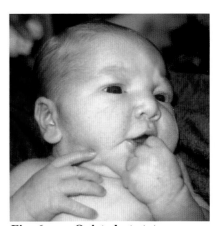

Fig. 6   Quiet alert state

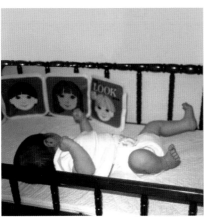

Fig. 7   Active alert state

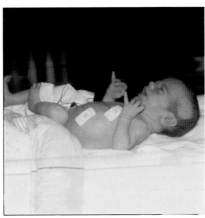

Fig. 8   Motoric stress cues -- finger splaying, stiffening, crying

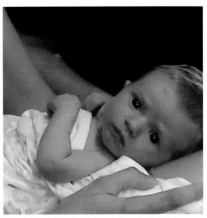

Fig. 9   An infant who is failing to thrive -- worried alert state

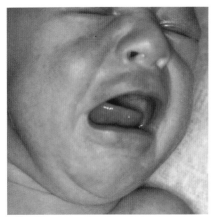

Fig. 10   Crying -- a significant
           infant stress cue

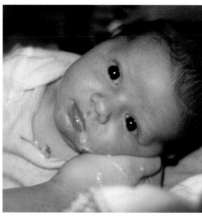

Fig. 11   Satiated appearance
           (wet burp)

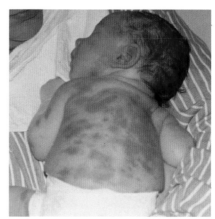

Fig. 12   Normal infant rash

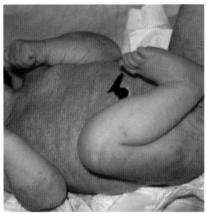

Fig. 13   Infant was ill -- rash
           may indicate sepsis

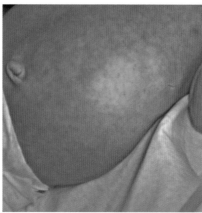

Fig. 14   Mottling on the trunk --
           an indication of cold stress

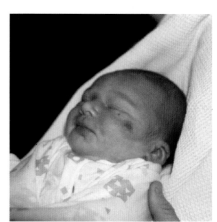

Fig. 15   Forceps bruise

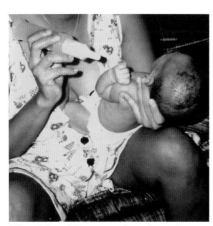

Fig. 16   Vacuum abrasion of
           the scalp

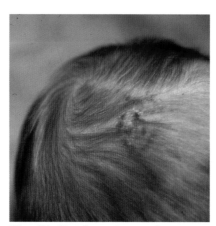

Fig. 17   Fetal monitor scab

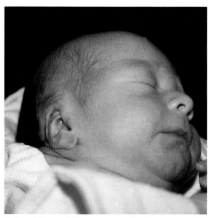

Fig. 18   Flat ear owing to
             breech position

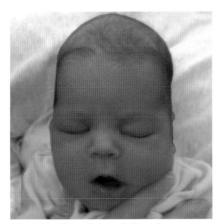

Fig. 19 Cranial molding (narrow head) in a newborn

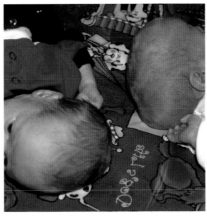

Fig. 20 Cranial asymmetry (premature fusion of cranial sutures)

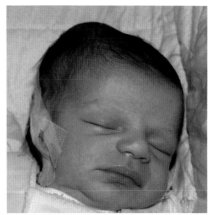

Fig. 21 Cephalohematoma

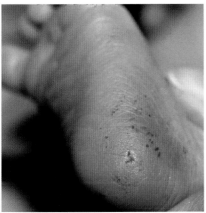

Fig. 22 Heel sticks

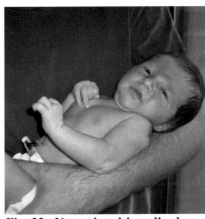

Fig. 23 Normal and jaundiced skin tones (4 day-old)

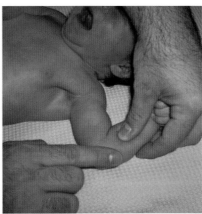

Fig. 24 Identifying jaundice -- press on the skin

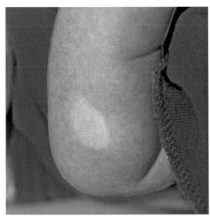

Fig. 25 Identifying jaundice -- observe underlying skin tone

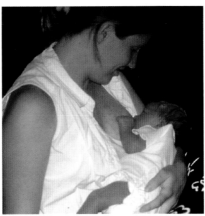

Fig. 26 Fiberoptic bili blanket -- portable phototherapy

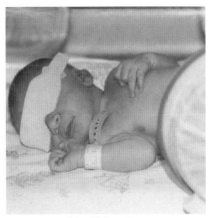

Fig. 27 Traditional phototherapy

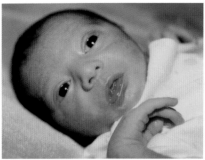

Fig. 28 Thin cheeks, flat philtrum --
36 week-old infant

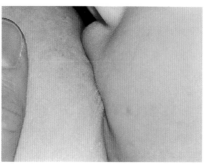

Fig. 29   Lip retraction

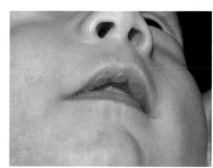

Fig. 30   Sucking blisters on the lip

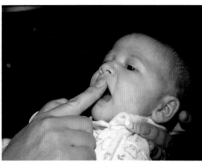

Fig. 31 Facial tone stimulation
exercise provided by parent

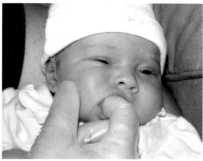

Fig. 32   Assessing thickness of
cheek fat pads

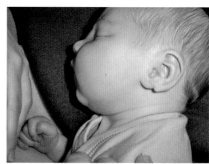

Fig. 33   Receding chin and ear
anomaly

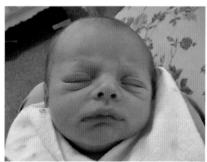

Fig. 34   Jaw asymmetry -- mouth
closed

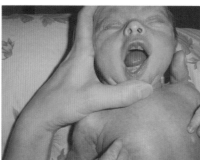

Fig. 35   Jaw asymmetry -- mouth
open

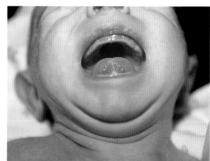

Fig. 36   Bubble palate and Stage 4
tongue-tie

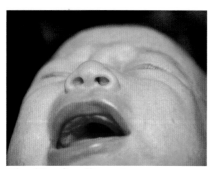

Fig. 37   Small nasal passages

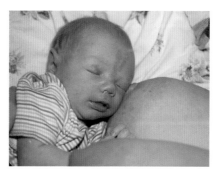

Fig. 38   "Stork bites" on forehead

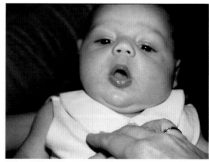

Fig. 39 Lip rounding -- normal
lip tone

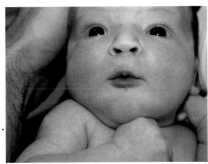

Fig. 40 "Purse string" lips -- excessive lip tone

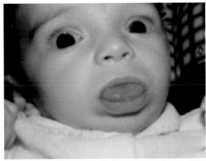

Fig. 41 Low facial tone -- Day 17

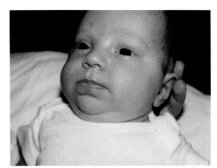

Fig. 42 Lip closure at 5.5 weeks after CST

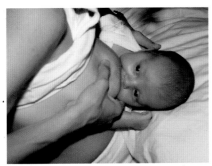

Fig. 43 Deep breast compression

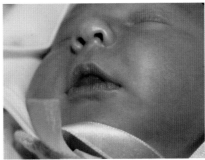

Fig. 44 Low tone -- tongue-tip elevation on Day 4

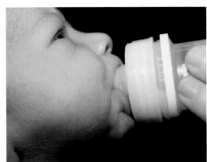

Fig. 45 Lip retraction while bottle feeding -- grimacing

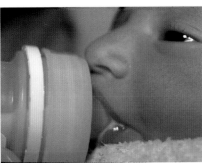

Fig. 46 Poor seal on bottle teat -- weak lip tone

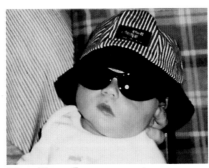

Fig. 47 Jaw asymmetry

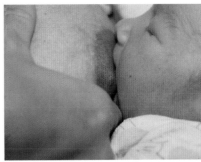

Fig. 48 Jaw support

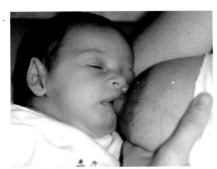

Fig. 49 Depressed rooting reflex

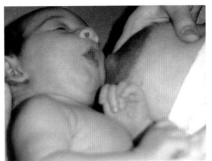

Fig. 50 Remove clothes to rouse

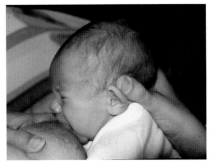

Fig. 51 Gag reflex

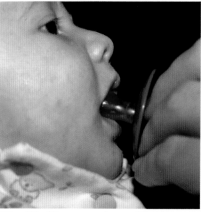

Fig. 52 Therapeutic pacifier use

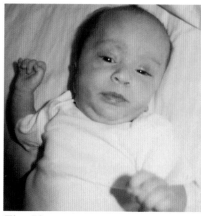

Fig. 53   Torticollis

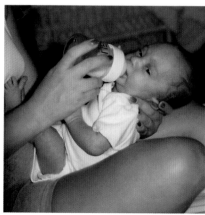

Fig. 54   Hip flexion to assist feeding -- torticollis

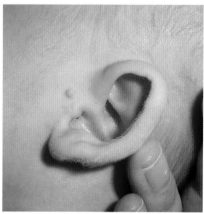

Fig. 55   Ear (auricular) skin tag

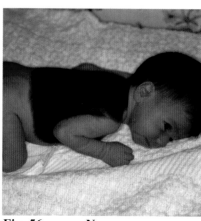

Fig. 56   Nevus

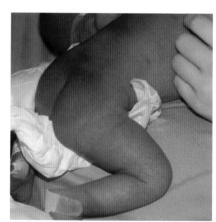

Fig. 57   Congenital dermal melanocytosis

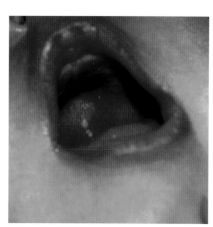

Fig. 58 Epstein's pearls (sometimes mistaken for thrush)

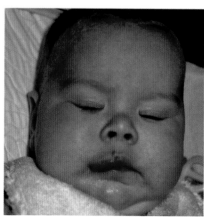

Fig. 59   Hemangioma of the lip

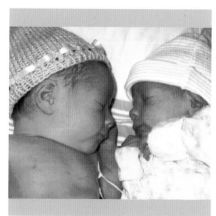

Fig. 60   Discordant twins (twins of different sizes)

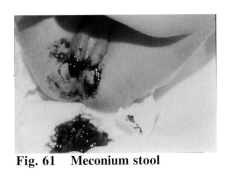

Fig. 61   Meconium stool

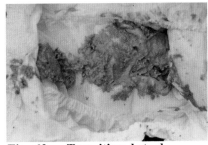

Fig. 62   Transitional stool

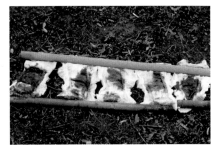

Fig. 63   Bowel output of a 3 day-
old breastfeeding infant

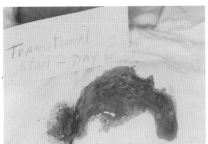

Fig. 64   Delayed transitional stool
on Day 6

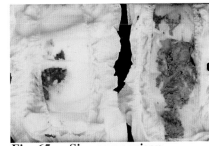

Fig. 65   Size comparison

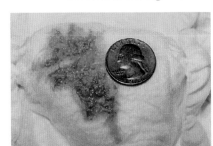

Fig. 66   Coin size comparison --
A US quarter is 24 mm

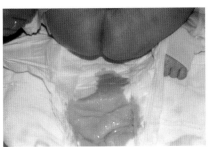

Fig. 67   Watery stool

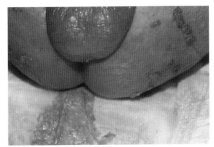

Fig. 68   Seedy stool

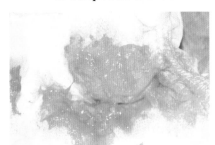

Fig. 69   Curd-like stool on Day 6

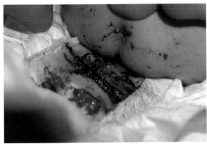

Fig. 70   Green stool

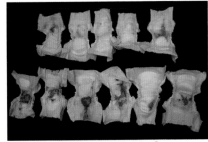

Fig. 71   24-hour output of an
8 week-old breastfeeding infant

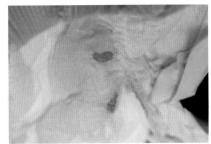

Fig. 72   "Brick dust" urine on
on Day 2

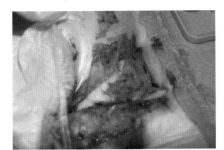

Fig. 73   Blood in stool

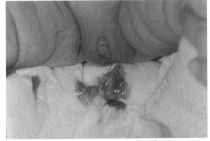

Fig. 74   Bloody vaginal discharge

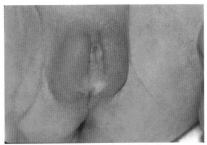

Fig. 75   White vaginal discharge

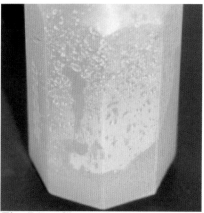

Fig. 76   Clear colostrum

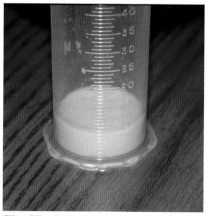

Fig. 77   Bright yellow colostrum

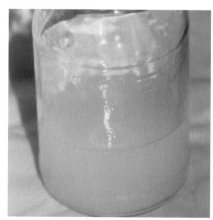

Fig. 78   White colostrum

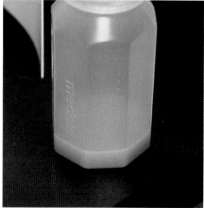

Fig. 79   "Rusty pipe" colostrum

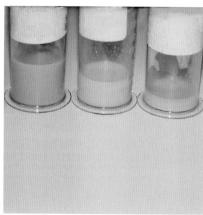

Fig. 80   Light brown colostrum

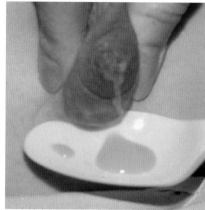

Fig. 81   The size of a newborn's swallow (0.6 ml)

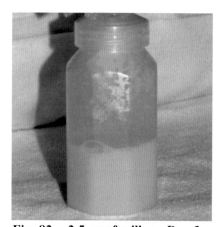

Fig. 82   2.5 oz of milk on Day 3

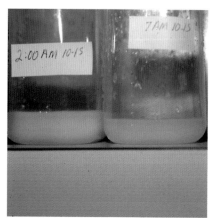

Fig. 83   Milk maturation color changes

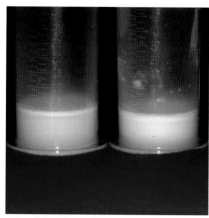

Fig. 84   Foremilk and hindmilk

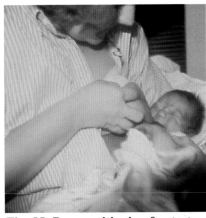

Fig. 85 Poor positioning frustrates
the baby

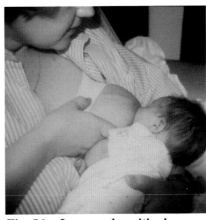

Fig. 86   Improved positioning

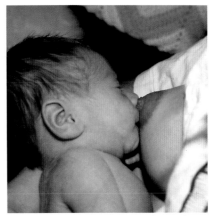

Fig. 87 Line up nose to nipple in
"sniff" position at start of latch

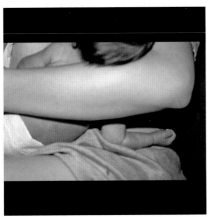

Fig. 88   Poor postural support --
lower arm stress for baby

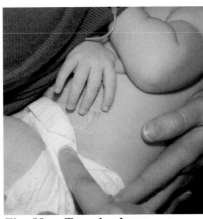

Fig. 89   Trapping lower arm
across the baby's body

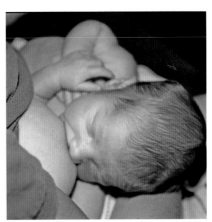

Fig. 90   Both arms are comfortably
positioned at the midline

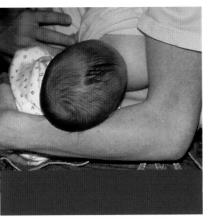

Fig. 91 Baby's head on forearm

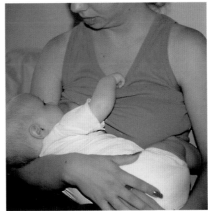

Fig. 92   6 week-old fits in the
crook of the arm

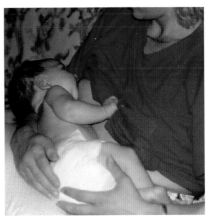

Fig. 93   Cradle hold -- 6 week-old

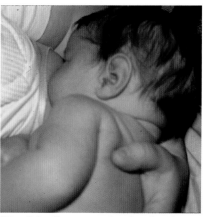

Fig. 94   Over-rotation buries face

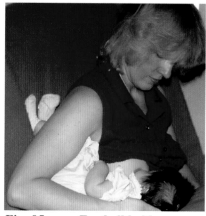

Fig. 95   Football hold

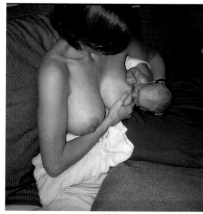

Fig. 96   Variation of football
            position

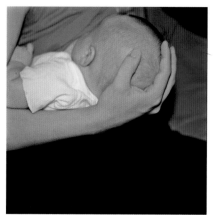

Fig. 97   Avoid hand on head
            flexing head forward

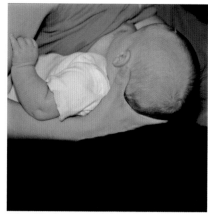

Fig. 98   Improved hand position
            lessens risk of flexing head

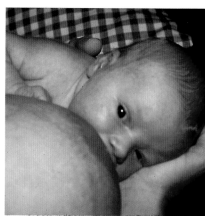

Fig. 99   Cross-cradle position

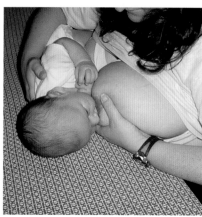

Fig. 100   Cross cradle with table
            for support

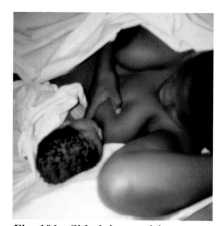

Fig. 101   Side-lying position

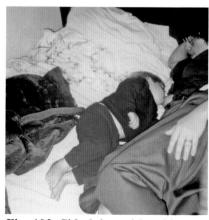

Fig. 102   Side-lying with a 22
            month-old

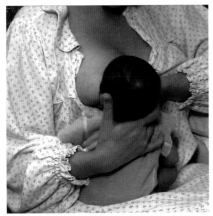

Fig. 103   Seated straddle position

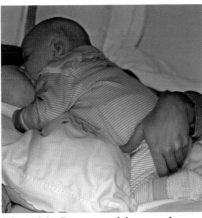

Fig. 104   Prone position -- also called "posture" feeding

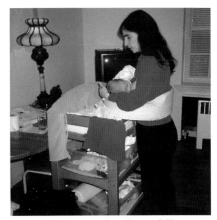

Fig. 105   Breastfeeding while standing

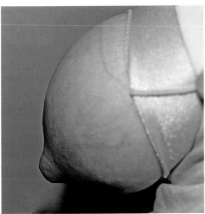

Fig. 106   Nipple located on down-hill slope

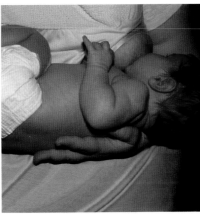

Fig. 107   Supine position to latch

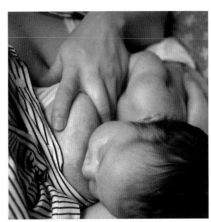

Fig. 108   Scissors hold

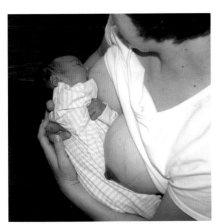

Fig. 109   Alternate cradle position with a small baby

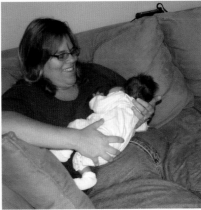

Fig. 110 Alternate cradle position with a larger baby

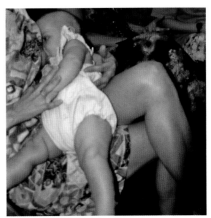

Fig. 111   5 month-old positioning herself

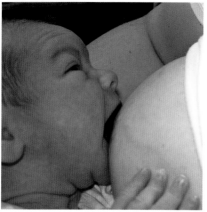

Fig. 112   Chin touches the breast

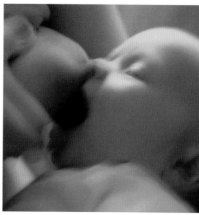

Fig. 113   Rest the breast on the lips and line up nipple to nose

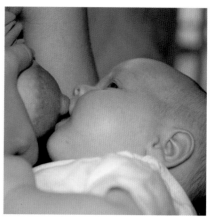

Fig. 114   Tilt the nipple to the palate

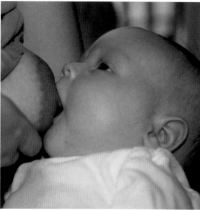

Fig. 115   Hugging the baby in close at the shoulders

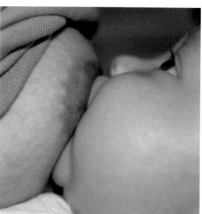

Fig. 116   Asymmetric latch

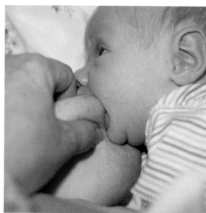

Fig. 117   "Breast sandwich" helps baby latch

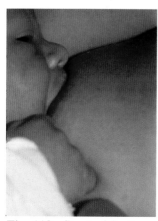

Fig. 118   Start of feed, tight fist

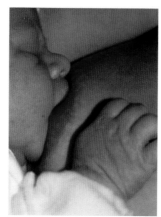

Fig. 119 Gradual relaxation

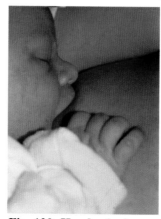

Fig. 120 Hand relaxing

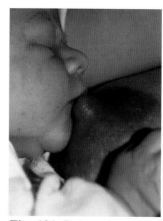

Fig. 121 Baby releases the breast

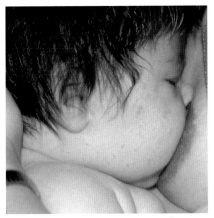

Fig. 122   Chin too close to chest --
face buried

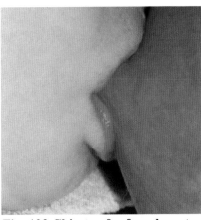

Fig. 123 Chin too far from breast --
jaw will close on nipple shaft

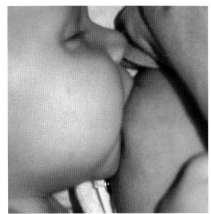

Fig. 124   Shallow latch -- depressed
feeding affect

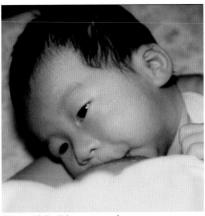

Fig. 125   Lip retraction -- narrow
gape

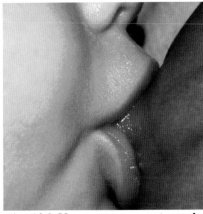

Fig. 126   Narrow gape -- note angle
at the corner of the mouth

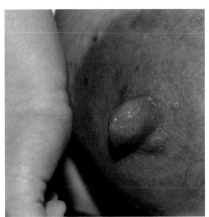

Fig. 127   Pinched nipple -- note
angle of the shadow

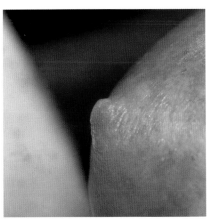

Fig. 128   Angled nipple face

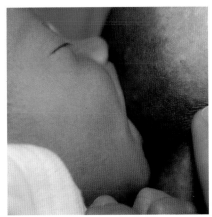

Fig. 129   Well latched newborn --
note wide angle of gape

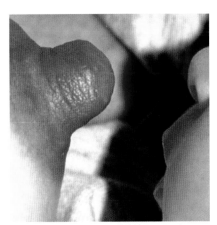

Fig. 130   Nipple undistorted after
breastfeeding

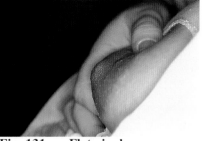

Fig. 131   Flat nipple

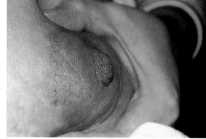

Fig. 132   Sandwich technique

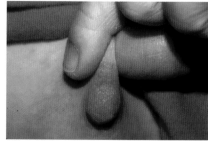

Fig. 133   Teacup or inverted
nipple hold

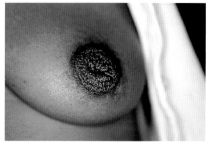

Fig. 134   Inverted nipple at rest

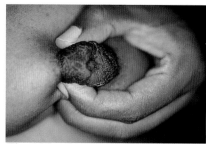

Fig. 135   Inverted nipple when
compressed

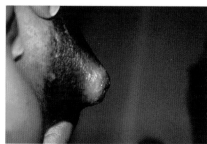

Fig. 136   Inverted nipple after
mom pulls back on areolar tissue

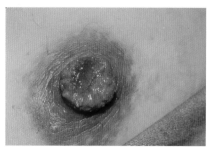

Fig. 137   Dimpled nipple immediately after pumping

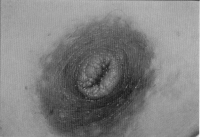

Fig. 138   Dimpled nipple retracted
2 minutes after pumping

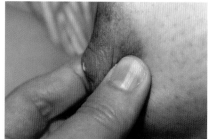

Fig. 139   Lack of breast elasticity
and a flat nipple

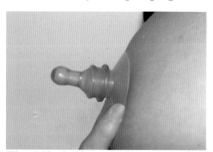

Fig. 140   Antique design of nipple
shield still being sold

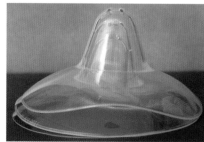

Fig. 141   Size comparison of 3
nipple shields

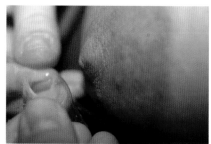

Fig. 142   Applying a nipple shield --
turning rim inside out

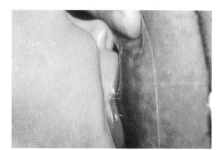

Fig. 143   Well latched on a
nipple shield

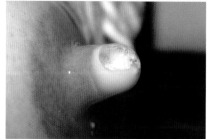

Fig. 144   Nipple drawn into shield --
note reservoir of milk

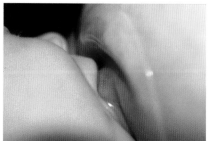

Fig. 145   Poorly latched onto
a nipple shield

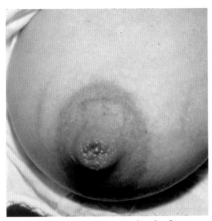

Fig. 146 Inflamed on nipple face --
Stage I damage

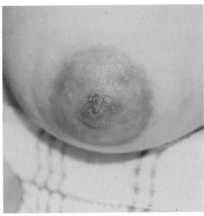

Fig. 147 Suction lesions on flat
nipple -- Stage II damage

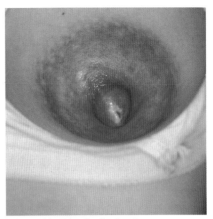

Fig. 148 Pinched nipple --
Stage II damage

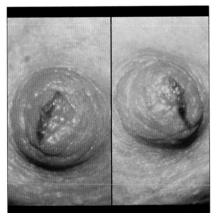

Fig. 149 Scabs from positional
stripes -- Stage II damage

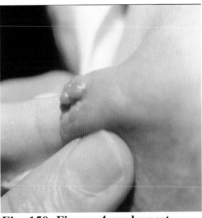

Fig. 150 Fissure 4 weeks postpartum -- Stage III damage

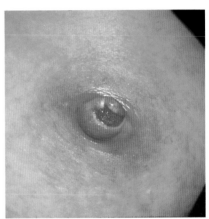

Fig. 151 Partial thickness wound --
Stage III damage

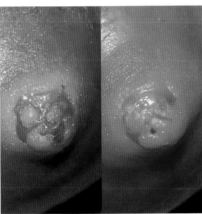

Fig. 152 Eroded and partially
healed nipple -- Stage III damage

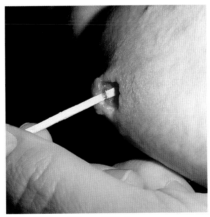

Fig. 153 Stage IV damage

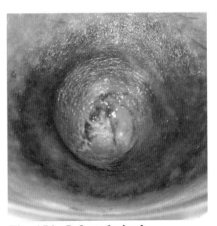

Fig. 154 Infected nipple

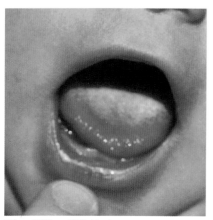

Fig. 155 White tongue

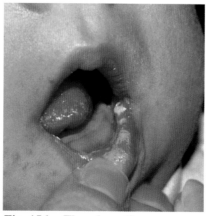

Fig. 156 Thrush on lips

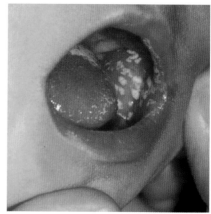

Fig. 157 Thrush on inside
of cheeks

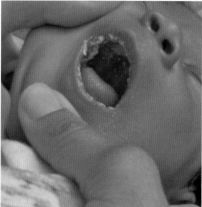

Fig. 158 Oral thrush

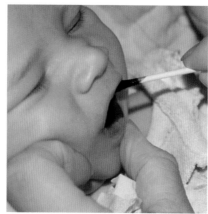

Fig. 159 Treating thrush with
gentian violet

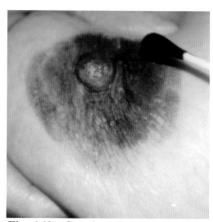

Fig. 160 Gentian violet to treat
nipple yeast

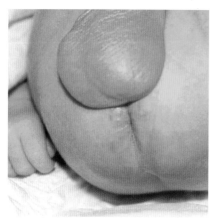

Fig. 161 Yeast diaper rash

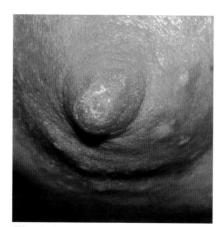

Fig. 162 Nipple yeast -- note
white material on nipple

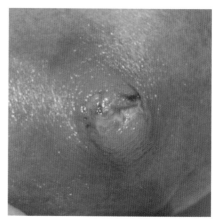

Fig. 163 Bacterial and fungal
infection

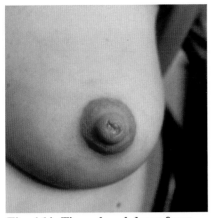

Fig. 164 Tissue breakdown from
untreated infection

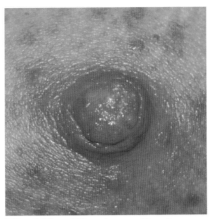

Fig. 165 Allergic reaction to
nipple cream

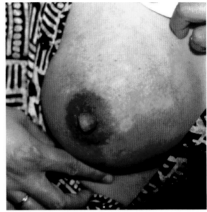

Fig. 166 Hives -- allergic reaction
to topical nystatin

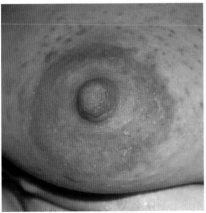

Fig. 167 Eczema

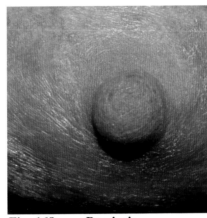

Fig. 168 Psoriasis

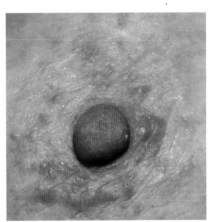

Fig. 169 Poison ivy

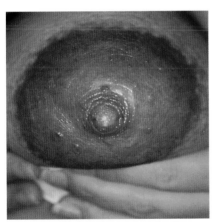

Fig. 170 White spot on nipple --
painful blocked nipple pores

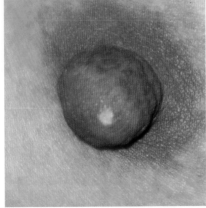

Fig. 171 White spot on nipple --
not painful

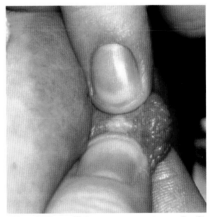

Fig. 172 Sebaceous cyst on shaft
of nipple

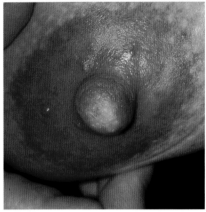

Fig. 173   Vasospasm

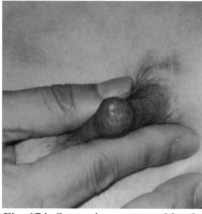

Fig. 174 Squeezing restores blood
flow and reduces vasospasm pain

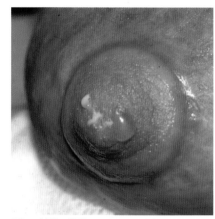

Fig. 175   Blister caused by
pumping

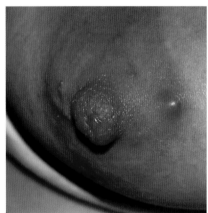

Fig. 176   Infected Montgomery
gland

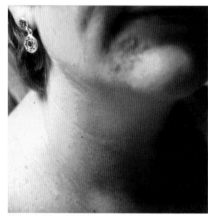

Fig. 177   Rash on chin spread
to her nipples

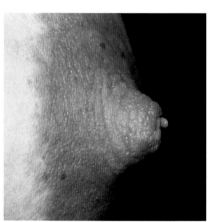

Fig. 178   Skin tag on nipple

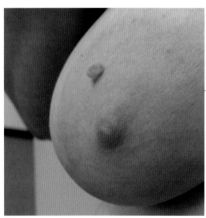

Fig. 179   Skin tag on breast

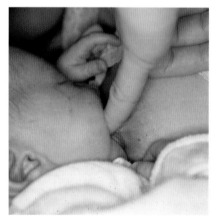

Fig. 180   Break suction
between gums

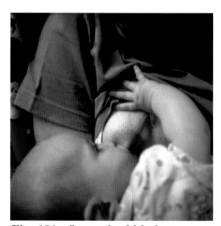

Fig. 181   5 month-old baby

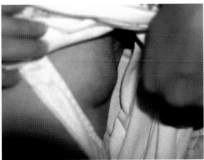

Fig. 182   Engorgement of the tail of Spence

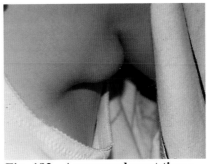

Fig. 183   Accessory breast tissue in the axilla 1 month postpartum

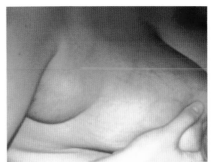

Fig. 184   Accessory breast tissue 4 days postpartum

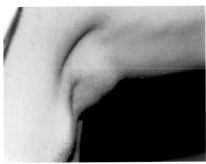

Fig. 185   Engorgement of accessory breast tissue

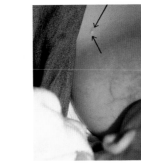

Fig. 186   Ectopic duct

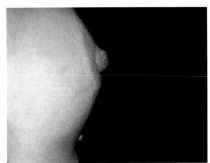

Fig. 187 Accessory (supernumerary) nipple in profile

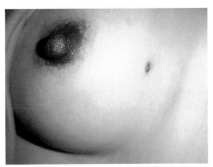

Fig. 188   Accessory nipple

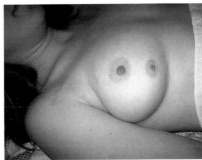

Fig. 189 Bilateral accessory nipples (Photo S. Gehrman)

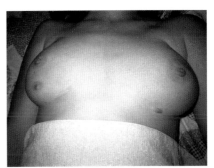

Fig. 190 Bilateral accessory nipples (Photo S. Gehrman)

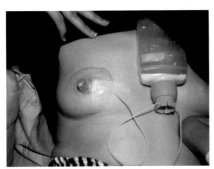

Fig. 191 Underdeveloped breast tissue (amastia)

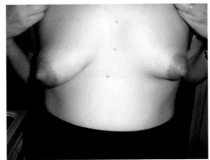

Fig. 192 Underdeveloped breast tissue (hypoplasia)

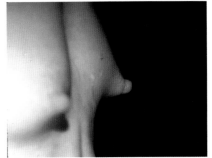

Fig. 193 Underdeveloped breasts (hypoplasia and amastia)

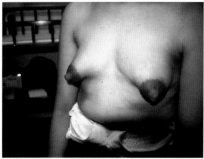

Fig. 194   Tubular breasts --
             impaired milk supply

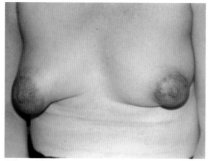

Fig. 195 Unusually shaped breasts --
         normal milk supply

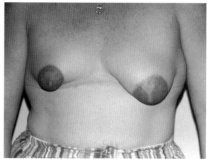

Fig. 196 Breast asymmetry --
          impaired milk supply

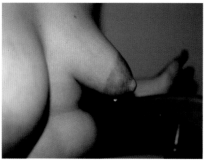

Fig. 197   Tubular breast with
             forward cone areolar placement

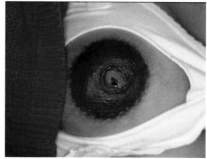

Fig. 198 Periareolar incision --
          impaired lactation

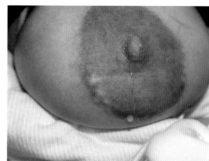

Fig. 199 Periareolar incision --
          evidence of normal MER

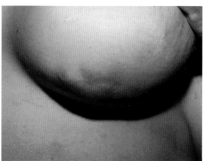

Fig. 200 Abscess at implant site

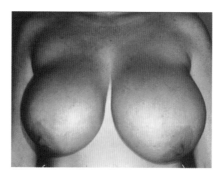

Fig. 201   Large breasts

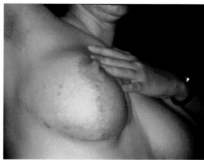

Fig. 202   After reduction
            mammoplasty

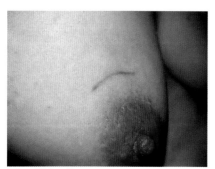

Fig. 203   Lumpectomy scar

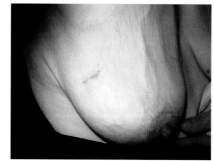

Fig. 204   Weaning breast --
            biopsy scar

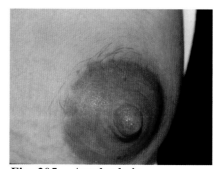

Fig. 205   Areolar hair

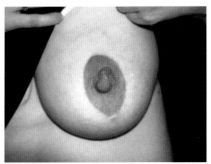

Fig. 206 Unusual nipple shape

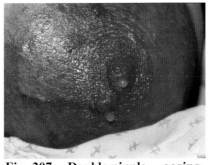

Fig. 207   Double nipple -- oozing milk from both sites

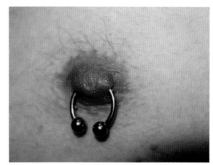

Fig. 208   Nipple ring

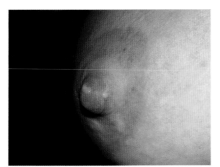

Fig. 209 Oozing milk from nipple ring holes 9 months pp

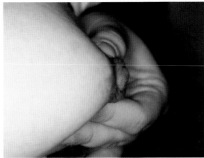

Fig. 210   Inverted nipple at rest

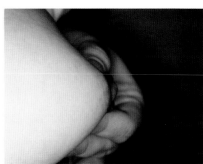

Fig. 211   Nipple inversion revealed when compressed

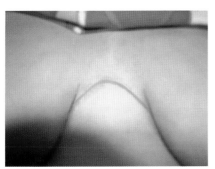

Fig. 212 Open heart surgery scar between her breasts

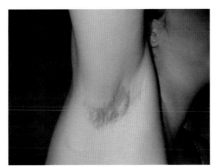

Fig. 213   Axillary scar

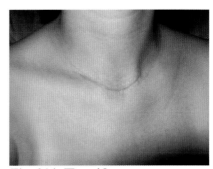

Fig. 214 Thyroid surgery scar

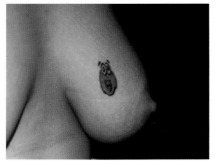

Fig. 215   Tattoo

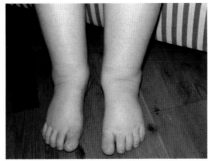

Fig. 216 Swollen ankles during the first week postpartum

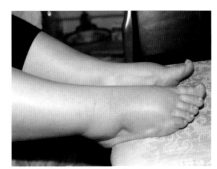

Fig. 217   Swollen feet

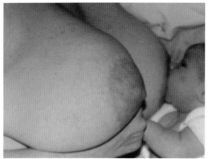

Fig. 218   Large breasts

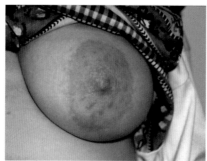

Fig. 219   Large areola

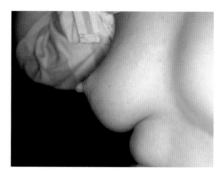

Fig. 220   Small nipple and areola

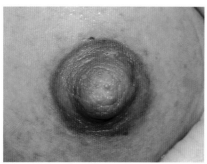

Fig. 221   Small areola

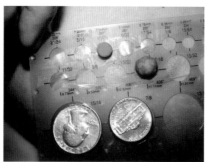

Fig. 222   Engineer's circle template
a tool for size comparisons

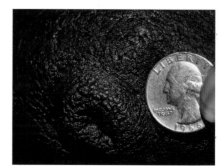

Fig. 223   Quarter-sized nipple

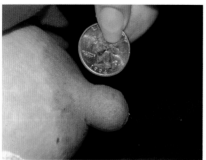

Fig. 224   Coin size comparison -
17 mm long nipple

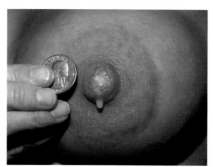

Fig. 225   Large nipple - evidence
of infection on Day 6

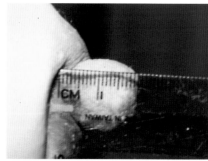

Fig. 226   Nipple length at rest is
2 cm (20 mm)

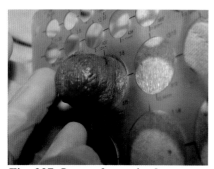

Fig. 227   Large, long nipple
(2 cm long)

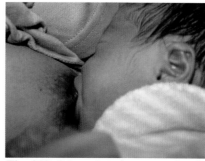

Fig. 228   36-week twin cannot latch
onto her large, long nipple

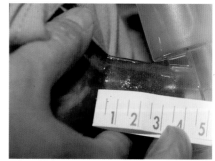

Fig. 229   Nipple 4 cm
at full extension

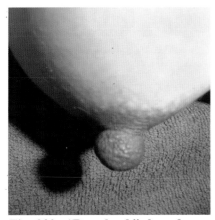

Fig. 230 "Door knob" shaped nipple -- note shadow

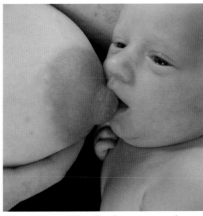

Fig. 231 Nipple size comparison with newborn's mouth

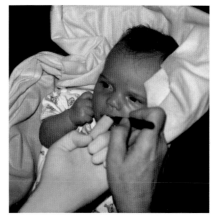

Fig. 232 Measuring oral reach -- palate length of 7-wk-old

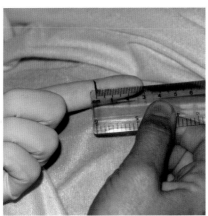

Fig. 233 Palate length of 3 cm

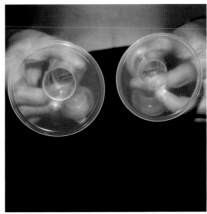

Fig. 234 Medela flange sizes
30 mm   24 mm

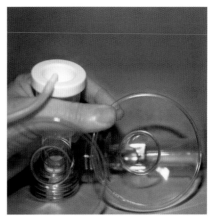

Fig. 235 Ameda (Hollister) flanges
25 mm   30.5 mm

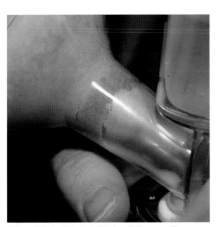

Fig. 236 Tight fit in 25 mm flange

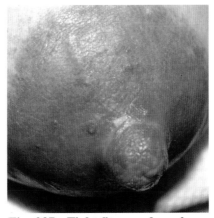

Fig. 237 Tight fit caused cracks at base of nipple

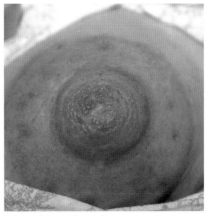

Fig. 238 Tight flange causes cracking and abrasion

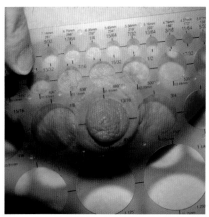

Fig. 239   Pre-pumping nipple
size 20.64 mm

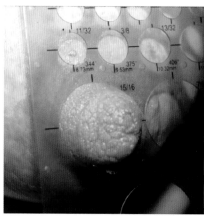

Fig. 240   Post-pumping size swells
to 23.81 mm

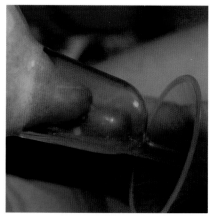

Fig. 241 Glass flange --
40 mm diameter

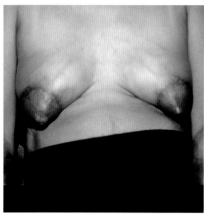

Fig. 242   Woman with PCOS

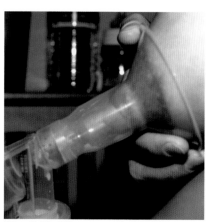

Fig. 243   Woman with PCOS
pumping with large flange

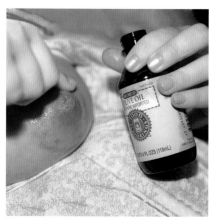

Fig. 244   Lubricating breast with
olive oil

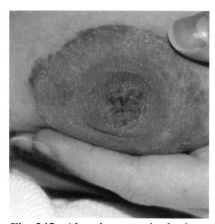

Fig. 245   Abrasions on nipple tip --
29 mm nipple using 24 mm flange

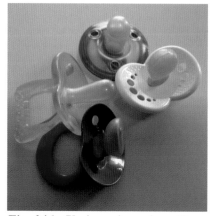

Fig. 246   Various sizes of pacifiers

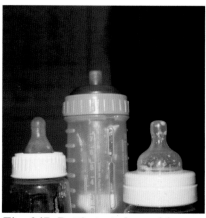

Fig. 247   Bottle teat shapes/sizes
have clinical implications

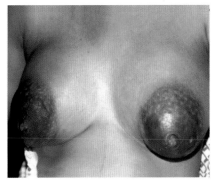

Fig. 248　Breast engorgement
　　　　　Day 3

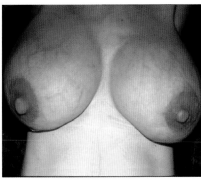

Fig. 249　Breast engorgement
　　　　　Day 8

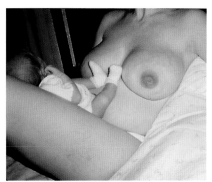

Fig. 250　Breast engorgement
　　　　　Day 6

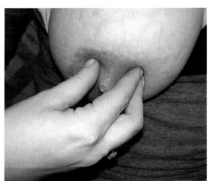

Fig. 251　Reverse pressure
　　　　　softening technique

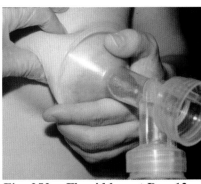

Fig. 252　Flaccid breast Day 12 --
　　　　　down regulation of supply

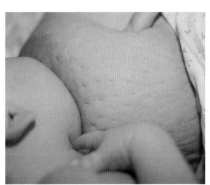

Fig. 253　Peu d' orange
　　　　　(pitting edema)

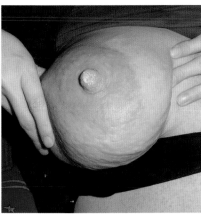

Fig. 254　Infected nipple, mastitis,
　　　　　peu d' orange (pitting edema)

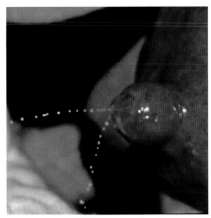

Fig. 255　Milk spray during
　　　　　let down

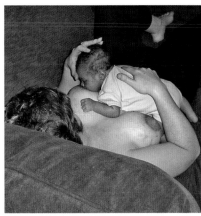

Fig. 256　Prone position
　　　　　for managing milk oversupply

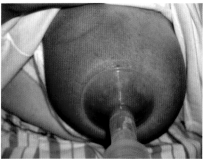

Fig. 257   Breast inflammation
            on Day 4

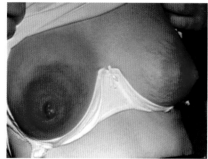

Fig. 258   Bilateral mastitis

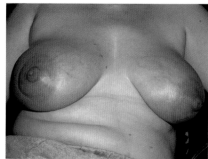

Fig. 259   Bilateral mastitis on
            Day 11

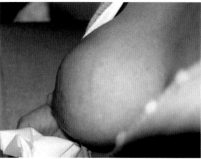

Fig. 260   Ripening abscess with
            induration of the nipple

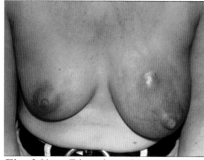

Fig. 261   Ripening abscess

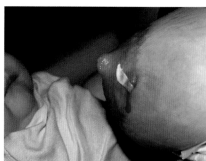

Fig. 262   Subareolar abscess with
            wick

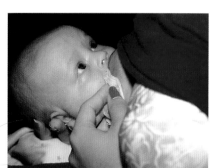

Fig. 263   Holding pad over
            draining abscess wound

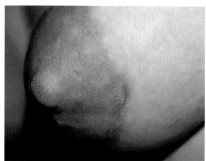

Fig. 264   Healed subareolar
            abscess

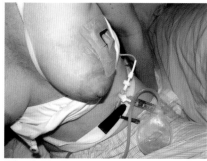

Fig. 265   Percutaneous drain for
            MRSA-related abscess

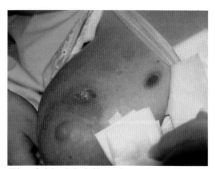

Fig. 266   Multilocular abscesses

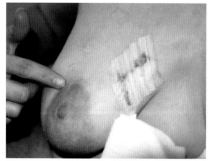

Fig. 267   Abscess scar and healing
            galactocele incision

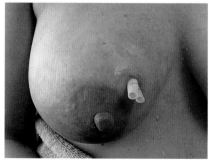

Fig. 268   Abscess drainage tubes

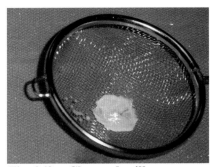

Fig. 269   Clumped milk
            during mastitis

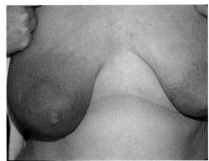

Fig. 270   Case report of MRSA
            breast infection

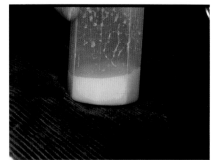

Fig. 271   Yellow milk pumped
            during MRSA infection

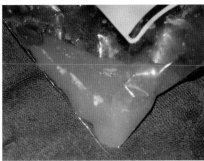

Fig. 272   Orange milk pumped
            during MRSA infection

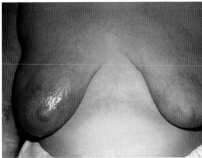

Fig. 273   MRSA infection damages
            connective tissue and skin

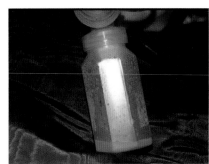

Fig. 274   Red milk pumped
            during MRSA infection

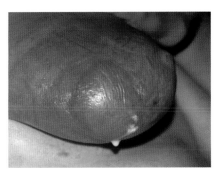

Fig. 275   Milk leaking through
            broken skin

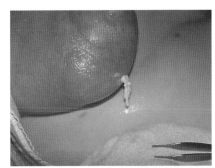

Fig. 276   Congealed milk pulled
            from original aspiration site

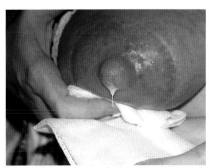

Fig. 277   Congealed milk observed

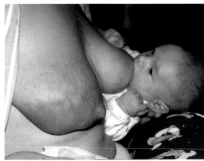

Fig. 278   Breastfeeding on
            unaffected breast

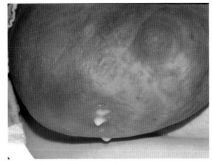

Fig. 279   Healing wound continues
            to leak milk

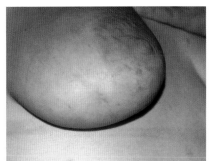

Fig. 280   Healed breast one
            year later

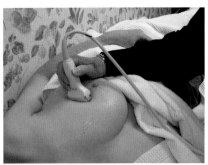

Fig. 281   Ultrasound scan of the
            breast

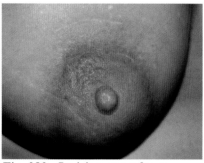

Fig. 282   Incision scars from
            biopsy and lumpectomy

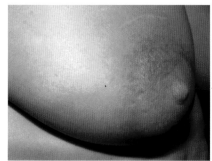

Fig. 283   Bronzed breast during
            radiation treatment

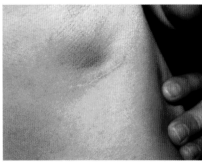

Fig. 284   Axillary node biopsy
            scar

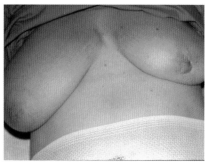

Fig. 285   Lumpectomy

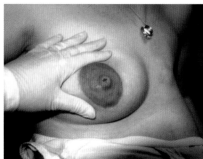

Fig. 286   Sore nipple on remaining
           breast after mastectomy

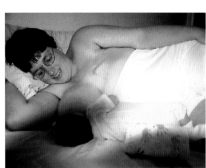

Fig. 287   Breastfeeding after
           mastectomy

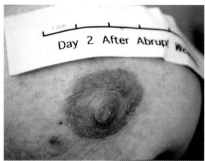

Fig. 288   Needle aspiration bruise
            on left breast at tumor site

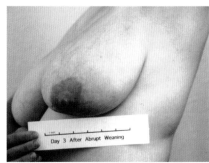

Fig. 289   Induration of the breast
           above the tumor site

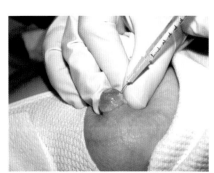

Fig. 290   Lidocaine injection prior
           to nipple biopsy

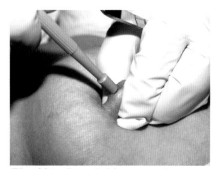

Fig. 291   Punch biopsy tool

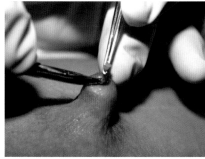

Fig. 292   Core biopsy to rule out
            Paget's disease of the nipple

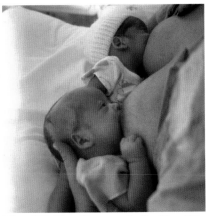

Fig. 293 Simultaneously feeding 36-week gestational age twins

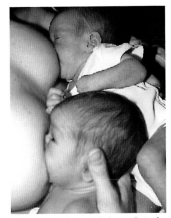

Fig. 294 Poorly positioned twins

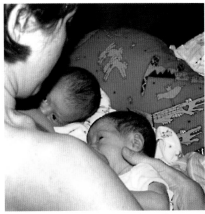

Fig. 295   Improved positioning

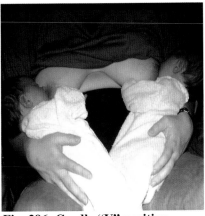

Fig. 296 Cradle "V" position

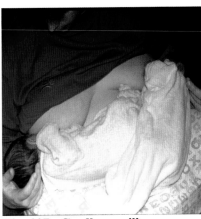

Fig. 297   Cradle on pillow

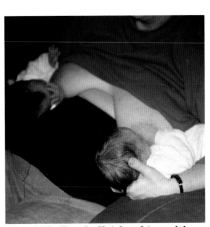

Fig. 298 Football (clutch) position

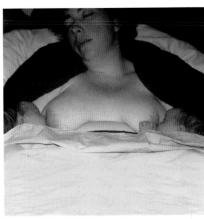

Fig. 299   Along the side in bed

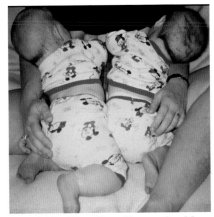

Fig. 300   Kneeling (5 month-old twins with chicken pox)

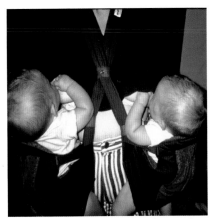

Fig. 301   Twin carrier, 8 months old

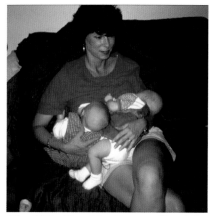

Fig. 302   Combination cradle and football holds, 3 months

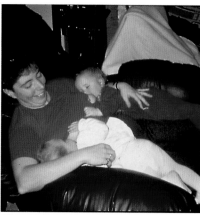

Fig. 303   Reclining along the side, 13 months

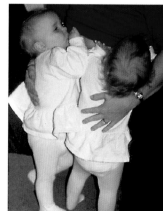

Fig. 304   Twins standing, 13 months old

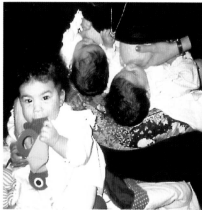

Fig. 305   Triplets, 8 months old

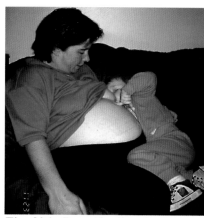

Fig. 306   Breastfeeding during pregnancy

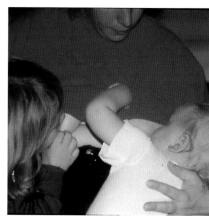

Fig. 307   Tandem breastfeeding 4 year-old and 16 month-old

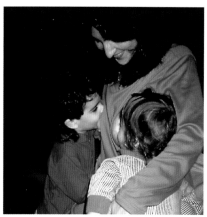

Fig. 308   Tandem feeding 4 year-old and 19 month-old

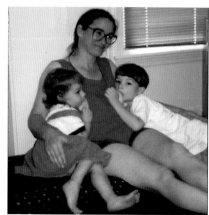

Fig. 309   Tandem feeding 4 year-old and 2 year-old

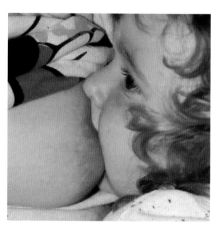

Fig. 310   Breastfeeding 3 year-old

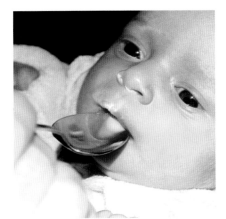

Fig. 311 0.6 ml of colostrum
delivered by spoon

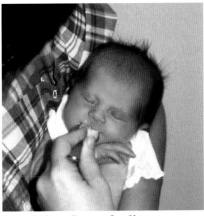

Fig. 312 Spoon feeding to rouse
sleepy baby

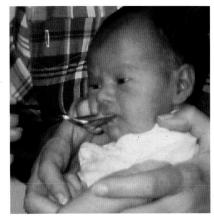

Fig. 313 Spoon feeding

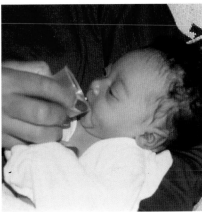

Fig. 314 Cup feeding

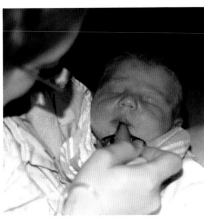

Fig. 315 Feeding with a paladai

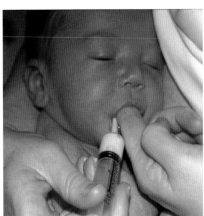

Fig. 316 Finger feeding with 12 cc
Monoject® curved-tip syringe

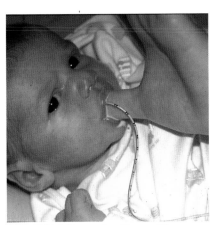

Fig. 317 Finger feeding with a
feeding tube along the thumb

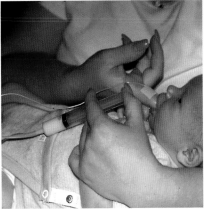

Fig. 318 Finger feeding with feeding tube on 12 cc syringe

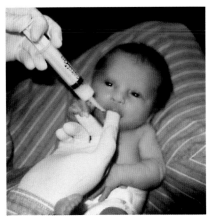

Fig. 319 Finger feeding FTT baby

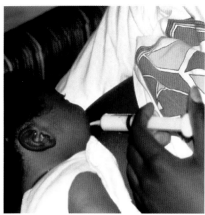

Fig. 320   Syringe feeding at breast

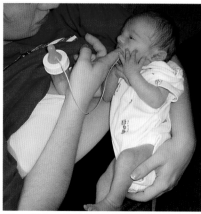

Fig. 321   Homemade feeding tube device

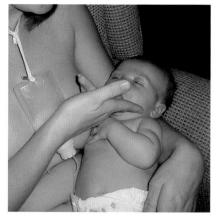

Fig. 322   Finger feeding with SNS ™ supplementer

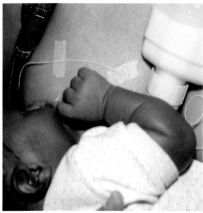

Fig. 323   Adopted infant at breast with an SNS ™ supplementer

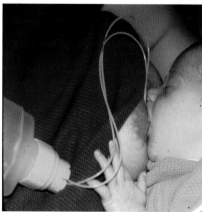

Fig. 324   SNS ™ with both tubes on the same breast

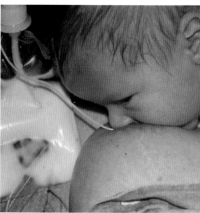

Fig. 325   Lact-Aid™ supplementer

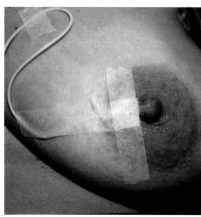

Fig. 326   Reverse taping of the feeding tube

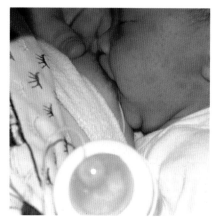

Fig. 327   At breast with tube positioned along the tongue

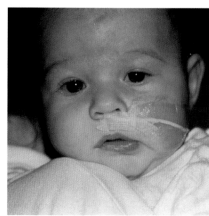

Fig. 328   3 month-old baby with a nasogastric tube

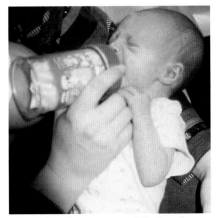

Fig. 329 Stress cue while bottle
feeding

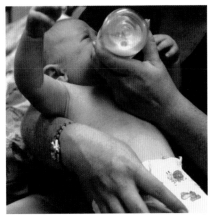

Fig. 330 Stress cue while bottle
feeding

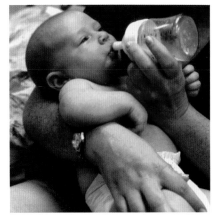

Fig. 331 Less stress when pacing
techniques are employed

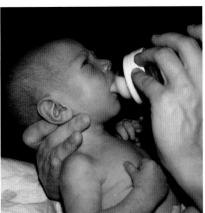

Fig. 332 37-weeker demonstrating
stress

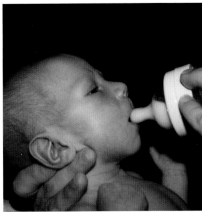

Fig. 333 Removing the bottle to
pace the feeding

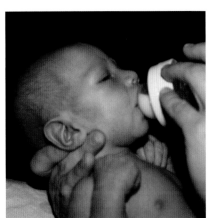

Fig. 334 Pacing results in more
organized feeding

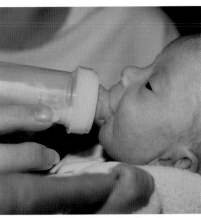

Fig. 335 Holding the bottle
horizontally to slow the flow rate

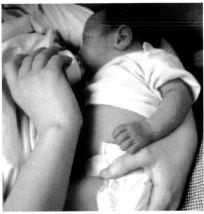

Fig. 336 Bottle feeding at the
breast

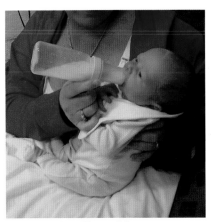

Fig. 337 Feeding with a
Special Needs™ feeder

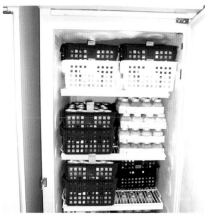

Fig. 338   Raw milk in the freezer

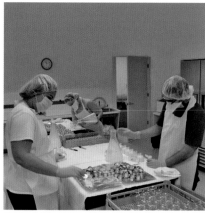

Fig. 339   Foss Milkoscan for
nutritional analysis

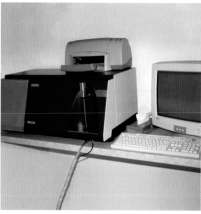

Fig. 340   Pasteurizing human milk

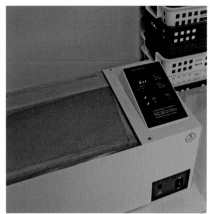

Fig. 341   Holder pasteurizer

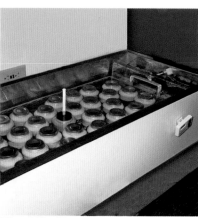

Fig. 342   Temperature control
during Holder process

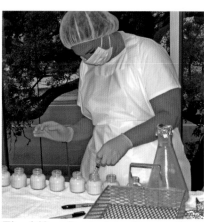

Fig. 343   Bacteriologic sampling
after pasteurization

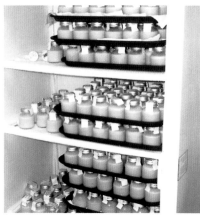

Fig. 344   Frozen pasteurized milk
awaiting bacteriological results

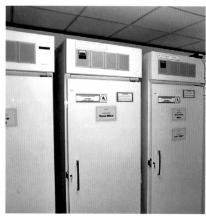

Fig. 345   Bank of freezers at a milk
bank - milk is ready to dispense

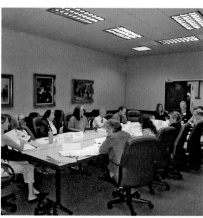

Fig. 346   Milk bank board of
directors

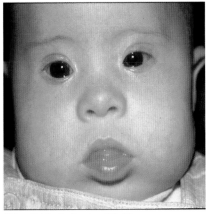

Fig. 347 Infant with Down
Syndrome -- 4 mo old

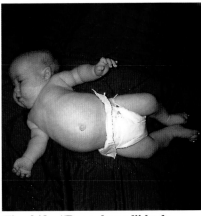

Fig. 348 "Pear-shaped" body

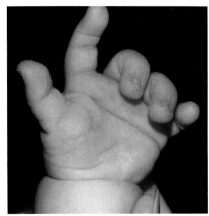

Fig. 349 Palmar crease

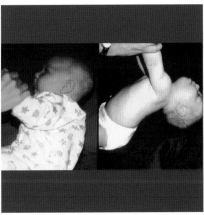

Fig. 350 Normal tone/ head lag in
infant with Down Syndrome

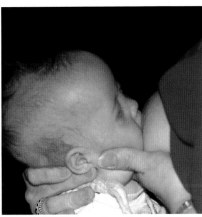

Fig. 351 Dancer hand position
stabilizes feeding

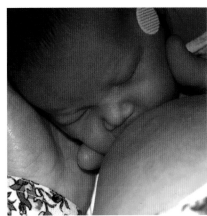

Fig. 352 Cheek counter-pressure
reduces intra-oral space

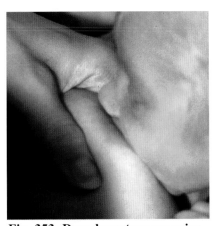

Fig. 353 Deep breast compression

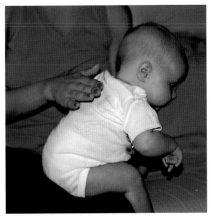

Fig. 354 Avoid increasing abdominal pressure in infants with reflux

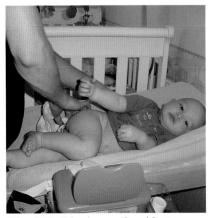

Fig. 355 Diaper on the side to
decrease abdominal pressure

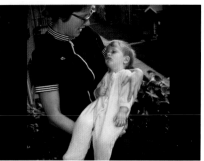

Fig. 356 Hypotonia as a marker
for illness

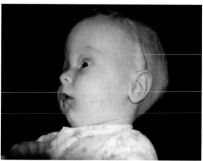

Fig. 357 Hydrocephalus -- shunt
to drain cerebrospinal fluid

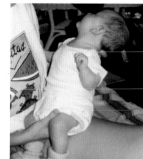

Fig. 358 Hypertonia -- arching
causes hyperextension

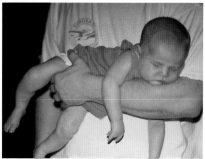

Fig. 359 "Colic hold" helps draw
baby into flexion

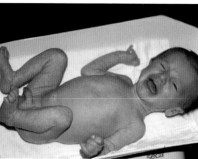

Fig. 360 FTT -- 35 day-old only
142 g above birthweight

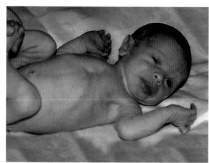

Fig. 361 FTT -- 18 day-old who
is 454 g below birthweight

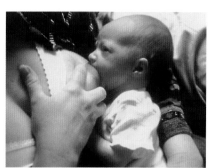

Fig. 362 FTT -- note retracted lips,
worried expression

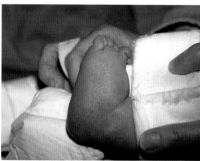

Fig. 363 Infant with Turner's
Syndrome -- unusually shaped foot

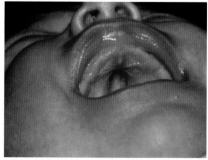

Fig. 364 Naturally occurring
grooved (channel) palate

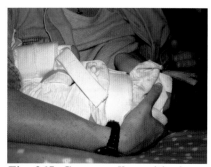

Fig. 365 Cross-cradle positioning
with hip cast for hip dysplasia

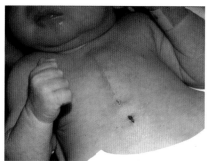

Fig. 366 Heart surgery scar
14 day-old infant

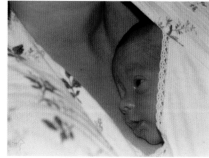

Fig. 367 Skin-to-Skin (Kangaroo)
Care benefits preterm infants

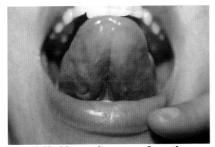

**Fig. 368 Normal range of motion --
tongue lift**

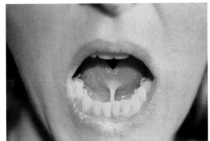

**Fig. 369 Tongue-tied adult
attempting to lift tongue**

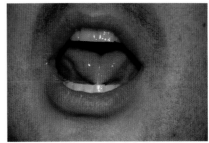

**Fig. 370 Tongue-tied father of
tongue-tied infant**

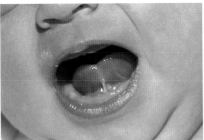

Fig. 371   Heart-shaped tongue tip

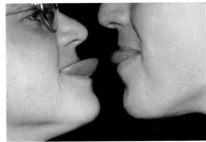

**Fig. 372   Variability of tongue
length -- short tongue on the right**

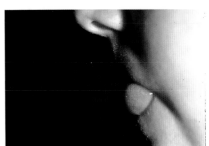

**Fig. 373 Tongue-tied 12 year-old --
limited extension**

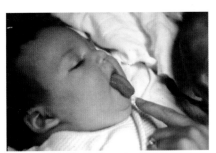

**Fig. 374   Tongue extension --
long tongue**

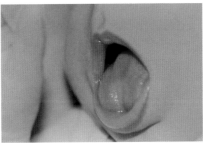

**Fig. 375   Tongue-tie -- distortion
during extension**

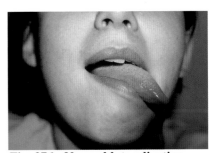

Fig. 376   Normal lateralization

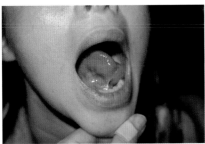

**Fig. 377   Limited ability to
lateralize**

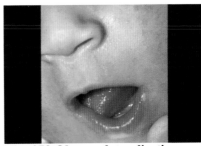

**Fig. 378 Observe lateralization
in infants**

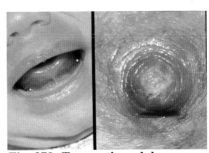

**Fig. 379   Tongue-tie and damage
to mother's nipple**

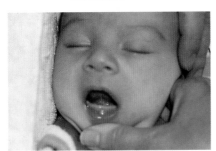

**Fig. 380   The infant's tongue lifts
to the upper gum ridge**

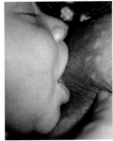

**Fig. 381   Normal tongue cups and
extends beyond gum ridge**

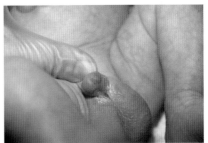

**Fig. 382   Hypospadius -- another
mid-line defect**

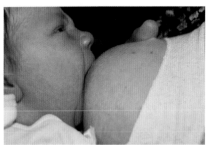

Fig. 383 Case study of FTT infant
with tongue-tie -- no latch

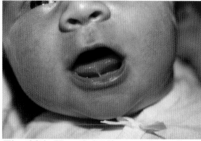

Fig. 384 Her tight lingual frenulum

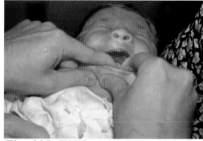

Fig. 385 ENT evaluates range of
motion of her tongue

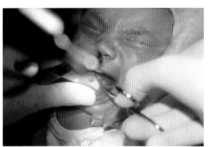

Fig. 386 Clipping the frenulum

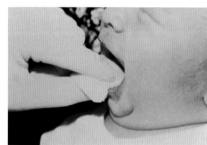

Fig. 387 Brief pressure with gauze
pad after frenotomy

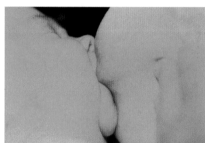

Fig. 388 Breastfeeding 10 minutes
after frenotomy

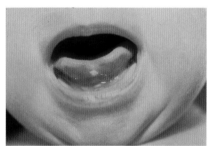

Fig. 389 Frenotomy site 1 week
later

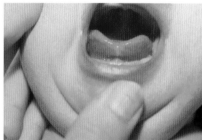

Fig. 390 Tongue healed at 2 weeks

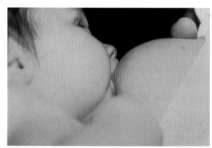

Fig. 391 Breastfeeding 3 weeks
after frenotomy

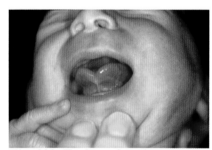

Fig. 392 Evaluate function not
appearance -- baby fed well

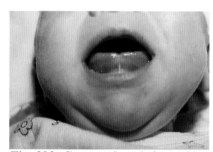

Fig. 393 Case study -- infant with
tongue-tie

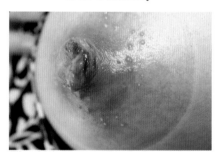

Fig. 394 Her mother's damaged,
infected nipple

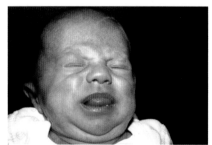

Fig. 395 The infant after frenotomy

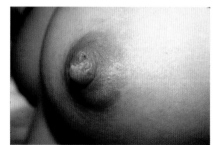

Fig. 396 Her mother's healing
nipple

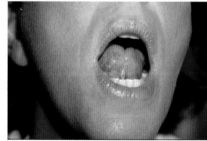

Fig. 397 Tongue-tied adult shown
in Fig. 369 after frenotomy

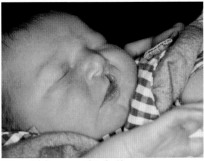

Fig. 398   Cleft lip

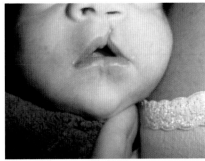

Fig. 399   Cleft lip

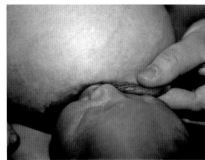

Fig. 400   "Teacup hold" to plug
the gap and help form a seal

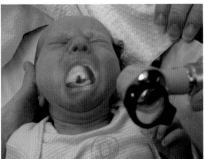

Fig. 401   Cleft of the soft palate

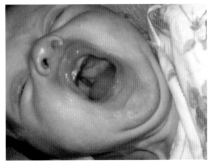

Fig. 402   Cleft of the soft palate

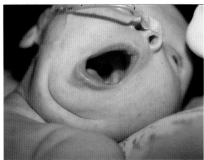

Fig. 403   Cleft of the soft palate --
A case study

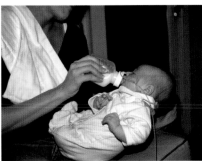

Fig. 404   Flexed at the hips to
prevent hyperextension

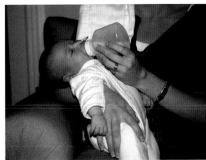

Fig. 405   Aversive feeding
behavior

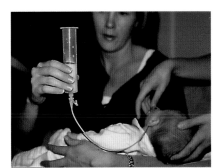

Fig. 406   Nasogastric tube-feeding
to protect growth

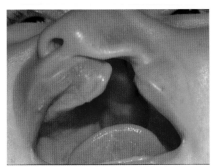

Fig. 407   Complete cleft of the
lip and palate

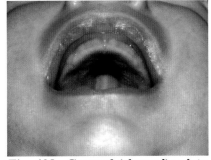

Fig. 408   Grooved (channel) palate

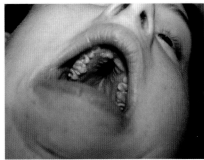

Fig. 409 Grooved palate in 12 year-
old with Down Syndrome

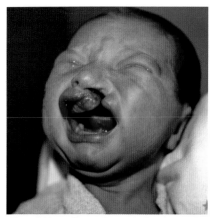

Fig. 410   Complete cleft of the lip
              and palate -- A case study

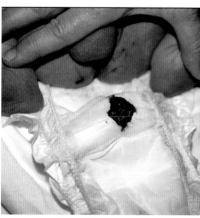

Fig. 411   Scant, dark stools on
              Day 4

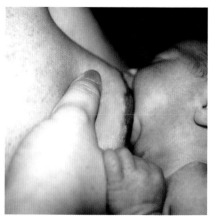

Fig. 412 Upright feeding position
            and breast compression

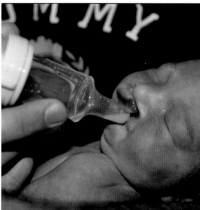

Fig. 413   Feeding colostrum with
              a Special Needs Feeder™

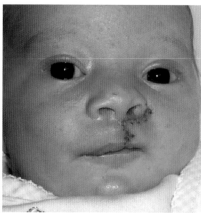

Fig. 414   After early repair of the
              cleft lip (courtesy K. Bird)

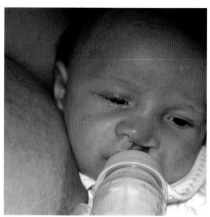

Fig. 415 Bottle-feeding at breast
            with the Pigeon Feeder™

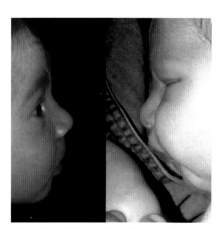

Fig. 416   Normal and receding
              chins

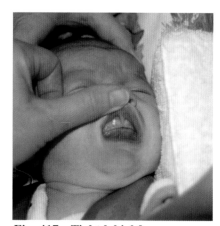

Fig. 417   Tight labial frenum

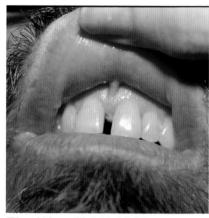

Fig. 418   Tight labial frenum --
              affects tooth spacing

Index

mandible: 14, **Figs. 33-35:** 160, **Fig. 416:** 196

mastectomy: 97, 98, **Figs. 286-287:** 184

mastitis: 50, 52, 66, 75, 77, 79, 82, 83, 89-90, 96, 99, **Fig. 225:** 178, **Fig. 254:** 181
    bilateral: 85, **Figs. 258-259:** 182
    inflammatory: 82-83, **Fig. 257:** 182
    MRSA-related mastitis: 87-88, 90-91, **Fig. 265:** 182, **Figs. 270-280:** 183
    Streptococcus: 85
    subclinical mastitis: 82, 83

maternal overweight: 35, 66, **Fig. 256:** 181

maternal stress (*See also stress*): 131

Mead cleft palate feeder: 150, **Figs. 404-405:** 195

meconium: 25, 151, **Fig. 61:** 163, **Fig. 411:** 196

menstruation: 58, 81

Methicillin-resistant *Staphylococcus aureus* (MRSA): 22, 50, 52, 87-88, 90, **Fig. 265:** 182, **Figs. 270-280:** 183

mid-line defect (*See also ankyloglossia, cleft palate, and hypospadius*): 143, 149, 154, 193

milk:
    banking: 117-122, **Figs. 338-346:** 190
    contamination: 89, 132, **Figs. 340-344:** 190
    cultures: 85, **Fig. 343:** 190
    flow rate: 14, 17, 76, 81
    production: 29, 30, 128
    storage: 120, **Figs. 338, 344-345:** 190

milk ejection reflex: 17, 33, 81, 125, 148, **Fig. 199:** 176, **Fig. 255:** 181

milk line: 61

Montgomery glands: 57, 144, **Fig. 176:** 174

motoric stress cues: 6, 8, 9, **Fig: 8**: 157, **Fig.330**: 189

mottling: 7, **Fig. 14**: 158

MRSA (See also Methicillin-resistant *Staphylococcus aureus*): 22, 52, 87

multiple birth (*See also twins and triplets*): 101, 104

mupirocin (Bactroban): 52, 85, 98

Myasthenia gravis: 18

N

narrow gape: 38, **Figs. 125-126:** 169

nasal:
    congestion: 124
    passages (nares): 16, 113, **Fig. 37**: 160
    regurgitation: 148, 150, 152

nasogastric tube-feeding: 112, 150, **Fig. 328:** 188, **Fig. 406:** 195

nasopharynx: 16, 124

necrotising enterocolitis (NEC): 102, 117

negative pressure: 73, 149

negative pressure wound therapy: 50

neurological dysfunction: 125

nevus: 21, **Fig. 56:** 162

nipple: 42, 67, 71, 72, 83
    cracked: 48-52, 83, **Figs. 148-154:** 171
    diameter: 44, 73
    dimpled: 42-43, 53, **Figs. 137-138:** 170
    doorknob shape: 74, **Fig. 230:** 179
    double: 67, **Figs. 206-207:** 177
    engorgement: 72, **Figs. 236-238:** 179, **Fig. 251:** 181
    everted: 42, **Fig. 130:** 169
    fit problems related to: 20, 71, 73, **Fig. 228:** 178, **Fig. 231:** 179
    infection: 51, 52, 54, 84, **Fig. 154:** 171, **Fig. 163:** 172, **Fig. 225:** 178, **Fig. 254:** 181, **Fig. 394:** 94
    inverted: 41-42, **Figs. 134-138:** 170, **Figs. 210-211:** 177
    long: 73, **Figs. 224, 226, 227-229:** 178
    pierced: 68, **Figs. 208-209:** 177
    placement on breast: 36, **Fig. 106:** 167
    ring: 68, **Fig. 208-209:** 177
    shapes: 67, **Figs. 206-207:** 177,
    size: 72, **Figs. 220, 223-229:** 178, **Fig. 230:** 179, **Figs. 239-243, 245:** 180
    supernumerary: 61-62, **Figs. 187-190:** 175
    undistorted: **Fig. 121:** 168, **Fig. 130:** 169

nipple cleansing (*See also soap*): 51, 85

nipple confusion: 41, 107, 113

nipple cream: 50, **Fig. 165:** 173

nipple on down-hill slope of breast: **Fig. 106:** 167

nipple shield: 15, 21, 43, 44, 48, 79, 81, 130, 133, 153, **Figs: 140-145:** 170

non-nutritive sucking (NNS): 6, 17, 76, **Fig. 4:** 157

nose (*See also nasal passages*): 16

nosocomial infections: 21, 84

nursing pillow: 35, 130, **Fig. 91:** 165, **Fig. 105:** 167, **Fig. 297:** 185

nursing strike: 58

nutritional analysis (of milk): 120, **Fig. 339:** 190

nutritive sucking: 17

nystatin: 54, **Fig. 166:** 173

O

obesity: 35, 66

obturator (palatal): 152

Occupational Therapist (OT): 13, 113, 148

odd posturing: 125, **Figs. 356-358:** 192

older baby: 58, 104, 105, **Fig. 181:** 174, **Figs. 300-301:** 185, **Figs. 304-310:** 186

olive oil: 76, **Fig. 244:** 180

open heart surgery scar: 68, **Fig. 212:** 177, **Fig. 366:** 192

oral anatomy: 13, 71

Z

Ziemer, M: 51
zinc deficiencies: 30